RESEAR
METHODS
for PUBLIC HEALTH

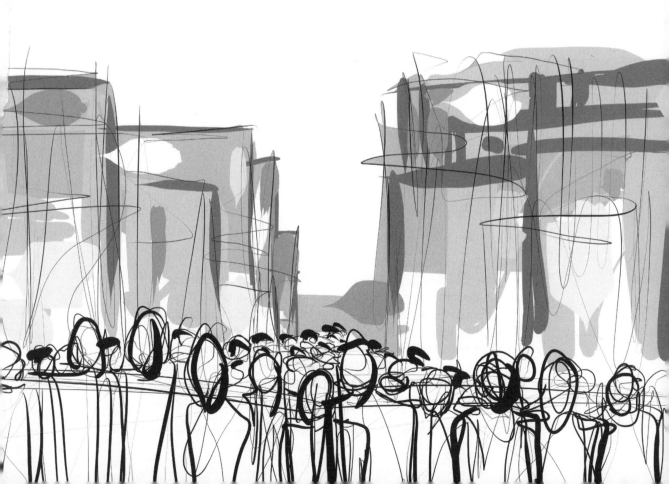

Sara Miller McCune founded SAGE Publishing in 1965 to support the dissemination of usable knowledge and educate a global community. SAGE publishes more than 1000 journals and over 800 new books each year, spanning a wide range of subject areas. Our growing selection of library products includes archives, data, case studies and video. SAGE remains majority owned by our founder and after her lifetime will become owned by a charitable trust that secures the company's continued independence.

Los Angeles | London | New Delhi | Singapore | Washington DC | Melbourne

RESEARCH METHODS
for PUBLIC HEALTH

Stuart McClean, Isabelle Bray, Nick de Viggiani,
Emma Bird and Paul Pilkington

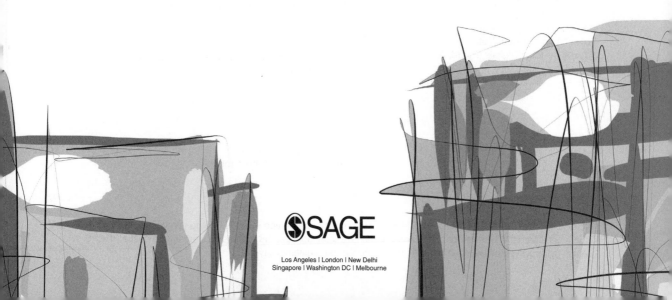

$SAGE

Los Angeles | London | New Delhi
Singapore | Washington DC | Melbourne

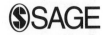

Los Angeles | London | New Delhi
Singapore | Washington DC | Melbourne

SAGE Publications Ltd
1 Oliver's Yard
55 City Road
London EC1Y 1SP

SAGE Publications Inc.
2455 Teller Road
Thousand Oaks, California 91320

SAGE Publications India Pvt Ltd
B 1/I 1 Mohan Cooperative Industrial Area
Mathura Road
New Delhi 110 044

SAGE Publications Asia-Pacific Pte. Ltd.
18 Cross Street #10-10/11/12
China Square Central
Singapore 048423

Editor: Alex Clabburn
Assistant editor: Jade Grogan
Production editor: Tanya Szwarnowska
Copyeditor: Clare Weaver
Proofreader: Rosemary McDonald
Indexer: Melanie Gee
Marketing manager: George Kimble
Cover design: Wendy Scott
Typeset by: C&M Digitals (P) Ltd, Chennai, India
Printed in the UK

Library of Congress Control Number: 2019934755

British Library Cataloguing in Publication data

A catalogue record for this book is available from
the British Library

ISBN 978-1-5264-3000-7
ISBN 978-1-5264-3001-4 (pbk)

At SAGE we take sustainability seriously. Most of our products are printed in the UK using responsibly sourced
papers and boards. When we print overseas we ensure sustainable papers are used as measured by the PREPS
grading system. We undertake an annual audit to monitor our sustainability.

CONTENTS

LIST OF TABLES

LIST OF FIGURES

ABOUT THE AUTHORS

Stuart McClean is a social anthropologist working at the University of the West of England (UWE Bristol), UK as a Public Health academic. Stuart is the author of *An Ethnography of Crystal and Spiritual Healers in Northern England: marginal medicine and mainstream concerns* (Edwin Mellen, 2006), co-editor of *Folk Healing and Health Care Practices in Britain and Ireland* (Berghahn, 2010), and the co-author of *Thinking About the Lifecourse* (Palgrave, 2014). Stuart leads the MSc Public Health Programme at UWE, specialising in qualitative research methods, particularly ethnography. His research interests are the wider health and wellbeing culture and the ways this manifests in varied wellbeing practices, forms of agency, innovation and creativity in Western societies. He is interested in describing how individuals and communities work at 'doing well' and 'being well', the interconnected nature of these experiences, and in explaining the current socio-cultural forces and trends that underpin it.

Isabelle Bray is a Senior Lecturer in Public Health at the University of the West of England (UWE Bristol), UK. She leads a module on Quantitative Health Research on the MSc Public Health and is involved in the supervision and examination of MSc dissertations in both Public and Environmental Health. Her research experience includes working on randomised controlled trials, cohort studies, case-control studies and cross-sectional surveys, with a particular interest in response rates. Much of this research has been in the field of mental health, from international comparisons of 'happiness' and 'life satisfaction' to suicide rates amongst military veterans. With a background in medical statistics, Isabelle's methodological expertise broadly involve the application of generalised linear models to assess associations between exposures and outcomes, including the analysis of complex interventions. Current research interests focus on the relationship between physical and mental health, with recent work being in the areas of childhood obesity, body dissatisfaction and predictors in childhood of eating disorders and risky behaviours in adolescence.

Nick de Viggiani is a Senior Lecturer in Public Health at the University of the West of England (UWE Bristol), UK. In 2003, he completed his PhD with the University of Bristol, having completed an ethnography involving men in prison, exploring prison masculinities as determinants of health. This led on to various funded research projects involving people in the adult and youth justice systems, including a Big Lottery funded three-year study involving young offenders, undertaken in partnership with a music charity. His research in the criminal justice health sector has involved developing relations with regional and national stakeholders across public, private and third sector agencies, and with colleagues across universities. He is particularly interested in working with hard-to-reach groups, sometimes described as 'challenging' or 'vulnerable', including male and female young offenders, older prisoners, sex offenders and foreign national prisoners, across different provider organisations. A key focus of his work has been to explore, explain and tackle health and social inequality. His publications include a range of peer reviewed outputs spanning prison public health, prison masculinities and the impact of economic austerity on prison health. He is a strong advocate for prisoner rights and for evolving just, humane and purposeful justice systems.

Emma Bird is a Senior Lecturer in Public Health at the University of the West of England (UWE Bristol), UK. Emma's research is focused on developing and evaluating public health interventions that aim to promote health behaviour change. Her research takes a socio-ecological approach, examining individual, social, and environmental factors that influence the health behaviours of a range of population groups in a variety of settings. Emma is an experienced lecturer, contributing to teaching across UWE Bristol and leading two modules: Health Promotion and Principles of Evidence Based Public Health. Emma is skilled in the utilisation of quantitative, qualitative and evidence synthesis research methods. She has published widely in international peer reviewed journals and presented her work at numerous regional, national and international conferences.

Paul Pilkington is a registered Public Health Specialist and Senior Lecturer in Public Health at the University of the West of England (UWE Bristol), UK. An experienced teacher and researcher, Paul has undertaken a wide range of research projects with impact in the field of healthy and sustainable environments, with funders including Wellcome Trust, NICE, NIHR, and Public Health England. His research and knowledge exchange activities have a particular focus on healthy planning and road danger reduction. Paul is a Fellow of the UK Faculty of Public Health. He has published widely in international peer reviewed journals and presented at numerous regional, national and international conferences.

ACKNOWLEDGEMENTS

There are many people we would like to thank. Firstly, thanks to our many colleagues at the Centre for Public Health and Wellbeing, University of the West of England (UWE), for their frequent advice, critical commentary and support. We are a very friendly and collegiate public health group at UWE Bristol, and we feel very lucky to have this support. We have also learned much from our discussions with colleagues over the years about all things methodological.

We want to thank all of our students, past and present, studying on the MSc Public Health at UWE Bristol, who have helped to continually challenge us about research methods, and have provided the inspiration to commit our ideas to paper. Our approach to *Research Methods for Public Health* has clearly been heavily influenced by the dialogue we have all had with our students over the last 10 years.

The team at Sage Publications, particularly Jade Grogan, Tanya Szwarnowska, and George Kimble, have been very supportive and have helped ensure we delivered the book. We would also like to thank our reviewers who have given their precious time to evaluate the contribution of our book to the wider public health research and teaching community. We are very grateful for their support and endorsements.

Finally, our deep thanks is due to our families who have supported us and tolerated our absences. It is to them that this book is dedicated.

PUBLISHER'S ACKNOWLEDGEMENTS

The publishers are grateful to the academic lecturers from the below institutions who reviewed the proposal for the book and draft material. Each reviewer provided critical feedback which has shaped the book for the better.

Lecturers

Jacques Oosthuizen, Edith Cowan University

Krishna Regmi, University of Bedfordshire

James Woodall, Leeds Beckett University

INTRODUCTION

Investigating Public Health and the Scope of Research Methods

Our approach

- The book is written by a multidisciplinary team of academics with strong research and publications profiles in public health and extensive experience of teaching and supervising postgraduate public health students.
- Our approach to public health research methods reflects the multidisciplinary postgraduate public health curriculum where the authors are located, where students are encouraged to develop research skills that translate into real-world impact.
- The book includes chapters on primary quantitative, qualitative and mixed methods research, evidence synthesis approaches, critical appraisal, research governance and ethics, and dissemination. This integrative approach combines methodologies in a format that is often missing from traditional, single-discipline research methods textbooks.
- The book is designed to be student-orientated, enabling the reader to reflect on how best to approach research problems from different standpoints, to develop research questions and to design and execute a research project.

Public health research has undoubtedly played a key role in advancing people's health and wellbeing. Recent successes in public health research are evident in celebrated achievements in health improvement and health protection, including advances in the control and management of communicable and non-communicable diseases, to healthier children and families, safer environments and more resilient schools, workplaces and communities (Gray et al., 2006; BMJ, 2018). Methodological innovations have helped contribute to the evidence underpinning these achievements, coupled with distinctive contributions of researchers and scholars from a broad range of subject disciplines. Our book offers a primer to this complex methodological field that embraces the diverse character of multidisciplinary public health. This book also represents a plea to public health researchers to integrate multidisciplinary learning into their methodological repertoire. In doing so, we believe you will be better equipped to meet the grand challenges, existing and emerging, of twenty-first century public health.

Our introductory chapter provides an overview of the book's content, and it presents our general approach towards research methods in public health. Here we set out the context for public health research and in particular the socio-ecological model of public health with a focus on health inequalities and social determinants of health. The book seeks to provide arguments and tools to enable public health researchers to meet the complex, contested health challenges encountered across local, national and international contexts. An approach to research is championed where conventional research methods are brought together to address complex issues in innovative ways. Real-world examples are presented to contextualise contemporary public health research, relevant to local and global scenarios.

Who is this book for?

The purpose of this book is to make the theory and practice of research methods more accessible to students, novice researchers and public health practitioners with an interest in research. We are a team of authors with academic and professional backgrounds in the social sciences, human sciences, life sciences and epidemiology. Since public health students and practitioners tend to come from diverse disciplinary or professional backgrounds, we have written this book for readers who may be new to public health research or new to a particular research method. It is primarily aimed at postgraduate students, novice researchers and public health practitioners who may be involved in public health-related research or evaluation, or who are especially keen to underpin their practice with good research evidence. It is recommended as essential reading and a core textbook for anyone undertaking a postgraduate course in public health (MSc Public Health or Master of Public Health [MPH]) where research methods are part of the core curriculum. It is also recommended for individuals preparing for the UK Faculty of Public Health Part A examination (www.fph.org.uk).

This book is also applicable to anyone studying or working across fields aligned with public health – health studies, environmental health, health protection, health promotion and improvement, health psychology, education, community development or primary care – and across voluntary, community and non-governmental organisations and agencies, local, regional and national government, such as planning, housing, urban regeneration, social care, international development, human rights and social justice contexts.

Multidisciplinary public health

While there isn't a universally agreed definition of public health, some definitions have emphasised action on the broad determinants of health, akin with a systems-orientated, socio-ecological model of health. Indeed, WHO (2002) defined public health as,

> ... all organised measures (whether public or private) to prevent disease, promote health, and prolong life among the population as a whole. Its activities aim to provide conditions in which people can be healthy and focus on entire populations, not on individual patients or diseases. Thus, public health is concerned with the total system and not only the eradication of a particular disease.

This definition underlines the importance of recognising that public health is concerned partly with people and with environments or settings. Fundamental to this approach is the principle of social responsibility for health – that environments are social spaces and not merely aggregates of individuals, that people and place are intimately connected in terms of health and wellbeing. The Ottawa Charter for Health Promotion (WHO, 1986) was pivotal in shifting emphasis away from individual responsibility ('victim blaming' individualism) towards the notion of supportive environments for health, the latter later expressed through the Sundsvall Declaration (WHO, 1991).

A second significant standpoint of public health is its commitment to tackle inequality and social injustice, a stance that reflects the values of the United Nations, and which prevailed for the last two decades of the twentieth century in WHO's 'Health for All' movement (WHO, 1978). This was more recently heralded by the Marmot Report, commissioned by WHO (2008), which emphasised the need to tackle social determinants of health and to reduce health inequalities. This was on the basis that economic and social conditions, as well as their distribution within and between populations, influence differences in health status. A broad public health perspective acknowledges the social and environmental contexts of health and wellbeing, and it is the position we take in this book. Our motivation is consistent with that of Donaldson and Rutter (2017) in terms of:

> ... protecting and improving the health of whole populations and communities [... and taking ...] a broader focus to understand and engage with the many factors (societal, behavioural, environmental) that promote or undermine health.

Public health, as a multidisciplinary strategy, thus represents the interplay of multiple factors, sectors and practices (Orme et al., 2007; Wright et al., 2014). Unlike Public Health Medicine, contemporary public health has multiple disciplinary drivers that transcend epidemiology, biomedicine, the social, environmental, human and political sciences, social policy and economics. The contemporary public health workforce reaches far beyond medicine to include the full spectrum of health and social care professions, and – in the spirit of the 1975 Lalonde Report and WHO's (1986) intersectoral vision – encompasses professions beyond the conventional health sector. Consequently, public health research has grown exponentially in recent years and become increasingly ambitious in its scope and reach across a range of human health concerns (Wright et al., 2014). Each of those subjects brings their own unique questions and forms of investigation to the public health field; together they provide a more integrative approach adopting the strengths of natural, health and social sciences, along with arts and humanistic approaches that transcend conventional public health.

Public health medicine was traditionally epistemologically situated within clinical and biomedical sciences, adhering to gold standard scientific research as its benchmark, and adherence to quantitative and epidemiological research conventions. With the gradual shift towards multidisciplinary public health, we have seen increasing acceptance of qualitative and mixed methods research, consistent with the incorporation of human and social sciences, but also with increasing necessity to address complex and intractable public health issues and grand challenges. In this spirit, we seek to provide balance in presenting and debating the broad church of methods and methodologies that can be employed by public health researchers.

(Re)Framing public health problems

Public health problems can be framed in different ways depending on one's disciplinary perspective. A conventional public health perspective would define global health in terms of burden of disease, measured by mortality and morbidity. From a multidisciplinary public health perspective, a socio-ecological interpretation of health and illness enables us to acknowledge that context is fundamental to understanding and interpreting the causes and distribution of disease and illness, especially since health is not merely the absence of disease but includes psychosocial factors.

The World Health Organization prioritises mortality as a key indicator of health, identifying ischaemic heart disease, stroke, chronic obstructive lung disease and lower respiratory infections as the top causes of mortality globally, and chronic diseases such as type-2 diabetes and dementia increasing year-on-year. Injuries are also recognised as a significant cause of premature death among males (WHO, 2018). Moreover, the WHO argues that to make progress towards the health-related Sustainable Development Goals (SDGs) requires intervention to tackle child mortality, maternal mortality and mortality due to non-communicable diseases, suicide, pollution, road traffic injuries, natural disasters and conflict (WHO, 2018). The Lancet's *Global Burden of Disease Study* (Lancet, 2018) suggests that rather than seeing greater resilience and improvements in health globally, we are witnessing increased fragility and fragmentation, with increases in mortality reflecting emerging new trends. Conflict and terrorism are identified as the two fastest growing causes of death, coupled with increases in violence, opioid dependence, non-communicable diseases and depression. Non-communicable diseases now account for three-quarters of all global deaths, half of these attributable to high blood pressure, smoking, high blood glucose and high body-mass index. Obesity prevalence has increased in almost every country in the world. Also significant in terms of mortality is the burden of preventable communicable disease, such as diarrhoeal diseases especially affecting children under 5 years.

Epidemiological data like these described above provide an essential basis for identifying patterns and causes of disease and disability within and across populations, and guide the development of national and international public health policy in terms of building resilient health systems. They also enable us to identify and begin to explain the distribution of ill-health with a view to redressing inequalities through galvanising governments and other key agencies and institutions. The epidemiological landscape is linked with broad underlying socio-economic, political and cultural conditions, creating ever-changing emergent problems that present as complex challenges for public health. The success of conventional programmes – for example, the development of vaccines to control and prevent infectious diseases – is dependent upon the combination of economic, political and social dilemmas that impede progress, where successful eradication requires system level change. The broad range of increasingly complex and intractable public health concerns of modern society – natural disasters, violence and war, migration, obesity, mental ill-health, drug and alcohol misuse, physical inactivity, ageing populations, and so on – present major challenges to our health systems and governments and, as such, require sophisticated research and development approaches.

We therefore advocate a 'horizontal' approach to public health research, one that considers and values different forms and sources of evidence, that isn't conventionally hierarchical or 'gold standard' driven. The ever-expanding, multisector international public health workforce must be able to respond to evolving public health issues with a repertoire of evidence gathering skills and capabilities. This means being able and ready to ask different research questions and to interrogate research problems from different standpoints. It requires public health researchers to have an open mind, able to interrogate complex issues, draw upon divergent bodies of knowledge, and employ different methods, sometimes in combination, to investigate the research problem. This means being able to embrace quantitative, qualitative, mixed methods and evidence synthesis approaches. Part of this 'journey' is the evolution of a shared language and understanding that doesn't prioritise one form of evidence over another.

A pragmatic approach to research methods

This book was conceived and written not to privilege one specific research tradition or approach over another but with the pragmatic view that public health research problems are best answered by methods most suited to the research question. As such, we do not recognise a conventional research hierarchy that positions one methodology or method above another, whether it be quantitative, qualitative, mixed methods or evidence synthesis. We recognise the value that different approaches and traditions bring to research, and that most public health issues can be examined in different – sometime complementary, sometimes alternative – ways, often drawing from the repertoire of available approaches. As we highlight throughout the book, the research question is an important starting point and should indicate the direction and nature of the research. The research context is also important as public health settings bring a whole range of challenges, especially those that involve human experiences. Moreover, being a team of authors from different academic disciplines, we routinely engage in primary research that involves working in multidisciplinary teams, often with different perspectives. Our particular methodological preferences influence how we think, and we acknowledge that our respective stances bring different contributions to discussions of public health research.

However, we firmly believe that multidisciplinary public health should be approached and taught with a preparedness to critique, question and subvert convention. In this regard, a student or researcher who is approaching a public health problem should face the problem with an open, critical and reflexive mind-set and endeavour to best fit the research methods and approach to the emerging research question, rather than the other way around. Public health researchers should not be 'methodologists' seeking a question, but an informed and curious investigator seeking the most appropriate methods available to address real-world problems.

Conducting public health research in a rigorous way requires researchers to demonstrate broad understanding of research approaches, and to approach public health problems in a methods-literate way. This means having a clear and competent understanding of research design, sampling or case selection, data collection and data analysis, and of how to ensure that rigour and quality are hallmarks of research processes and outputs. Each approach has its own strengths and limitations, research questions and focus that they are most suited to, while mixed methods approaches can offer interesting and creative ways to answer different and discrete research questions within the same study.

Students or novice researchers also commonly have research preferences, based on their disciplinary backgrounds, personal values and interests, skills and capabilities, and mind-set. We don't discourage following one's instinct in this fashion as it is challenging, for instance, for a person who is experienced in quantitative research to take up ethnography or phenomenology, while a qualitative researcher might equally find it challenging or disconcerting to undertake a randomised controlled trial. We will show how quantitative and qualitative approaches require different ways of thinking about research problems, but we do urge anyone venturing into public health research to consider the value different approaches bring to investigating public health issues.

Thinking critically about the 'hierarchy of evidence'

The traditional *hierarchy of evidence* (or *evidence pyramid*) – which features prominently within biomedical research literature – prioritises certain methodological approaches and forms of evidence above others. However, it is also assumed that for any study the research question concerns *effectiveness* of an intervention. If assessing effectiveness is indeed the aim, then the most appropriate 'gold standard' methodology is a 'randomised controlled trial' (we discuss this approach in more detail in Chapter 1). Public health research questions can certainly be oriented towards testing interventions; take, for example, the question, 'Can a smoking cessation intervention for pregnant women lead to a higher quit rate than standard advice given at antenatal appointments?' A randomised controlled trial would be ideal in this case. If several such trials had already been conducted, then a systematic review and meta-analysis would be even higher up the 'hierarchy of evidence'.

However, if the question asked, 'What proportion of pregnant women smoke?', in order to estimate prevalence of smoking in this population, then a randomised controlled trial would not answer the question, and the hierarchy of evidence would become inverted because the best-suited study design – a cross-sectional study – is situated near the bottom of the traditional hierarchy. Another related research question, 'Does becoming pregnant increase the chance that a smoker will successfully quit?' could not be answered by either a cross-sectional study or a randomised controlled trial because it is impossible to randomise women to pregnancy, so instead would require a cohort study. This is a serious point because in public health we are interested in more than effectiveness that can be randomised, or even interventions more broadly; rather, we are interested in an array of factors – biomedical, social, cultural, environmental, etc. – that cannot be randomised. At best, they may be considered as a 'natural' (e.g. non-randomised) experiment. Examples include studies of the effects of restricted diet during pregnancy (e.g. Ramadan fasting – van Ewijk (2011); Dutch hunger winter – Painter *et al.* 2005).

Furthermore, if public health is to make a difference, it must be able to investigate what drives people, what factors influence their behaviour and what the best approaches are to promote health in different populations. To design effective interventions to help pregnant women quit smoking, it is necessary to understand first why some pregnant women continue to smoke. This might include trying to understand why they choose not to engage with services already provided. The qualitative approaches required to answer these questions do not even feature in the traditional evidence hierarchy. A systematic review of randomised controlled trials is certainly not the answer.

Key features of this book

- It provides a straightforward and pragmatic approach to developing a public health research project.
- It explains methodological conventions in an accessible format that are directly relevant to a public health readership.
- It explains how to apply methodological approaches and methods in practical and realistic ways.
- It provides examples and case studies relevant to a UK and international public health student readership.
- The book is informed by a socio-ecological model of multidisciplinary public health that is relevant to a multidisciplinary readership, making it distinctive from more conventional research methods textbooks.

Organisation of this book

The book is organised into four parts that in turn cover quantitative methods, qualitative methods, mixed methods and evidence synthesis, and applications to public health practice.

Part I: Quantitative Methods for Public Health. Chapter 1: Epidemiology introduces the subject of epidemiology and basic principles of applying epidemiology to public health. The first part of the chapter deals with the key epidemiological issue of whether an observed association is causal. The most commonly used epidemiological study designs are then described, with examples to illustrate the situations in which they are used. Challenges in applying epidemiological study designs to real-world public health research questions are discussed. Chapter 2 (Sampling) outlines key sampling approaches in quantitative research (e.g. quota sampling, random sampling, stratified sampling, cluster sampling), and discusses the pros and cons of each. The practicalities of sampling are explored using real-world examples, particularly drawing on experiences of supervising students who have undertaken surveys in different settings. Chapter 3 (Collecting Quantitative Data) discusses methods of primary data collection for quantitative studies, including observation, interview (face-to-face, telephone, online), self-completed questionnaire (hardcopy and online) and other digital methods. The suitability of these methods for different situations, including pros and cons of each, is illustrated using real-world examples, drawing on the authors' own research experiences. Chapter 4 (Quantitative Data Analysis) discusses the use of descriptive statistics, graphs and disease atlases, followed by measures of risk (relative and absolute) and measures of association. A brief guide to appropriate statistical tests (parametric and non-parametric) for different types of data is provided, and further references are provided for more advanced statistical analysis. Chapter 5 (Quality and Rigour) addresses quality and rigour in primary quantitative research, in particular the key concepts of validity and reliability. A pragmatic approach is presented that is relevant to public health research contexts. This chapter also explores quality and rigour in secondary data analysis and critical appraisal of epidemiological studies. The key tools for appraising quantitative research are introduced and potential for developing bespoke tools is explored.

Part II: Qualitative Methods for Public Health. Chapter 6: Methodological Approaches and Basic Principles introduces the primary methodological approaches used in qualitative research – grounded theory, ethnography and phenomenology. Particular focus is provided on how each methodological approach can enhance public health knowledge, along with discussion of the strengths and limitations of each. Chapter 7 (Accessing and Selecting Cases) highlights fundamental differences between thinking about sampling in quantitative and qualitative research. It explores issues of access and recruitment and provides some debate on the definition of sample and case. It then explains the key sampling approaches used with different qualitative research methodologies. Chapter 8 (Collecting Qualitative Data) examines the character of 'data' in qualitative research before discussing the most common approaches to primary data collection – participant observation and interviewing (one-to-one and group). The suitability of these methods for different situations and challenges associated with them are discussed. Chapter 9 (Qualitative Data Analysis) considers the basic principles of qualitative data analysis and explores how data analysis techniques can be used to ensure rigour. Specific qualitative data analysis strategies are alluded to, with specific discussion of thematic and framework analysis. Chapter 10 (Quality and Rigour) explores quality and rigour in qualitative research, including discussion of methods employed to build trustworthiness and reflexivity into the research designs.

In **Part III: Mixing it Up: Combining Methods and Evidence Synthesis in Public Health. Chapter 11: Mixed Methods Research and Evaluation Design** introduces mixed methods approaches, discussing the value and efficacy of mixed methods research in terms of what it offers beyond purely quantitative or qualitative designs. Here we highlight the importance of adopting a pluralistic or pragmatic approach to research design. We discuss different mixed methods designs, including sequential and concurrent approaches. Chapter 12 (Evidence Synthesis Approaches: Systematic Reviews) introduces evidence synthesis, with a specific focus on how to apply traditional systematic review methodology and methods. Chapter 13 (Evidence Synthesis Approaches: Meta-ethnography and Realist Synthesis) explores two alternative approaches to evidence synthesis for public health research: meta-ethnography for qualitative synthesis and realist synthesis. It debates terminology and choice of method when undertaking synthesis of published research evidence and use of non-standard sources.

Part IV: Applying Research to Public Health Practice. Chapter 14: The Ethics of Public Health Research highlights a range of emerging ethical issues in relation to public health research and practice. Contemporary and historical examples of global public health research are examined, and the relationship between medical ethics and public health is explored. Chapter 15 (Writing up, Dissemination and Publication) provides guidance for students and novice researchers in public health about the process of moving from 'project dissertation' to 'publication'.

PART 1
QUANTITATIVE METHODS FOR PUBLIC HEALTH

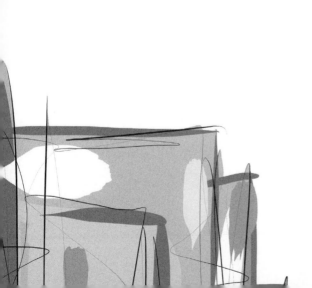
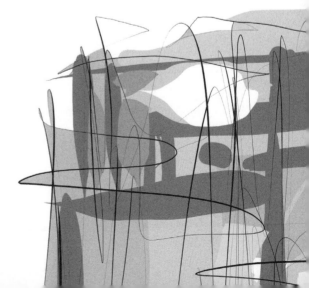

1 EPIDEMIOLOGY

=== CHAPTER SUMMARY ===

This chapter is divided into two sections. The first introduces the subject of epidemiology in the context of public health, and the key concepts of **chance, bias, confounding** and **causation**. The second describes the most common **epidemiological study designs**, and finishes by considering how these can be applied to the complex interventions and settings often encountered in public health.

Introduction to epidemiology

A classic definition of epidemiology is 'the study of the distribution and determinants of health-related states or events in specified populations and the application of this study to the control of health problems' (Last, 2001: 55). This definition stresses that we are interested in the health of populations rather than individuals, and the factors associated with health outcomes. Epidemiology provides the evidence for evidence-based healthcare, by using numbers to estimate and compare risks, either for different subgroups of the population or according to different levels of exposure. More broadly, epidemiology is a quantitative approach to answering questions relating to population health.

Public health research often uses both qualitative and quantitative analysis, and epidemiology is just one of several tools available to public health researchers. For example, an epidemiological approach to determining whether hip protectors are effective in preventing fractures among older people in residential care might select an appropriate study design, such as a randomised controlled trial (RCT) in which half of a sample of nursing homes are provided with hip protectors and half are not. If a large RCT concluded that there was only limited evidence of effectiveness in this population, you might jump to the conclusion that this is not a good use of resources, and rule out this intervention. But you don't have the full picture – what if the people offered the hip protectors don't want to wear them, and are therefore not complying with the intervention being tested? Then some qualitative work is needed to understand the experience of older people wearing hip protectors, and barriers to their use. This could inform further research into alternative designs with potentially higher rates of compliance. Assuming different designs come at different costs, then a comparison of the relative cost-effectiveness of each would be useful. Other tools, such as qualitative research and health economics, are therefore required to complement epidemiology (Bowling, 2014).

Framing a question

Before we can consider the most appropriate epidemiological study design in a particular situation, we have to be clear about our research question. A useful framework for doing this is PICO. In public health, P stands for 'population' (rather than 'patient' as in traditional evidence-based medicine). This highlights the key difference between public health and clinical professions – we are considering whole populations rather than individual patients. I stands for 'intervention' (or 'exposure' in non-experimental studies). C stands for 'comparison' (having a control or comparison group is a key characteristic of epidemiological studies), and O stands for 'outcome'. So, in any epidemiological study we are considering the effect of an exposure or intervention on a particular health outcome, but we also need to define what this is being compared to and in which particular population.

BOX 1.1   PICO: POPULATION, INTERVENTION, COMPARISON, OUTCOME

Using the hip protector example given above:

P   Older people (e.g. 65+ years) living in residential homes in the UK
I   Provision of hip protectors
C   No provision of hip protectors
O   Fractures

In this example, we have compared the provision of hip protectors to no provision, but it could be that we want to compare the provision of a new type of hip protector with the current market leader. Then the comparison would be with another intervention, rather than no intervention.

In epidemiology, the intervention or exposure is sometimes referred to as the independent variable, explanatory variable or risk factor, while the health or social outcome that we are interested in may be described as the dependent variable. So, an epidemiological study uses quantitative techniques to assess the effect of a particular exposure or intervention on a health outcome of interest in a defined population by comparing groups with different levels of exposure. Before going on to describe the main epidemiological study designs in further detail, we will consider some common problems in epidemiology which researchers must be aware of. These topics of chance, bias and confounding are dealt with in greater depth in epidemiology textbooks such as Gordis (2013) and Rothman (2012).

Chance

Epidemiological studies are usually based on samples drawn from the population of interest, because it is not normally possible to measure exposures and outcomes on the entire population. For example, if I want to assess whether open-water swimming is a risk factor for a particular waterborne illness in the southwest of England, I am unlikely to be able to gather information on frequency of open-water swimming for every individual in this population, but I can survey a sample. The next chapter will focus on different methods of sampling. If, in my sample, I find that there is evidence of an association, in other words that open-water swimming does appear to increase the risk of the illness, then how confident should I be that this association is real? Is it possible that if I took a different sample then I might get a different result? Most people intuitively trust results based on a large sample more than those derived from a small sample. So, if I told you that I had surveyed 10 people on this issue and found an association, you might be dubious. If I told you I had surveyed 1,000 people and found an association between open-water swimming and waterborne illness, you would probably be more inclined to believe me. This is correct; larger samples are more reliable. Statistics can be used to quantify how confident we should be in the study's results. Confidence intervals can be calculated for our results, which take into account the size of the sample, and other characteristics of the study design and sample. 'p-values' are sometimes also calculated to quantify the probability that the difference we observed is due to chance (how likely is it that we would have got the observed difference, or a larger difference, if there was actually no association between open-water swimming and waterborne illness?). Since p stands for 'probability', it is on a scale of 0 to 1, and it is important to interpret the p-value as a value on a continuum, to describe the strength of the evidence, rather than using an arbitrary cut-off for the p-value to determine whether a result is 'statistically significant' or not. Traditionally, this arbitrary cut-off has been set at 0.05 (or 5%), and used to interpret a p-value of less than 0.05 as 'significant' (in other words there is evidence of an association or a difference) and a value greater than 0.05 as non-significant (no evidence of an association/difference). When presenting your own research, it is good practice to present confidence intervals (Gardner and Altman, 1986), and if p-values are also used then the actual p-value should be given (rather a statement about the statistical significance or otherwise of the results). When reading or critiquing published research, remember to take into account the width of the confidence intervals rather than focusing on the overall estimate, because they will often indicate a very wide range of likely values, in other words a lack of confidence about what is actually going on in the population.

Bias

Bias refers to a systematic error in the way a study is conducted, analysed or reported, which means that the results cannot be trusted. There are many different types of bias, as illustrated by the following examples. In the case of the study looking at open-water swimming and waterborne illness, the study could be biased if it were conducted at a particular time of year when the waterborne pathogen of interest was particularly prevalent – this might over-estimate, and therefore exaggerate, the risks more usually associated with open-water swimming. This is a form of sampling bias, in that the sample was not taken at a representative time. Imagine next that I am surveying patients about their satisfaction with a smoking cessation service. It seems sensible to wait until patients have completed all planned sessions before asking them to evaluate the service. But if half the patients drop out before completing all sessions, and so do not get surveyed, it is reasonable to assume that my results will be positively skewed by not including those who did not complete, and quite likely were less satisfied with the service, in other words the results are biased by attrition. In the case of a trial of hip protectors in residential settings for older people, the researchers might find a reduction in risk for pelvic fractures but no evidence of a reduction in risk for hip fractures associated with the intervention. If only the results for pelvic fractures are presented, then this will give an overly optimistic view of the effectiveness of the intervention, and this is known as reporting bias. Taking this example a step further, if it were the case that ten such trials have been conducted in the last five years, and imagine that half have found evidence of a protective effect of providing hip protectors and half have not. If the five 'negative' finding studies are not published in peer-reviewed journals (either because the authors do not think it is worth writing up, or because this is not a sufficiently interesting finding to find its way into a journal), but the five 'positive' finding results are accessible in journals, then any review of the subject will conclude that the evidence for providing hip protectors in residential settings for older people is much stronger than it really is. This is due to publication bias, the extent and implications of which are further discussed by Dwan et al. (2013). There are many other forms of bias beyond those mentioned here. The key thing is for researchers to be alert to possible sources of bias in their own research, and in published studies (see, for example, Lundh et al., 2017).

Confounding

Confounding is actually a form of bias, but is so important in epidemiology that it is usually considered as a separate problem. It refers to the very common situation in which the association of interest between an exposure and an outcome is biased by some other factor. This other factor, known as a confounder (or confounding factor), is associated with both the exposure and the outcome.

Consider a study looking at the association between dietary vitamin supplementation and breast cancer, to test the hypothesis that dietary supplementation reduces the risk (see Figure 1.1a). If a negative association is found (i.e. supplementation is associated with lower rates of cancer), then this could be taken in support of the hypothesis. This apparent association is denoted by the dotted arrow in Figure 1.1a. However, it is quite likely that those people in the sample who take vitamin supplements are more health conscious than those who don't, and therefore engage in other health behaviours likely to reduce their risk of cancer (in terms of diet, and alcohol and tobacco use). This association is denoted by the double-headed solid arrow in Figure 1.1a.

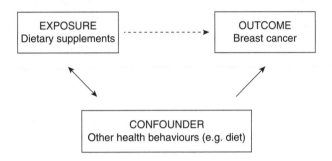

Figure 1.1a   **Example of confounding by health behaviours**

It may be these other health behaviours that reduce the risk of breast cancer (denoted by another solid arrow), rather than the dietary supplementation. Another example is the apparent association between breastfeeding and the subsequent body mass index (BMI) of the child (see Figure 1.1b). Breastfeeding in the UK is socially patterned (solid double-headed arrow). Since higher socio-economic status is associated with a range of dietary and lifestyle factors which are likely to lead to lower BMI (also denoted by a solid arrow), it appears that breastfeeding is associated with lower BMI in children (dotted arrow). Interestingly, this social patterning does not exist in every country, and data from Brazil has been used to demonstrate that in the absence of an association between breastfeeding (the exposure) and socio-economic status (the confounder), there is no evidence of an association between breastfeeding and child BMI (Brion et al., 2011).

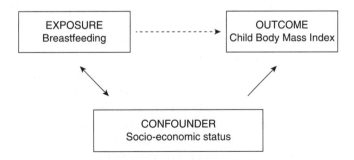

Figure 1.1b   **Example of confounding by socio-economic status**

Common confounders in epidemiology are age, gender, socio-economic status and ethnicity. While Figure 1.1 shows one confounder operating at a time, in reality there could be several confounders operating at once, including other more specific confounders for the particular association under study. When considering possible confounders, always ask whether it is (or could plausibly be) associated with both the exposure and the outcome. If not, then it is not a potential confounder.

Epidemiology has various methods to deal with confounding at both the study design stage and the analysis stage (and both will be discussed later), but these generally require us to identify and measure these variables for our study population. If we are unaware of certain confounders then we cannot measure them, and this is a problem (though one which is largely overcome by RCTs, as we shall see later). Another problem with most epidemiological study designs is that even though they allow confounders to be measured and taken into account, there is often a degree of 'residual confounding'. This is because when we try to measure confounders, we often end up with a poor proxy, so our adjustment for confounding is only partial. While age and gender are fairly straightforward to measure, the construct 'socio-economic status' is less clear cut and harder to measure. Should we base it on income, and if so is this the income of the individual in the study (who may not be in paid employment) or the household income, and should it take into account capital wealth, perhaps looking at home ownership or the estimated value of the property? You might decide that it would be easier to measure educational level, in which case how should vocational training such as apprenticeships be scored in relation to academic qualifications, and how do we take into account changes in grading systems over time (as has recently happened to school leavers' exams in the UK)? It is clear that any such attempts to quantify socio-economic status for individuals are inadequate, and therefore so is our ability to control for confounding by socio-economic status. For other examples see Kozuki et al. (2013) and Hulse et al. (1997).

Causation

If we observe an association between two variables (in epidemiological terms an exposure and an outcome), does that mean that the exposure is causing the outcome, in other words that the relationship is causal? Imagine a report that claims a correlation between ice-cream sales and cases of unexpected collapse. It doesn't take much to work out that the ice-cream is unlikely to be causing people to collapse, and that any association is due to both ice-cream sales and collapses (due to heat stroke) occurring in warmer weather. Here, temperature is a confounder, which leads to an apparent but spurious relationship between ice-cream sales and people collapsing. So we can see fairly easily that this is not a causal relationship. But taking a less trivial example, consider the results of a lifestyle survey, which finds a strong positive association between levels of physical activity and mental health. Those with higher levels of physical activity have better mental health. It is tempting to jump to the conclusion that there is a causal relationship such that exercise improves mental health. While this is very likely to be the case, we cannot assume, based on a cross-sectional survey, that exercise is influencing mental health in this way. It is equally possible that mental health is affecting peoples' motivation to take exercise. Those who are more depressed are perhaps less likely to go to the gym, or go out for a walk. This is an example of reverse causation, because the causation is happening in the opposite direction to what we expected. Next imagine a news report claims that drinking at least three cups of coffee a day improves longevity. This is not a case of reverse causation, because dying earlier is not going to make you drink less coffee. Does that mean we can trust it, and start drinking lots of coffee to improve our life expectancy?

When an association is observed between an exposure and an outcome, there are three things that must be considered before going on to assess the likelihood of a causal relationship. These are chance, bias and confounding, all of which have been introduced above. If these can be ruled out, then the Bradford Hill criteria are useful in further examining whether or not the association is causal. The criteria outlined by Hill (1965) are shown in Table 1.1. While it is not necessary that all these criteria clearly apply for an association to be deemed as causal, they assist us in judging the likelihood of a causal relationship.

Table 1.1 The Bradford Hill criteria

Criteria	Interpretation	Application
Temporal relationship	Are we sure that the exposure happened before the outcome?	It sounds obvious that this has to be true if the relationship is causal, but in many study designs it is not clear whether it is the case.
Biological plausibility	Does it make sense biologically that the exposure causes the outcome?	It is possible for an epidemiological study to identify that a particular exposure causes an outcome before science can explain why it does so, but some sort of understanding of the causal mechanisms is helpful.
Consistency	Are similar results found in different populations and using different study designs?	A study in the UK found a relationship between breastfeeding and offspring BMI, but this was not supported by a similar study in Brazil, so it is unlikely to be causal. Cohort studies of vitamin supplementation and cancer find that supplementation is protective (reduces the risk), but the same results are not found in trials.
Strength	How big is the apparent effect of the exposure on the outcome?	If the study suggests a very strong effect, such as a doubling or halving of risk, then this is more likely to be real than a smaller effect. Note that this is not referring to statistical significance.

(Continued)

Table 1.1   (Continued)

Criteria	Interpretation	Application
Dose-response	Does the size of effect vary in accordance with the magnitude of the exposure?	The more people smoke, whether that is measured in terms of number of cigarettes smoked per day or the number of years they have been a smoker, the greater their risk of developing lung cancer. This is an example of a dose-response relationship.
Specificity	If an exposure increases the risk of one outcome but not others, then the relationship is specific.	In reality, this type of one-to-one relationship between exposure and outcome rarely exists. For example, smoking increases the risk of a wide range of cancers. An example of a more specific relationship is between hair dyes previously used by hairdressers and bladder cancer.
Reversibility	Does the removal of the exposure lead to a reduction in the health outcome of interest?	We know that smokers who subsequently give up have a reduced risk of lung cancer, compared with those who do not give up. So the relationship between smoking and lung cancer is, to some extent at least, reversible.

Key epidemiological study designs

There are two important classifications that can be made of epidemiological study designs. First, in observational studies we do not intervene, but simply observe exposures and outcomes in a sample from the population, while in intervention studies we are testing an intervention by giving it to some people and not others, then monitoring the outcome – in other words, we are experimenting. Second, some studies collect information on exposures before the outcome is known (these are prospective studies) while others collect data on outcomes before exposures (these are retrospective studies).

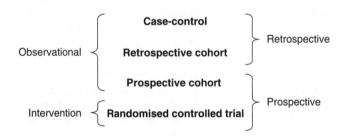

Figure 1.2   Characteristics of key epidemiological study designs

Figure 1.2 shows the key epidemiological study designs, and classifies them as either observational studies or intervention (experimental) studies, and as retrospective or prospective. It is worth noting that cross-sectional studies, such as surveys, collect data on exposures and outcomes at the same point in time. Although survey methodology plays an important role in epidemiology as a data collection tool (see Chapter 3), and cross-sectional studies are useful for descriptive epidemiology, they do not help in understanding causal relationships between exposures and outcomes. For that reason they are not discussed further in this chapter.

Case-control studies

As can be seen in Figure 1.2, case-control studies are retrospective and observational. The defining feature of a case-control study is that participants are selected based on either being a 'case' (see Figure 1.3) or a 'control'. A case is someone who has the health outcome of interest, and a control is someone who does not. Most commonly, we take an equal number of cases and controls and they are 'matched' to be similar in terms of potential confounders (such as age, sex, ethnicity), but this does not have to be the case. We then look back in time at exposures that occurred before the onset of the disease or health outcome of interest. Comparing the proportions of cases and controls who were exposed to potential causes of the disease, we can assess which exposures, if any, appear to be associated with the outcome of interest. The strength of the association is measured using an 'odds ratio' – this is explained in more detail in Chapter 4.

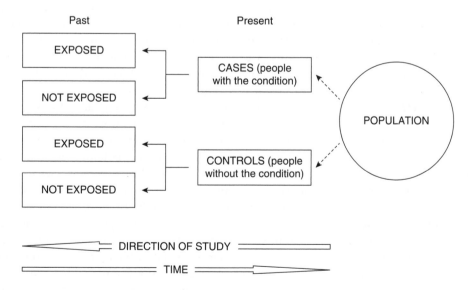

Figure 1.3 Case-control study design

The most obvious drawback of this approach is that we are asking participants to recall exposures that happened in the past. The accuracy of this data will depend on the exposure we are interested in, and how long ago it occurred. For example, consider how well you would expect participants to answer the following questions: a) how many cups of coffee did you drink in the last week? and b) how many children have you given birth to? Our memories are fallible, so the data is not accurate – in other words, there is measurement error of the exposure. But, more than that, our memories are affected by our own particular viewpoint, including life-changing experiences. So, if an individual has been diagnosed with a terminal illness, and they know that the exposure you are asking them to recall (say a particular medical procedure they may have previously undergone) is a potential risk factor for that illness, then they are more likely to recall it than someone who is well, even if they both had the same level of exposure. This is called 'recall bias' and is a particular problem in case-control studies that rely on participant recall for measuring exposures. In the example given here, it might be possible to corroborate self-reported exposure to the medical procedure with data from medical records. Of course, administrative records can be incomplete or inaccurate, but they do not suffer from recall bias, and comparison of the two would improve the quality of the exposure data in this case.

It might seem that with this study design we can be sure that the exposure happened before the outcome (the first of the Bradford Hill criteria described above), but the following example illustrates that this may not always be the case. Consider a case-control study looking at dementia (the outcome) and social networks (the exposure). If we ask cases (who have recently been diagnosed as having dementia) and controls (with no dementia diagnosis) about levels of social contact 10 years ago, we might find that the cases report lower levels of social contact than controls, and therefore conclude that social contact is protective against dementia. It is possible, however, that those who have recently been diagnosed with dementia have for some time been experiencing symptoms which have limited their social interactions. In this case the exposure did not happen before the onset of dementia, and our study suffers from reverse causation (in other words, it is the early symptoms of dementia which are causing a reduction in social contact).

The advantages of case-control studies are that they are relatively quick to carry out, because there is no follow-up period, and they are suitable for rare diseases. They are used extensively for outbreaks of infectious diseases because it is important to identify the source quickly and prevent further spread. This illustrates another potential problem with this study design that is worth being aware of, in that those selected as cases may actually be controls who are not yet symptomatic. Imagine I select all ten cases in a town who have been diagnosed by a doctor, based on their symptoms, as suffering from salmonella poisoning. I then select ten controls from the same town, matched on age, sex and residential street. A dietary questionnaire is administered to both cases and controls, to identify foods which may be causing the infection. In this situation, it is possible that some of the controls are carrying salmonella, but have not yet reached the symptomatic stage. This inaccurate classification of cases and controls (measurement error of the outcome) will make it harder for us to identify the source of the infection.

Cohort studies

Cohort (or longitudinal) studies can be either retrospective or, more commonly, prospective. Prospective cohort studies are generally considered to be superior to case-control studies, mainly because they do not suffer from recall bias. As shown in Figure 1.4a, they begin by selecting a cohort of people, measuring exposures (before the outcome of interest has occurred) and then following up and measuring outcomes at a later point in time, sometimes many decades later. This has the benefit of ruling out recall bias and helps to define a temporal relationship. It is worth pointing out that this is not an efficient method to study a rare disease or outcome, because even among a relatively large cohort, an inadequate number of cases will accrue to draw reliable conclusions from the study – so for rare outcomes a case-control study may be preferable. However, a major advantage of cohort studies over case-control studies is that they can be used to examine a multitude of outcomes as well as numerous possible exposures. (In contrast, a case-control study is restricted to one particular outcome of interest.) A drawback is that they rely on long-term follow-up of participants, which is expensive, and that some participants will choose to drop out or will be lost to follow-up, creating attrition bias. This occurs because those people who drop out or are lost are likely to be different to those who remain in the study. For example, we know that women and people with higher educational levels are more likely to continue to contribute to a longitudinal study, and it seems likely that those with chaotic lifestyles are more likely to be lost to follow-up, through frequent changes of address for example. To illustrate the importance of attrition bias, consider a cohort study of HIV patients that sets out to describe prognosis. If, by the end of the follow-up period of 10 years, those who dropped out did so because they became so ill that they could no longer get to follow-up appointments or respond to questionnaires, then prognosis would

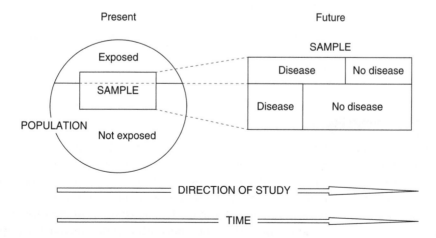

Figure 1.4a **Prospective cohort study design**

look better than it really is. If, on the other hand, those who drop out did so because they are not yet symptomatic and are therefore less motivated to take part in the study, then prognosis would look worse than it really is.

Retrospective cohort studies work the other way round, and try to create past exposure data for an existing group of people. Like case-control studies, retrospective cohort studies generally rely either on participant recall or on administrative records to measure previous exposures, neither of which is ideal. If the former, then recall bias is a possibility, as with case-control studies. It is sometimes difficult to differentiate between case-control studies and retrospective cohort studies. It helps to remember that case-control studies start by selecting two separate groups of participants based on disease status – cases and controls – while retrospective studies take a whole cohort of participants then establish disease status for the whole cohort. Both then seek to ascertain past exposure data for all participants, but the cohort study is more likely to include longitudinal data on a range of exposures at different points in time.

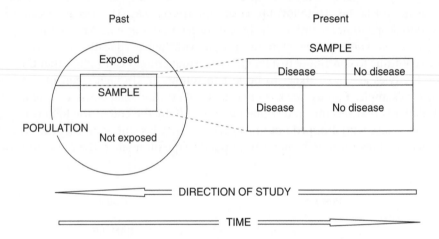

Figure 1.4b   **Retrospective cohort study design**

Randomised controlled trials

The theory of RCTs developed around drug trials. It can be challenging to apply this in practice to public health interventions, but to illustrate the process let's take an example of a school-based physical activity intervention designed to reduce childhood obesity. As illustrated in Figure 1.5, a group of eligible children is randomised to one of two groups, the intervention (exposure) or not (control group). The outcome of interest (body mass index) is measured after randomisation, then the intervention group receive the physical activity programme and the control group do not, and body mass index is measured again at the end of the follow-up period. The average change over time for each group is compared to see whether the intervention helped to reduce body mass index. The major advantage of this study design over observational study designs is that it deals effectively with confounding. Although there are methods for dealing with confounding (such as using matched controls in case-control studies, and controlling for potential confounders in the analysis of cohort studies), the risk of residual confounding means that the results of any observational study must be treated with caution.

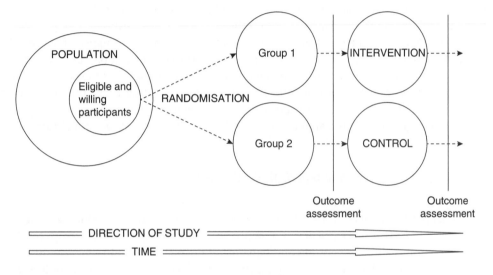

Figure 1.5   Randomised controlled trial design

To see the benefit of randomisation, consider the previously discussed example of dietary supplementation and risk of breast cancer. Let's say that in a cohort study the role of dietary supplementation in reducing breast cancer risk is confounded by other lifestyle factors. So, on average, the women who took supplements also took more exercise, drank less alcohol, smoked less and had a healthier diet, and it is these factors, rather than the supplements, that reduced the risk of breast cancer. If we are not aware of these as confounders, and able to measure them all, then we will draw the wrong conclusion based on this study. Now imagine a RCT in which a large group of women are randomised to two groups. The intervention group will receive dietary supplements and the control group will not. On average, the two groups will be quite similar with respect to their lifestyle choices, because they have been allocated at random rather than through personal choice or any sort of selection process. That means that if at the end of the follow-up period we see a difference in breast cancer rates between the two groups, it cannot be due to exercise, alcohol, smoking or dietary differences. In other words, it is not confounded. Better still, if there are other confounders that we are unaware of (and therefore cannot measure) then these also will be approximately equally distributed between the two arms of the trial.

Of course, if the randomisation process does not result in roughly similar groups (which is more likely to occur when there is a small number of participants) then confounding is still possible, but we can check for the distribution of known confounders, and deal with these at the analysis stage if necessary. Bias is a potential problem with RCTs and this is because the participants and anyone else involved in assessing their outcomes could well be biased by knowledge of whether they received the intervention or the control. If it is possible to 'blind' both the participants and the assessors to the treatment group, in other words to hide from them which group the individual is in, then the chance of bias will be reduced. To achieve this, it helps to give a 'placebo' to the control group. This is something that is as similar to the intervention being tested as possible, that is not expected to have any effect other than the 'placebo effect'. In the context of drug trials, this would be a sugar-coated pill made to look like the active drug. The use of placebos in trials of public health interventions, and the application of RCTs more generally, is less straightforward.

Summary of key epidemiological study designs

The importance of the classification of study designs (see Figure 1.2) relates to the important concepts of bias and confounding. Only experimental studies can eliminate the role of confounding. This is a particular problem with cohort studies, which attempt to identify associations between exposures and outcomes, which are distant in time – many other factors will have influenced the study participants between these two time points, and some of these will be potential confounders. But if they are not measured, then we cannot control for them in the analysis, and we may not even be aware of them as potential confounders. Retrospective studies are more prone to bias than prospective studies (because they often rely on recall of previous exposures, which may be affected by the health outcome of interest). But even prospective studies can suffer from bias, such as a trial in which blinding of participants is not possible, and the outcome is self-reported. So, for any epidemiological study, it is important to consider whether bias and confounding are likely to have occurred, to attempt to describe the likely effect of bias or confounding, and to deal with it at the analysis stage if possible.

Complex interventions

Public health interventions rarely consist of a simple intervention such as a drug capsule, which can be easily replicated by a placebo capsule, dealing with confounding and bias in a standardised study design such as that described in Figure 1.5. Interventions in public health typically involve programmes involving a range of components, targeting various levels (such as individuals and communities), with multiple outcomes to be measured at different time points. These are known as 'complex interventions'. These present challenges in terms of conducting RCTs, because it is difficult to blind someone as to whether or not they are participating in a physical activity session or a smoking cessation intervention, for example. Finding appropriate placebos is much more challenging than in more medical trials. There are also problems of 'contamination' with these types of interventions.

One approach, which is commonly used in public health, is to randomise whole clusters of people rather than individuals. This is often done for practical reasons, as well as to avoid contamination. If we were to plan a trial to test a new method of providing clean drinking water to households in rural Bolivia, for example, it would not be practical to randomise individuals to receive the new water purification system being tested, as it will apply to the water source for the whole family. And randomising individuals to interventions in the healthcare setting can be difficult practically and even ethically for the professionals involved; for example, offering one level of care to one patient on a ward and a less intensive intervention to the patient in the bed next to them could be difficult for staff on the ward, even if as researchers we have no objections to randomisation as a way to test interventions.

BOX 1.2   COMPLEX INTERVENTIONS AND THE PROBLEM OF 'CONTAMINATION'

Assume that a health promotion intervention delivered in schools to improve children's knowledge and behaviour around healthy eating is to be assessed through a randomised controlled trial (RCT).

If the children in a school were randomised to receive the intervention or not, you would expect to find in some families that some siblings would receive the intervention and others would not.

If one of the aims of the intervention is to encourage children to discuss with their parents healthy meals, thereby influencing meals eaten at home as well as at school, then this will have an effect on the whole family. Similarly, within friendship groups, if some children receive an intervention aimed at increasing levels of physical activity while others do not, then you might expect friends in the control group to be influenced by the intervention, through their friendships.

This will dilute the apparent effect of the intervention, because the control is being *contaminated* by the intervention.

One of the greatest problems faced by those trying to use RCTs in public health is that any attempt to randomise individuals to receive an intervention is perceived as 'playing God' or inherently unfair, and that cluster randomisation results in a postcode lottery. Two simple solutions can be applied to this problem. The first is to ensure that everyone receives the intervention eventually, in other words the control group receive it after the trial has concluded. The second applies in situations of scarce resources – if it is the case that we cannot give all eligible participants the intervention anyway (perhaps we are offering a number of free childcare places), we might as well randomise the allocation and get good quality evidence about the effect of this on outcomes (which may be child development, for example). See Chapter 14 on ethics for further discussion of these issues.

There are other adaptations of the textbook RCT that are useful in public health, namely natural experiments and stepped wedge designs. Natural experiments make the most of naturally occurring levels of exposure (either over time or in different locations), so that the intervention is not actually randomised. A good example would be the comparison of children's tooth caries in three distinct areas: a) no water fluoridation, b) naturally fluoridated water and c) artificially fluoridated water (Jones et al., 1997). Another would be comparison of coronary events, before and after the introduction of national smoke-free legislation (Sebrié et al., 2012), also known as a 'before-and-after study'. Finally, stepped wedge designs suit the situation in which an intervention is gradually introduced across an area or population, with a pilot followed by staged roll-out, such as the introduction of 20 mph limits within a city (Bornioli et al., 2018). Though not so straightforward to administer and analyse as the standard RCT, these methods are invaluable to generate high-quality evidence in public health.

Conclusion

In conclusion, epidemiology provides a set of quantitative tools to study risk factors and health outcomes at a population level, and associations between them. However, before an observed association is assumed to be causal, it is important to consider whether it could have been caused by chance, bias or confounding. The Bradford Hill criteria are useful in judging whether an observed association is likely to be causal. Epidemiological study designs include case-control studies, cohort studies and RCTs. The strengths and weaknesses of each have been considered. In particular, the difficulty in applying RCTs in public health has been highlighted, and some alternative designs introduced.

Further reading

Bonita, R., Beaglehole, R. and Tord, K. (2006) *Basic Epidemiology*. Geneva: World Health Organization.

Gordis, L. (2013) *Epidemiology*. Philadelphia: Saunders.

Hennekens, C.H. and Buring, J.E. (1987) *Epidemiology in Medicine*. Boston: Little, Brown.

Rothman, K.J. (2012) *Epidemiology; an introduction* (Second edition). Oxford: Oxford University Press.

2 SAMPLING

============ **CHAPTER SUMMARY** ============

This chapter will start with the reasons for **sampling** from a population when conducting research, touching on the issue of **inferential statistics**. The concept of a **sampling frame** (with relevant examples) and key approaches to sampling in **quantitative research** will be outlined. This includes both **probability** and **non-probability sampling**, with the strengths and limitations of each approach discussed. Rather than emphasising the differences between sampling techniques used in qualitative and quantitative research, we will seek to use a common language that matches that used in Chapter 7 on qualitative sampling, explaining which techniques are most appropriate, when, and why. The practicalities of sampling will be explored through real-life examples from public health research.

What is sampling and why do we do it?

One of the first considerations for students when undertaking quantitative research is to identify the population that they are planning to do their research on. This population could be groups of people with particular characteristics (such as children diagnosed with asthma), or it could be non-human units of interest, such as geographic sites from which air quality tests, or traffic counts will be carried out.

The population of interest is of course defined by the research question that the researcher is seeking to answer. For example, 'What are the attitudes of UK-based MSc Public Health/MPH students towards issues relating to climate change?' would require a focus on those studying public health at the postgraduate level in the UK. But would a student seeking to answer this question survey all students who are currently undertaking postgraduate MSc/MPH study in public health? In the UK alone, this would be a significant task, given the large number of providers of public health master's courses. Usually for those undertaking public health research as part of their dissertation, or in practice, there are significant limitations in time and other resources, most notably research costs. And although the advent of online survey tools has made it easier and cheaper to target larger and more disparate populations, there are still resource issues for students and small-scale researchers when taking a whole population approach. This includes the need to deal with a larger number of gatekeepers or facilitators (who will help you to access your targeted population and encourage response to the survey), such as programme leaders. What if your research question was not limited to UK postgraduate public health students, but included those throughout North America and Australasia too? Hopefully, it is clear that you wouldn't aim to send out your survey, even an online survey, to every public health postgraduate student undertaking an MSc Public Health/MPH across those territories!

The good news is that to answer research questions such as the one above, we don't need to target the whole of a population. Sometimes, under certain circumstances, this is done, and we will discuss this below. However, usually it is not necessary, or even preferable, to target every member of a specified population in order to answer a research question. In normal practice, we select a sample, and make 'inferences' from this sample back to the whole population of interest.

From sample to population – considerations when selecting an approach

A sample of a population, in its simplest terms, represents a sub-set of the whole population from which that sample was taken. The means by which we obtain the sample can be varied, and these will be discussed in the remainder of this chapter. So too will be the strengths, limitations and other implications associated with each approach to selecting a sample. As with lots of public health research, the chosen approach is often guided by the research question under consideration, tempered by resource constraints and speckled with a dose of pragmatism!

Wherever possible, the sample should represent the population from which it is taken. This then allows us to make inferences about the results from the sample, applying the findings back to the wider population. Certain sampling approaches are better than others at maximising the generalisability of the sample gained, and this will be noted in the chapter.

The sampling frame

Once we have decided on the population from which we want to select our sample, the next question we need to ask ourselves is this – is there a clear sampling frame from which to select our sample? A sampling frame is the means by which we can select those people (or non-human units such as geographical locations) to be in our sample. It is the 'list' of the population under study, from which you can then sample. The sampling frame, both its existence and its quality (including completeness and detail) determines *how* we can select our sample. We will come on to the *how* in a moment.

So what about an example of a sampling frame? Going back to the example of postgraduate public health students and their attitudes towards climate change, how can we obtain a list of all students from which to take our sample? We know that universities hold the records of all students on electronic systems, usually identified by unique Student ID numbers and organised by home Faculty/School/Department, course programmes registered on, modules studied and other administrative groupings. So, in this case, the sampling frame is the list of students registered on the MSc Public Health/MPH, as detailed by the university student registration system. The list of students, acting as the sampling frame, then enables us to select our sub-set, our sample, on which we do research and then make inferences from the findings back to the whole population.

In the case of the university students, there is an identified sampling frame, which is complete and accurate. This is obviously the ideal scenario, but sometimes the sampling frame is not always so straightforward.

When we don't sample

Before we turn to the *how* of sampling, it's worth mentioning occasions when we don't need to sample. Probably the most famous piece of survey work that targets a whole population approach in the UK is the Census (see Box 2.1). Indeed, the word census refers to an activity that obtains details from all of the population.

BOX 2.1 UK HOUSEHOLD CENSUS

This questionnaire-based survey is sent to every household in the UK, for the head of that household to complete. The last census data was collected in 2011.

The exercise is vast and expensive. It takes places once every ten years, gaining socio-demographic details from households that is then fed into planning and used for research.

Census data is collected around the world with some countries like Australia, Canada, and Japan collecting census data every 5 years.

There are question marks over the future of the census, given the huge cost involved, as well as the practical difficulties of reaching (and engaging) the whole population.

Source: Office for National Statistics: www.ons.gov.uk/census

There might be occasions when, even as part of a dissertation or small-scale service public health research project, you might choose to target the whole population. The most obvious scenario where this might happen is if the total population is small enough to target in its entirety, even with the limited resources available. In that situation, it is sensible to take a whole-population approach, as all things being equal, using the whole population is better than inferring results from a sample to that same population.

Approaches to sampling

Once we have our sampling frame, as outlined in the previous section, the decision needs to be made as to how we sample. There are broadly two approaches to sampling: probability and non-probability sampling. Before we talk in more depth about these two approaches, and the sub-approaches within them, it's worth focusing on an important issue: representativeness. If we wish to make inferences from our sample to the general population, the more that we can ensure the people in our sample are representative of the wider population from which they were taken, the better. Ideally, the sample will be the 'population in miniature', including the same spread of people in terms of characteristics such as age, sex, ethnicity, socio-economic status, etc. How well this is achieved determines not only how representative the sample is of the wider population, but how representative the *findings* are from our research and, in turn, how generalisable they are to that wider population. The way we select our sample, and the results of that selection in terms of the characteristics of the sample, are therefore crucial. An unrepresentative sample will lead to problems when inferring results to the wider population. We'll discuss some of these problems later in this chapter.

What is probability sampling?

Probability sampling, done well, is the best way to ensure that you gain a representative sample from your population of interest. In probability sampling, every member of the target population has an equal chance (probability) of being selected for inclusion in the sample. Selection is made based on chance, free from value judgements of the researcher. This value-free method of selection should ensure that the sample that is selected is representative of the total population of interest. There are several approaches to probability sampling, which we will now discuss.

Simple random sampling

Simple random sampling is the most straightforward approach to probability sampling and, if done correctly, is extremely effective at ensuring the selected sample is representative of the wider population – if the sample is large enough. Assuming we have our sampling frame, a simple random sampling method then selects a number of individuals from the population list using a means of random selection. This can be through the use of random number tables (a traditional method) or more recently by using random number generators that are available online. Each member of the population must be identifiable by a number that is generated randomly. So, for example, a spreadsheet of all the MSc Public Health/MPH students across universities in the UK could be extracted from the student records systems (forming the sampling frame), and each of these students could be assigned a number, from 1 to however many students there are in the total population. If it has been decided to sample 300 of these students (more about sample size later!), then 300 random numbers would be generated to form the sample.

Systematic random sampling

Systematic random sampling is a variation of simple random sampling. The sampling frame is ordered, before a random selection is made of the first individual in the sample. For example, this might be the fourteenth person on the list of students. Selection of the remaining 299 students is then made by selecting every 'nth' person on the list – so, for instance, every fifth person after the initial individual who has been selected. This method of probability sampling might be problematic if there is some particular ordering of the individuals in the sampling frame; for example, an alphabetical order that results in those from certain ethnic backgrounds to cluster around one point in the list. If this is the case, it may result in an unrepresentative sample. Caution is therefore needed when undertaking a systematic sampling approach, to ensure that ordering of the list is free from such issues. One example of this approach is a study which examined the content of initiatives that the alcohol industry implemented to reduce drink-driving (Esser et al., 2016). The researchers arranged the initiatives alphabetically by title and then selected every third for analysis.

Stratified random sampling

Stratified random sampling is used when the researchers want to ensure that the sample contains a representative spread of individuals based on a particular characteristic. Although simple random sampling should ensure this happens, sometimes, through chance, the resulting sample might under-represent certain types of individuals. For example, in the survey of UK-based MSc Public Health/MPH students, a simple random sampling approach might, just by chance, result in a sample that under-represents students from a particular institution, based on how many students are studying there in relation to the total number of UK-based postgraduate public health students. In order to ensure that there is a representative spread of students from across the institutions, we could stratify the sampling frame – that is, to split the sampling frame into strata. In this example, the strata would be institution, with the list split by institution of study. A set number of students at each institution would then be randomly selected for inclusion in the sample. The number of students selected per institution could be set to ensure that the same number of students are included in the sample for each institution, or it could be set to reflect the proportion of students in the total population from each institution. This would then ensure that the resulting sample is representative in terms of institution. However, it does not guarantee it is representative in other ways, such as the population distribution by age, sex, ethnicity and whether they are UK or international students. It is possible to stratify by more than one characteristic, so for example by institution and by sex, or even three or more characteristics. The decision of whether to stratify, and by how many strata, depends on how important it is to ensure that a particular characteristic is represented in the sample. It also depends on the information that is available in the sampling frame, to enable the characteristics to be identified.

BOX 2.2   STRATIFIED RANDOM SAMPLING (POPE ET AL., 2015)

A key example of a stratified sampling approach is that from Pope et al. (2015), a study of how quality of green space can improve mental wellbeing and alleviate psychological distress.

In this study, a random sample of people on a local GP list, *stratified by age and sex*, was selected to explore the relationship between access to and quality of green space and mental wellbeing.

By stratifying by age and sex, the researchers sought to ensure that their sample was representative on these two key demographic factors.

Cluster sampling

Cluster sampling involves random sampling not of individuals, but clusters of individuals. For example, common clusters used in research include schools and workplaces. One example of a study that took a cluster sampling approach is that by Lyons et al. (2008), where local authority areas were the cluster unit. As part of a randomised controlled trial, the researchers sampled local authority areas (and then electoral wards within them) to either receive a road safety intervention or not, to determine whether this impacted on efforts to improve pedestrian injuries at local levels. The researchers did not want to have intervention and control wards in the same local authority, which is why the cluster sampling approach was taken. As with this example, cluster sampling is often used as part of a multi-stage random sampling strategy.

Multi-stage random sampling

Multi-stage random sampling, as its name suggests, involves more than one sampling stage. For example, we may decide in our study that, for pragmatic reasons, we do not wish to sample students across all UK MSc Public Health/MPH courses. A first stage then would be to list all the institutions in the UK who provide masters courses in public health, and randomly select a specified number of these institutions to be included in the study (cluster sampling). Once these institutions have been selected, a second stage could be to randomly select students from those institutions, either through simple random sampling or a stratified approach. This would be a two-stage random sampling approach. Such an approach might be preferable to a dissertation student as it would reduce the number of institutions that they would have to engage with, thereby targeting their energies and other resources at a smaller group of programme leaders, or whoever else they might want to assist them with their study.

If done well, the resulting sampling should still represent the wider population of UK-based public health students.

What is non-probability sampling?

Non-probability sampling is an approach to sampling whereby members of the population under study do not have an equal chance of being selected for inclusion in the sample. Unlike probability sampling, selection is not the result of chance, value-free selection. The sample will not therefore be representative of the wider population in terms of key demographic and other characteristics. For this reason, non-probability sampling is not the best approach to take if you wish to generalise the findings from the sample to the wider population. As generalisation is usually the aim of researchers, wherever possible a probability approach to sampling should be taken. However, there are situations where a non-probability method of identifying individuals for inclusion in the study sample could be justified. One valid reason is where no comprehensive sampling frame can be identified. In this scenario, it may not be possible to randomly select individuals as there is no list from which to select, and therefore a non-probability approach may be the only option. The limitations of such an approach should always be recognised and discussed, and these limitations will be noted in the sections below.

Convenience sampling

Convenience sampling is an approach to sampling where pragmatism is at the forefront of decision making. For example, given resource limitations a student may decide that they want to focus their research locally, on a sample of individuals who are more easily accessible to them and/or more willing to participate in the research. For instance, in the study of student attitudes, an MSc Public Health student at the University of the West of England (UWE) may decide to survey their cohort classmates about attitudes towards climate change. Let's say there are 50 students on the MSc, and of those students, 45 complete and return the survey. The student undertaking the research is pleased with the response, given that only five students failed to participate. They analyse the results and write up their findings, summarising attitudes towards climate change, and generalising the findings to all UK-based postgraduate public health students. Is this sensible? Hopefully it's clear that such an approach isn't sensible. Students on the course at UWE might differ in important ways from the wider UK-based student population – currently UWE has a strong focus on sustainability and climate change in the curriculum, and across the university, so this would possibly lead to a cohort that is more aware of climate change issues and their links to public health. Or at least the faculty would hope so! It would be more appropriate to amend the research question so that the focus was restricted just to exploring attitudes among UWE public health students. But that would limit the wider applicability of the research, and hinder any attempts to publish from the work by applying the findings more widely.

BOX 2.3 CONVENIENCE SAMPLING: STUDY OF 20 MPH (32 KPH) SPEED LIMITS IN CITIES

In this example of convenience sampling, a student wishing to investigate attitudes among the population of Bristol, UK to 20 mph speed limits might decide that the most convenient way for them to gain a sample of the population would be to stand in a busy part of the city centre and approach passers-by.

Would this result in a representative sample of the Bristol population?

The likelihood is that it would not, because the choice of *who* to approach would be made by the *researcher*, and their choice of person might be influenced by any number of factors, such as whether the passer-by looks friendly, or whether they are male or female, of a certain ethnic background, or whether they seem busy!

This human influence in the selection of the sample would be likely to lead to a biased selection. We will talk more about bias later in this chapter.

Snowball sampling

Snowball sampling is an approach where sample members are recruited based on contacts or recommendations from other sample members, with the size of the sample increasing like a snowball picking up snow as it rolls down a hill. It is more commonly used in qualitative research; however, it can be useful in quantitative research in certain circumstances. The most common reason for taking a snowball sampling approach in quantitative research is where there is no clear sampling frame from which to carry out probability sampling. It may be that the population is particularly difficult to reach and/or identify from any official lists or registers, either because of a lack of routine data or because that particular population chooses to stay outside the system. For example, if a researcher wanted to explore the issue of local networks of drug users, to gain access to that population they would need to first find a way in, and then build trust among that group – a snowball sampling approach may be the best (and only!) way to do this.

Snowball sampling usually begins with a focus on a small group of the population of interest, who can be accessed by the researcher. These contacts are then used to identify and access other members of that population, and so on, until the researcher decides that they have enough people in their sample. Because of the method of identifying sample members, through recommendations and personal contacts, it is highly unlikely that the resulting sample will be representative of the wider population. For this reason, it isn't an ideal approach in quantitative research, and shouldn't be used where probability sampling is possible. But, as said, there are circumstances where it is the best approach.

Quota sampling

Quota sampling has traditionally been used in the field of market research, for example when companies want feedback on new products from a range of demographics. Market researchers have a quota for each sub-group of the target population, such as those of different ages, sex and ethnicity, and survey the population until the quotas are reached. While this might resemble stratified random sampling, the key difference is that with quota sampling, participants are not randomly selected. Methods of gaining individuals for the sample often include high street recruitment, as with the example used for convenience sampling. And even though the quota approach ensures a representative spread of individuals in the sample, based on the selected demographics, this does not rule out bias in selection of participants by other factors such as perceived friendliness.

Online sampling

With development in technology, particularly the existence of the Internet, ways of identifying and reaching populations are changing. Increasingly, the Internet presents opportunities for researchers to access populations, often through online surveys. For example, a survey investigating the attitudes of pregnant women towards smoking and use of electronic cigarettes during pregnancy might use the forum of an online mother and baby website to recruit participants. In some ways, this is a form of convenience sampling. Often the denominator is not known, and as with other forms of non-probability sampling the characteristics of non-responders is also unknown because the researcher does not have a comprehensive sampling frame.

Email distribution lists are also a good way of accessing potential participants, if you receive permission from the list holder. In this situation, the denominator is known (the number of people on the email list), so you can calculate a response rate. However, this assumes that all those on the distribution list receive the email, which may not be the case – some people may neglect to open it, while others might never see the message as it could be redirected to their junk mail folder.

Minimising and recognising sampling error and bias

What is sampling error?

A researcher wanted to find out the mean (average) height of male students in their university. They used the student record list as the sampling frame and a simple random sampling approach to select their sample. The height of every male student in the sample was recorded, and the mean height calculated, which revealed an average height of 175.2 cm. However, a second student mirroring this sampling approach to obtain their own sample of male students found an average height of 175.5 cm from their sample. A third student found 174.5 cm, and a fourth student 174.8 cm. All four students have used the same probability sampling approach to obtain a representative sample. So why do the sample means vary, and which one is correct?

The truth is that all are correct, but none may have found the true mean height of male students at the university. Although, as noted earlier, a well-conducted probability sampling approach should result in a sample that is representative of the wider population from which that sample was taken, findings from samples are subject to what is known as 'sampling error'. Sampling error relates to the fact that values derived from any one sample are likely to vary from the true value of that variable among the total population. This is because a sample will usually differ slightly from the total population, in terms of the characteristics of the people in the sample.

BOX 2.4   SAMPLING ERROR

Multiple samples of the same population will reveal variation in the sample values, but these values will all be near to the true population value.

This 'sampling variation' of all the sample estimates, if plotted for many repeated samples of the same population, would take the form of a normal distribution (a bell-shaped curve) around the true population value.

So, in our example, the true mean height of male students might be 175 cm, with all four sample values being close to this true value.

The variation of the sample values around the population value is known as the Standard Error (SE). So, the standard error tells us about the variability we would find between samples, if we took more than one sample from our population.

A large standard error indicates that the estimate from the sample is imprecise, while a smaller standard error indicates a greater level of precision. We obtain a more precise estimate (the standard error is reduced) if the size of the sample is increased, and if the variability of values for individual observations across the population is less – so, in our example, it depends on how much height varies across the UWE male student population. It is because of this standard error that our sample values will often not be equal to the true population value. So, what can we then say about the true population value?

Accounting for sampling error – standard error and confidence intervals

The fact that the sampling distribution – the variation of sample values around the true population value – takes the form of a normal distribution is important as it enables us to use inferential statistics to make more informed estimates of how our sample value is likely to relate to the true population value. In the case of our example, first we obtain a mean height of 175 cm from our sample, and calculate the standard error. We know, because of the properties of the normal distribution, that by multiplying this standard error by 1.96

and then adding and subtracting this from the sample mean (sample mean +/- 1.96*SE) will give us a range of values that will contain 95% of all sample values from that population. This calculation gives us what is known as a confidence interval, which is a range of values around the sample value that expresses the uncertainty we have around the estimate gained from our sample. In our example of heights among male university students, if the 95% confidence interval around our sample estimate of 175 cm was 174 cm to 176 cm we usually interpret this as meaning that while our sample value was 175 cm, we are 95% confident that the true population value (the mean height) lies between 174 cm and 176 cm. As the confidence interval is calculated from the standard error, the width of the confidence interval (and, in turn, the precision of our estimate) is dependent on the size of the sample and the variability of the observations within the population. This raises the question of how big samples should be, discussed in the section below.

Sample size considerations

One of the most common questions, and concerns, for students undertaking a piece of research that involves sampling, is: how large should the sample be? There are calculations that can be done to provide guidance as to an adequate sample size. However, such sample size calculations are most appropriate for studies that are interested in one main outcome measure, and specifically differences in that outcome measure between two or more groups within the population of interest. So, for example, in a randomised controlled trial examining the effectiveness of art therapy at improving levels of mental health and well-being among those diagnosed with depression, the researcher may wish to determine the differences in changes in levels of mental health and wellbeing (as measured by a validated scale) between a group who has received art therapy compared to those who received normal care. The researcher should ensure that the number of people in those two groups is sufficient (has the necessary 'power') to detect a statistically significant difference in levels of mental health and wellbeing, should a difference truly be present in the wider population. The sample size calculation, taking into account the difference in the primary outcome measure that the researcher thinks may exist between the two groups, provides the researcher with a number of people to recruit to their study. There are plenty of statistics books that talk through how to calculate sample size, and if you have access to statisticians in your organisation or institution, they can advise.

The ability to calculate sample size and generate a number to aim for can be comforting to the novice researcher, but it is usually unnecessary and sometimes unhelpful. The reality is that most quantitative research, particularly involving surveys, does not have one single outcome of interest – the researcher is interested to explore many different issues within the population, comparing across several different sub-sets of that population. It doesn't therefore make sense to base the sample size on one outcome. Also, as noted already in this chapter, students undertaking dissertations, or those in practice undertaking small-scale research, are likely to have important resource limitations. The issue of what is feasible and practical, while still being of value, should therefore inform the decision of how many to include in a sample for any given research project. This does not mean that the sample size does not matter. Size of sample does have an impact on the precision of the estimate that is gained from the sample as related to the wider population from which it was taken. Within reason, the larger the sample that can be taken, the better. So, how many is enough? Again, this is not a straightforward question. There will come a point when the effort and expense of increasing the sample will have diminishing returns on your research outputs, in terms of its ability to infer results to the wider population. Interestingly, the important factor here is the absolute size of your sample, not the size proportionate to the total population under study: so a survey of the UK population with a sample of 500 is as powerful statistically as a survey of students at the University of the West of England with a sample of 500. Maybe the key message here is don't worry too much about the size of your sample, but instead aim for the maximum number that is feasible for you given your resources. The way you obtain your sample, in terms of the quality of the sampling approach, is much more important than the total number in your sample.

What is non-sampling error?

Having talked about sampling error, it is also worth noting issues that often are categorised as *non-sampling errors*. This includes the issue of response rate. Even in the case of a probability sampling approach, if there is a lack of response among those sampled (for example, individuals not completing questionnaires) this can lead to an unrepresentative sample being obtained for your research. This is particularly an issue if there is some pattern to that non-response – for example, if in our survey of postgraduate public health students, home students are more likely to complete the questionnaire than international students. If this happened, the findings we obtain from the sample regarding attitudes towards climate change might not be generalisable to MSc Public Health/MPH students as a whole, and instead only be applicable to students from the UK. To minimise errors like this, it is important to make attempts to maximise the response rate with any sample and, if possible, to examine any differences between responders, non-responders and the total population. The ability to do this depends on whether there is a clear sampling frame, and if there is, what quality of information there is about the individuals within it. For example, if the sampling frame contains details about a person's age, sex and ethnic background, we can use this to assess whether there are any important response patterns by those sociodemographic characteristics. If the sampling frame does not include such details, it can be difficult to assess responder bias. And if there is no clear sampling frame, even determining a response rate is impossible. Other forms of non-sampling error to be aware of include issues when collecting and analysing data. For example, if data is collected in a biased way by the researcher – most notably if the researcher collects data from different people in the sample in a different way, depending on things such as age and sex. A way to avoid this is to use standardised methods of data collection, such as questionnaires, as well as having clear protocols for how information is gathered. Data should also be analysed in the same way for all individuals in the sample, irrespective of their age, sex, ethnic background, etc.

Conclusion

This chapter has outlined the reasons for sampling from a population when conducting research, discussed the concept of a sampling frame and examined key approaches to sampling in quantitative research. Probability and non-probability sampling have been introduced, using examples where appropriate, with the strengths and limitations of each approach discussed. We see how sampling is a vital stage in the research process, as it affects the generalisability of the work and its usefulness for public health.

Further reading

Bryman, A. (2016) *Social Research Methods* (Fifth edition). Oxford: Oxford University Press.
Diamond, I. and Jefferies, J. (2009) *Beginning Statistics*. London: Sage.

3 COLLECTING QUANTITATIVE DATA

================ CHAPTER SUMMARY ================

This chapter considers different methods of **quantitative data collection**, with a particular focus on the use of **self-completed questionnaires**. In addition to questionnaire-based surveys, the chapter also considers other forms of quantitative data collection, such as through the use of **structured observation, diaries, activity trackers** and **smartphone-based apps**. As with the preceding chapters, the focus is on the practical application of tools and techniques to assist you with your public health research.

Data collection from secondary data sources

Sources of routine data

Before we explore methods of primary data collection, it is useful to first note the many sources of secondary quantitative data that can be accessed. For those working in public health, routine data can be separated into two main areas: health and non-health related data. These will be discussed below.

Health data

Health data includes data on mortality – that is, deaths that have occurred in an area over a specified period. Mortality data is usually collected via death certificates, completed by clinicians at the time of death. Cause of death is coded using a global standardised system, the World Health Organization (WHO) International Classification of Disease (ICD), which enables comparisons of deaths from specific causes across areas and time periods. Data on causes of deaths, once collected at the local level, is then collated centrally and cleaned by Government agencies, before being made available publicly. If you are undertaking a piece of research that aims to explore incidence of deaths, then this is an invaluable source of routine data. Although it only represents the tip of the iceberg in terms of disease morbidity, it is sometimes used as an indicator of this, often because it is the most reliable or most easily available data on that particular health condition.

Data on morbidity (disease, disability and ill-health in the population) has improved significantly in recent years. This is because more systems have been put in place to ensure better surveillance and monitoring of the health of the population. Such data, as well as being used for health service and public health planning, is often now available to researchers. In the UK, for instance, data collected in primary care includes prevalence of health conditions such as diabetes, high blood pressure, asthma and more, through the maintenance of disease-based registers.

BOX 3.1   HEALTH DATA: THE CLINICAL PRACTICE RESEARCH DATALINK (CPRD)

- Clinical Practice Research Datalink (CPRD) is a UK Government research service, jointly supported by the National Institute for Health Research (NIHR) and the Medicines and Healthcare products Regulatory Agency (MHRA).
- CPRD provides access to anonymised NHS data for observational and intervention-based public health research. It is a fantastic resource that collects de-identified patient data from a network of hundreds of GP practices across the country.
- Primary care data from over 35 million patients are linked to a range of other health-related data to provide a longitudinal, representative UK population health dataset.
- It has been used to support both retrospective and prospective public health and clinical studies.

Source: www.cprd.com

Another major source of health data is that relating to admissions to hospital. Although the completeness and quality of such data varies significantly across countries, the best systems routinely record the number and reasons for hospital admissions and provide this data for planning and research purposes. In the UK, the data is known as Hospital Episode Statistics (HES) data, and can be accessed via a dedicated website. The HES database contains details of all admissions, accident and emergency attendances and outpatient appointments (those not requiring admission to a hospital bed) at NHS hospitals in England.

Non-health data

In public health, we recognise the role of the wider determinants of health – that the health of populations is affected by a huge range of factors, including those relating to the built and natural environment, transport, housing, education, the economy, as well as health-related behaviours such as smoking, consumption of alcohol and other drugs. This means that public health projects often need to collect non-health data. The range of sources of such data is too vast to cover here, but a major source of such data includes local, regional and national government. Therefore, explore government sources at all levels as a first step. Other sources include the emergency services (police, and fire and rescue) and charities. There is growing access to such data, provided in helpful ways such as through interactive dashboards that allow users to explore data in various ways. One example of a public health research project that used non-health data was work exploring the social context of road traffic crashes among young people (Pilkington et al., 2014). This study used coroners' data, which includes witness statements, police reports, and records from inquests, to assess social factors that could have led to the crash occurring.

Notable sources of secondary data

In addition to sources of routine data, there are notable sources of secondary data that are part of ongoing studies. These have the advantage of being designed for research purposes, and such studies can provide an extremely useful source of data for those undertaking public health research.

Surveys

Existing surveys can provide an excellent source of data for those wishing to collect data for public health research. For example, the Health Survey for England (HSE) is an annual survey, which has been carried out in the UK since 1991, which examines changes in the health and lifestyles of the population. Each year around 8,000 adults and 2,000 children are randomly selected to take part in the survey, to form a representative sample nationally. Information is collected by interview (using a standardised questionnaire) in addition to clinical measurements taken by specially trained nurses. Results from the survey are summarised and published each year. Data is also made available on the UK Data Service Catalogue, which is home to the UK's largest collection of digital social and economic research data. It is worthwhile to explore whether surveys have already been undertaken in your area (topic and country) of interest, and if so, in what form data is available. Summary data could help to set your research in context, while availability of raw data from surveys could enable you to undertake further analysis.

Cohort studies

Cohort, or longitudinal studies, can provide a great source of data that has often been collected over a long period of time. For example, the Avon Longitudinal Study of Parents and Children (ALSPAC) is a birth cohort study, which has been running since 1991. Over 14,000 pregnant women were recruited into the study and these women, their children, and their partners have been followed up over two decades. Using questionnaires and clinical measurements, it provides an extremely rich resource for the study of environmental and genetic factors that affect a person's health and development. The opportunity to use data from cohort studies for your own research will very much depend on the arrangements put in place by those leading the research. In the first instance, such studies will often have websites that explain data availability issues. Contacting the study team can also then clarify whether, and on what basis, data can be accessed for research purposes.

Primary data collection via questionnaire surveys

If you are not able to access existing secondary data to answer your research question, then it is appropriate to collect primary data. The most common way to do this in public health research is through questionnaire surveys, which will be the focus of the following section.

Introduction to questionnaire surveys

Questionnaires offer the ability to collect data in a standardised way and, if conducted well, generalise results from the sample selected to the wider population. It is easy to produce a bad questionnaire, which will then lead to bad research. Careful consideration is needed at all stages of development, to ensure that the questionnaire enables the researcher to meet their aims. The following sections examine these stages in detail.

Defining the survey aims and objectives

In the preparation of survey research, it is vital to determine the aims and objectives of the survey at an early stage (Oppenheim, 2001; Weisburg et al., 1996). Once these are determined, the researcher can then begin to develop the sampling strategy, identify and formulate questions for the survey, and decide on how the data is to be analysed, to ensure that the survey instrument meets the research aims and objectives (Oppenheim, 2001). Having clear aims and objectives also helps to ensure that the researcher remains focused on the task at hand, rather than being distracted by linked but irrelevant areas of interest (Oppenheim, 2001; Rodeghier, 1996).

In order to develop the aims and objectives, you will first need an in-depth understanding of the topic area, usually by conducting a literature review. This will help you to identify any key issues that could be investigated through the survey questionnaire. For example, if you wished to carry out a study to examine attitudes and behaviour of school children towards energy drinks, you would first undertake a review of the literature to identify any other quantitative and qualitative studies that have taken place (which may help you to formulate questions) and also increase your understanding of the key debates that you might wish to aim to explore in your research.

Determining the sampling frame

Sampling has already been discussed in detail in Chapter 2. As a reminder, when preparing to collect data, it is crucial to identify a clear sampling frame, as this not only guides the development of the research process but also helps to ensure that the sample under study is representative of the population to which the results are to be generalised. The sampling frame relates to the population that is to be sampled, and the means by which sampling will take place (de Vaus, 2002; Oppenheim, 2001; Rodeghier, 1996). The first step is to identify the population you want to target with your survey, and then decide how to target them. Again, using the example of the study exploring behaviour and attitudes of school children to energy drinks, your preferred sampling frame may be to target all school pupils in the UK using a random sampling method, whereby all eligible pupils would have a known, non-zero chance of being included in the study (Oppenheim, 2001; Rodeghier, 1996). Targeting pupils across the UK would ensure that the survey was generalisable on a national level, while a random sampling technique would enable you to gain a representative sample of that population, while also keeping the numbers needed to be surveyed to a manageable level given your research constraints (de Vaus, 2002).

However, such an approach would require the co-operation of gatekeepers, including schools. And there would be serious logistical and cost issues with collecting data at a national level, particularly in the context of a student project, where time and money is restricted. It is more likely that your sampling frame will balance feasibility with generalisability, possibly confining research to a more local level.

A more pragmatic approach to simple random sampling would be to take a cluster sampling approach, where you would sample clusters (in this case schools). After selecting schools, you may then randomly sample children from those selected schools. For a student project, it is likely that you would restrict your sampling to local rather than national schools.

Questionnaire content

The designing of valid and reliable questions is crucial when constructing a questionnaire (Boyton and Greenhalgh, 2004; Oppenheim, 2001; Schuman and Presser, 1996). A reliable question is one that is answered in the same way each time by the same respondent; a question that fails to achieve consistent responses by the same individual is unreliable (de Vaus, 2002). Validity concerns whether an instrument (the questionnaire) actually measures what it aims to measure (Bowling, 2005a). Within the overall concept of validity you should be interested in ensuring both content and face validity. Content validity relates to the extent to which the instrument as a whole (the questionnaire) addresses comprehensively the aims and objectives of the survey. Face validity relates more to each individual question, assessing whether each question is unambiguous and measures what it purports to measure (Bowling, 2005a). Face validity is particularly important in self-completed surveys, as there are no real opportunities for clarifying the meanings of questions

(Abramson and Abramson, 1999; de Vaus, 2002; Oppenheim, 2002). Both validity and reliability are usually tested during the pre-testing and pilot stage of the survey design process.

Validity can be achieved more effectively by obtaining previously validated questions from pre-existing questionnaires (Abramson and Abramson, 1999; Alreck and Settle, 1995; Czaja and Blair, 1996; Fowler, 1993; Fowler, 1995; Oppenheim, 2001; Rodeghier, 1996). As previously noted, conducting a literature review can help to identify potentially relevant questions that may be included in your questionnaire. Some questionnaires may be from national surveys and others developed by researchers for individual pieces of work. Where possible, contact the authors of the studies to try and obtain a copy of their original questionnaire.

BOX 3.2 LOCATING SURVEY QUESTIONS: UK DATA ARCHIVE

A great resource for finding survey questions is the UK Data Archive website. Founded in 1967 as the Social Science Research Council Data Bank, the UK data archive curates high-quality research data for analysis and reuse.

The data archive provides access to the UK's largest collection of social, economic and population data, across a vast range of topics.

The site also allows users to access the data collection tools. For example, if you would like to view questions used in the Health Survey for England for any given year, you can access the questionnaire that was used.

Source: www.data-archive.ac.uk

Extract potentially relevant questions that relate directly to the objectives of your survey, and then consider whether the question measures what you want it to measure, and if its inclusion would actually add something new to what is already being measured by the other questions. Also give consideration to how each question can be coded and analysed, as this is a vital part of the design process (de Vaus, 2002; Oppenheim, 2001; Rodeghier, 1996).

Where possible, use questions from existing surveys, as this will enable you to compare your findings with that of other studies. Often, however, the pre-existing questions will not adequately meet all the objectives of the survey. Therefore, in addition to questions taken and adapted from other surveys, it is often necessary to construct original questions. For these newly created questions in particular, pre-testing and piloting is crucial. Do ensure that you keep a careful record of where you have sourced your questions, as well as any questions that you have created. Having this careful record will enable you to demonstrate how the data collection tool was constructed.

Questionnaires will often include both 'closed' and 'open' questions. Closed questions have a pre-defined, set number of answers, usually answered by selecting a single response item. Open questions allow the responder to answer in any way they like, for example in a comments box. Closed questions are easier and quicker to answer than open questions, can be much more efficiently coded and processed, and are best suited for quantification, making group comparisons, and testing hypotheses (de Vaus, 2002; Oppenheim, 2001). However, closed questions cannot probe in depth, they can be too crude, and there is the potential that respondents may feel frustrated at the limited choice of answers (Oppenheim, 2001; Rodeghier, 1996). Having an open question at the end of the question-naire enables respondents to write down anything that they may have liked to say at other points in the questionnaire, had they been given the opportunity. It can also generate issues that you may not have thought of that could be explored in any follow-up research.

Questionnaire design and production

Questionnaire design and production is extremely important, as it can affect response rates, impacts on accuracy of answers, and determines how easy it is to code and enter data from each questionnaire (de Vaus, 2002; Rodeghier, 1996).

In order to maximise response, questionnaires should be as aesthetically pleasing and professional as possible (Boynton and Greenhalgh, 2004; Edwards et al., 2002; Oppenheim, 2001; Rodeghier, 1996). A more professional-looking questionnaire can hold the attention of the potential respondents better (Edwards et al., 2002). For those on a budget, it's unlikely that you will be in a position to have your questionnaire professionally designed, but if you are using a paper-based questionnaire, it is worth the time to make it look as professional as possible. For example, consider producing the questionnaire as a pamphlet, with staples down the middle of the document. Online questionnaire software can also be used to produce paper questionnaires.

Think carefully about the order of questions, the commands for skip questions, the format and content of the front page, the coding of responses, and the names and number of section headings. All these aspects should be tested in pre-testing and piloting.

Determining the distribution methods

Questionnaires can be used to collect data in a number of ways, with the main methods being postal, face-to-face and online.

Postal surveys

Traditionally, the most common distribution method for self-completed surveys is postal. Postal questionnaires have several advantages. They offer a relatively cheap way of collect-ing and processing large amounts of data, they avoid interviewer bias, and they can reach respondents who live in widely dispersed locations (Bowling, 2005a; Bowling 2005b;

Oppenheim, 2001). Postal questionnaires are, however, unsuitable for populations with literacy problems, and they offer no real opportunity to correct misunderstandings about questions (Bowling, 2005a; Bowling 2005b). There is also no control over the order in which questions are answered and even whether respondents complete the questionnaire themselves or not (Oppenheim, 2001).

One major disadvantage with postal surveys is that they can produce lower response rates (de Vaus, 2002; Oppenheim, 2001). A low response rate may indicate that the respondents are atypical of the population sampled, which could introduce significant bias into the results (de Vaus, 2002; Edwards et al., 2002). Although there are no agreed-upon standards of what constitutes a good response rate, response rates of 70% or above are aimed for (de Vaus, 2002). Attention should be paid to maximising the response rate, including planning a second mail-out, organising posters to advertise the questionnaire on notice boards, etc., and ensuring that the letter and information sheet that accompanies the questionnaire is worded in the best way possible. These activities are associated with increasing response rates in questionnaire surveys (de Vaus, 2002; Edwards et al., 2002).

When assessing the impact of the response rate it is important to compare responders and non-responders where possible, to see if they differ in any important characteristics (de Vaus, 2002; Oppenheim, 2001). If possible, obtain basic demographic data from your sample before the mail-out stage (such as age and sex of those sampled) to compare responders and non-responders. However, you may not be able to obtain this data, as gatekeepers may not allow access to individual's details because of confidentiality reasons.

When distributing a questionnaire by post, doing so directly (by having the names and addresses of those who are to be sent a questionnaire) rather than relying on a third party will give you more control over the mail-out process (timescales, etc.), and will also enable you to use ID codes on the questionnaires linked to a database, to identify non-respondents. This would then enable you to target the non-respondents with a second mailing of the questionnaire. However, as with the demographic data, the gatekeepers may not be prepared to give you the contact details of their population list, for confidentiality reasons. You may also find that the ethics committee recommends that the gatekeeper sends out questionnaires on your behalf. A gatekeeper might be prepared to send out the questionnaires and keep track of individual responses via an ID code (such as a number or barcode), but it does represent an amount of work for them. Although using an ID number on the questionnaire is useful for monitoring respondents and retargeting, it may affect the response rate, because of concerns from potential participants that their answers may not be anonymous. This could be a particular concern in studies concerning sensitive issues, such as surveys of employees about working conditions, who might be worried about repercussions of any criticisms of their employers should their responses be revealed. Even when participants are reassured that their answers are anonymous, they may express concern that the ID enables the researchers to link them to their answers. Even if this concern is not expressed, it may well affect the honesty of their responses. For this reason, an approach which enables the participant to generate their own code (based on their date of birth and surname, for example), which they then add to the questionnaire and keep a record of themselves, is preferable and still enables them to request withdrawal of their data. It does not, however, allow for targeted reminders.

A decision to send out questionnaires completely anonymously has important implications. It means that if you want to conduct a second mailing of the questionnaire, it would have to be sent to all your sample, including those who had already responded. The potential problem with that approach is that people in your sample could respond twice. A second full mail-out may also cause irritation among those who have already replied. Despite these problems, however, you may still decide to send out a second mailing to everyone, as second mailings are shown to significantly increase response rates for postal surveys (de Vaus, 2002; Edwards et al., 2002; Oppenheim, 2001). To try and combat the possibility that people might respond twice, you can try and identify duplicate responders at the data analysis stage, using an appropriate statistical package such as SPSS. This can identify responders who match for key variables, such as age and sex, to spot duplicate responders. You can also try to minimise duplicate responders by starting the second mailing by saying 'Thank you to those of you that have already replied', both to acknowledge that this is the second copy of the questionnaire they will have received and you have received replies, and also to act as a reminder not to complete it again.

Face-to-face surveys

Paper-based surveys can also be conducted in a face-to-face manner. Face-to-face surveys can help to minimise any misunderstandings with questions and clarify other aspects of the questionnaire, as the person completing the questionnaire can ask the researcher. However, there are disadvantages with a face-to-face approach. The first is that unless the data collection is being carried out by a large number of researchers (which will not be the case for unfunded student research), for logistical and feasibility reasons participants can only be recruited from limited geographical areas and over relatively short periods of time. For example, a face-to-face survey of university students involving one researcher would result in data being gathered from specific areas of the campus at certain times. It might result in an unrepresentative sample. Therefore, before deciding to do a face-to-face survey, consider whether you might be able to reach your target population in a less time-intensive way. If cost or other factors prohibits you from carrying out a postal survey, then consider alternatives such as via pigeon-holes of employees or students. A second disadvantage with face-to-face surveys is that they can be affected by interviewer bias, both in terms of how participants are selected for inclusion in the survey (who the interviewer chooses to approach) and also how the questions are asked. For this reason, it is important to have clear criteria about approaching possible participants, as well as ensuring that participants are questioned in the same way, sticking to a script.

Online surveys

In recent years, the use of online methods of data collection has increased in popularity. Usually, potential participants would be presented with a weblink to complete the survey, which they would receive either directly via an email, or see via other means such as via a newsletter, advertisement or posting on a web forum. Clicking the link would take participants to the online questionnaire (hosted by an online survey tool provider), which they can choose to complete or not. The data from each questionnaire is then compiled by the online survey tool.

Online survey tools such as Survey Monkey and Qualtrics offer several advantages over paper-based postal distribution methods. The obvious advantage is that the costs of conducting an online survey are much less than by post, as there are no costs associated with printing questionnaires or posting out to potential participants. Online survey tools also enable the researcher to produce a professional-looking questionnaire with relative ease, including skip questions that ensure that respondents are only presented with questions that are appropriate to them. Online survey tools also enable you to include the participant information sheet and consent statements as part of the survey process, so participants can understand what the survey is about and give their consent in one document.

Online survey tools usually also enable researchers to produce basic descriptive statistics from within the package, which can be helpful in having an initial look at the data. For more detailed statistical analysis, using an online survey tool that enables you to export your data directly into a statistical software package such as SPSS is invaluable. With a paper-based survey you will need to enter all the data manually, which takes a long time, but exporting from an online survey tool means that data will be populated in the format of the statistical software package. You will still need to clean the data, and ensure that the data is labelled appropriately, but being able to export data directly will save days of time and effort. It also reduces problems associated with reading participants' responses, and eliminates data entry errors.

The main disadvantage of an online method of data collection is that people may simply ignore, or forget about, the survey invitation email that arrives. People receive so many emails a day that it is possible that the email with the link to your survey may be missed. And even if the email is read, unless the recipient clicks on the link and completes the survey there and then, it might slip down their email inbox and be forgotten about. Unlike paper-based surveys there is no obvious permanent visual reminder for people, such as an unanswered paper questionnaire sitting on top of their desk. For this reason, sending a reminder is crucial for online surveys; so too is very careful preparation of the email invite, including the subject heading to be used. You need to maximise the possibility that the recipient will first notice your email, then open it, and then click on the weblink to take part in the survey.

Another limitation with online methods of distribution is that it is often impossible to determine the response rate of your survey. This is because the variety of ways in which people can access your survey means that there is no single list of people to whom the questionnaire was sent, and therefore no clear denominator. Although you could restrict your survey invitations to a defined list of people, and therefore have that clear number of people targeted, there is the possibility that your weblink might be passed to others, who may then complete your survey. This means you still cannot be sure of your denominator. And often, you will not want to restrict, or maybe are not able to restrict yourself to a single list because of accessibility issues. For example, if you want to conduct an online survey to explore the views of pregnant women towards use of e-cigarettes while pregnant, your only feasible way of reaching large numbers of such women may be through an online forum for pregnant women. Such a strategy, while potentially reaching your target population, means that you will not know how many potential participants declined to participate. Similarly, an online survey link that is cascaded by gatekeepers from national, to regional, to local levels would mean that it would be very difficult to tell how many people received the weblink.

The inability to calculate a response rate would historically have been seen as a big problem, especially if you were seeking to publish your research in a peer-reviewed journal. This is because without the ability to determine how many of those who were eligible to complete your questionnaire did so, you cannot assess whether there is likely to be responder bias. However, with the increasing use of online surveys, there is growing recognition that in some cases, the need to reach certain populations in ways that are feasible means that being able to identify a denominator, while ideal, is not always possible. In such cases, researchers would, if possible, be expected to estimate the potential denominator, to come to some conclusions about how representative those taking the survey might be. This could be, for example, finding out the number of people who are registered on the forum where your weblink has been posted, or asking gatekeepers how many people are likely to have received a cascaded email. Another strategy to try to assess representativeness is to compare the demographics of your respondents against the demographics of the wider population to whom they belong. So even if you don't have the denominator, you may be able to make an assessment of whether the characteristics of those people who completed your survey are different in some way from the wider population to which they belong.

Pre-testing and piloting

Pre-testing and piloting are key stages in the development of a questionnaire survey (de Vaus, 2002; Oppenheim, 2001). Pre-testing, which is strongly recommended, is a continuous process of testing throughout the design of the questionnaire, and should involve a wide range of people, starting from friends and colleagues, and then focusing on the target population (de Vaus, 2002; Oppenheim, 2001; Rodeghier, 1996). Throughout the development of the questionnaire you should test ideas, questions and layout with a variety of people. This process can help to ensure that the questionnaire has gone through a number of revisions before the piloting stage.

Piloting of questionnaires is seen as a time-consuming but crucial process. It is more formal than pre-testing, and should pilot every aspect of a survey in order to make sure that everything works as intended. Piloting should not just involve piloting the questions in the questionnaire, but also the introductory letter, the ordering of questions, coding of questions and the method of distribution (de Vaus, 2002; Oppenheim, 2001; Rodeghier, 1996).

During the main pilot stage, issues of validity and reliability can be assessed. Each question should be answered in the same way by the same person on different occasions (reliability), and the questions should measure what they are intended to measure (validity). It is a good idea to separate your pilot testing into two sections: one focusing on the target population and the other using academic colleagues (these could be your supervisors, co-workers or fellow students). The pilot with the target population (possibly two or three individuals) can address issues around specific questions, seeing if the wording makes sense to them. It can also assess their views on the length and structure of the questionnaire and any accompanying materials such as an information sheet or introductory letter. The pilot work involving academic colleagues can check the face validity of the questionnaire against your survey objectives. It can also elicit comments on questions and layout.

Once you are satisfied that you have had sufficient feedback, it is time to finalise the questionnaire in preparation for distribution. Before this, it is sensible to show the finalised questionnaire to one or more of your pilot testers, for a final check. Once the questionnaire has been sent out, it is too late to make changes or clarify things, so try not to rush the final stages in the development of your data collection tool.

Survey distribution

Once your questionnaire has been finalised, the time has come to distribute it to your target population. The steps at this point will of course depend on your distribution method, be it postal, face-to-face, telephone, or online (see previous section). However you do choose to distribute it, plan the process carefully so as to maximise the response you receive and minimise any errors. If your survey is being distributed by post, it is highly recommended to include a pre-paid envelope to encourage response. You should also consider designing posters to be put on notice boards if you are targeting a population that works in or visits specific locations such as workplaces or health centres – there is evidence that such forewarning can increase response rates (de Vaus, 2002; Edwards et al., 2002).

BOX 3.3   ENCOURAGING PARTICIPATION IN YOUR STUDY

- Consider how you can use language to motivate people to respond – for example, being positive about the benefits of participating, and possibly appealing to altruism. Explain what participants may gain from participating in your study.
- Although this information should be included in the participant information sheet (as an ethical requirement – see Chapter 14), it is worth also including it in an introductory letter and/or email.
- You may also consider adding in an incentive (or a token of thanks) to participate, such as inclusion in a prize draw to win gift vouchers for anyone who responds and provides their contact details.

If a gatekeeper offers to distribute the questionnaires on your behalf, volunteer to assist with the mail-outs. This will help to ensure you retain control of the distribution process as much as possible to ensure that everything runs to plan. Gatekeepers should be happy for you to help out, as it will reduce the workload for their staff. As well as helping with the mail-out, you can retain control of the process by preparing the questionnaire packs yourself. If using a postal method, this would involve ensuring that envelopes contained a copy of the questionnaire, information sheet, introductory letter and reply envelope. Envelopes can be sealed before being delivered to the offices of the gatekeeper, where addresses can be added before being sent out. For online questionnaire surveys, preparation would involve penning the email to go with the link to the online questionnaire, and providing this to the gatekeeper, ready for emailing out.

Data entry and cleaning

Once the data collection stage has been completed, it is time to enter the data and clean it, ready for analysis. As noted previously in the chapter, if you are using one of the online survey tools, you can export your data directly into a statistical software package such as SPSS. If your survey is paper based, then you will need to enter the data manually. Hopefully, if you have coded the answers to each question carefully, this should make the manual data entering process as straightforward as possible. Whether you enter the data manually or import it, you will need to ensure that you label your data correctly in whatever software package you are using. This will enable you to analyse the data properly. You will also need to clean the data; that is, check the data for accuracy and completeness. A basic descriptive analysis of the data set can help you to identify where there may have been data entry or coding errors – for example, where you may have typed in the value 33 instead of 3. Once you are confident that your data is clean then it is time for the analysis.

Primary data collection through other methods

A major issue with quantitative data gained from questionnaire surveys is the self-reported nature of the data. Self-reported data can be problematic, especially for questionnaires that ask about behaviours such as levels of physical activity and diet. So-called social desirability bias means that people often over-estimate positive health behaviours and under-estimate negative actions. For instance, a person might say that they undertake 30 minutes of exercise, three times a week (rather than the reality of 20 minutes, once a week), as they want to portray a healthy lifestyle to others. There are ways of collecting quantitative data that do not rely on self-reported measures, and some of these will be covered below.

Structured observation

Structured observation is a method for directly observing and recording activity/behaviour in a structured way, using a set of pre-defined categories (Bryman, 2016). This deals with the limitations of using self-reported data, as the researcher can see for themselves what is happening. Bryman (2016) describes the aim of structured observation as 'to ensure that each participant's behaviour is systematically recorded so that it is possible to aggregate the behaviour of all those in the sample in respect of each type of behaviour being recorded' (pp. 269–270). An example of structured observation would be to observe the behaviour of drivers, pedestrians and other road users in shared space areas of town centres. To record the behaviour in a systematic way, it is necessary to develop an observation schedule, which is similar in ways to a questionnaire. This will help to ensure that data is recorded in a structured way that can then be collated for quantitative analysis.

Activity trackers

Activity trackers are increasingly used in public health research to provide an objective measure of physical activity. Wearable technology such as a pedometers and accelerometers can measure activity in several ways. Pedometers measure the number of steps taken, or at least an estimate of the number of steps. Pedometers are available with varying levels of sophistication. The most basic models are of course less accurate than more expensive designs, which measure steps in a more sophisticated way. Accelerometers measure accelerations, rather than steps, and are recognised as being a more accurate way of measuring physical activity. Such devices have been used in numerous studies, although they do have their limitations, including the cost associated with purchasing or hiring the equipment, and issues with accuracy if devices are not worn properly. For student projects, the use of such technology might not be feasible, either for cost or logistical reasons. However, if you are interested in undertaking work that investigates physical activity, it is an option worth considering. One solution is to utilise the smartphones of participants to record activity – many smartphones now have built-in activity trackers. This does also have implications, in that participants would need to own such a phone, and keep it on their person during the period of measurement. However, it is certainly worth considering.

Other methods of data collection

Although this form of data collection is self-reported, the use of diaries can be a way of trying to improve the accuracy and completeness of recording behaviour by participants. As with other forms of quantitative data collection, it is important that data collection is structured, so that data from individuals can be collated easily. For instance, a study of the dietary habits of participants could involve those participants having a structured food diary with a list of foods that would be used to record their eating habits. Traditionally, this approach has placed quite a high burden on participants. However, smartphones are making it much easier to collect data (e.g. on mood) from participants at regular intervals.

Conclusion

This chapter has considered different methods of quantitative data collection, with a particular focus on the use of self-completed questionnaires. In addition to questionnaire-based surveys, the chapter also noted other forms of quantitative data collection, such as through the use of structured observation, diaries, activity trackers, and smartphone-based apps. It is hoped that the focus on the practical application of tools and techniques will assist you with your public health research.

Further reading

Bryman, A. (2016) *Social Research Methods* (Fifth edition). Oxford: Oxford University Press.
Fowler, F.J. (1995) *Improving Survey Questions: Design and evaluation*. London: Sage.
Oppenheim, A.N. (2001) *Questionnaire Design, Interviewing and Attitude Measurement*. London: Continuum.

4 QUANTITATIVE DATA ANALYSIS

========== CHAPTER SUMMARY ==========

This chapter provides an overview of the techniques used to analyse and present **quantitative** (e.g. numerical) **data** in public health research projects. It may well be that the project also uses qualitative data, in which case it is a 'mixed methods' project. Techniques for analysing mixed methods projects are described in more detail in Chapter 11. This chapter divides **quantitative analysis** into **descriptive** and **aetiological**. Descriptive analysis seeks to describe data (in terms of time, place or person) while aetiological analysis also looks at relationships between potential risk factors and the outcome of interest (in other words, to understand disease aetiology). First, we revisit the different types of data that we might be analysing, as this will inform the method of analysis. We then consider methods of descriptive analysis, including population-level measures of risk such as prevalence, incidence and mortality rates, before moving on to methods of aetiological analysis.

Types of data

Quantitative data are either *categorical* or *numerical*. Categorical data is any variable that can be described using categories (e.g. ethnicity, marital status, age group). Of these, ethnicity and marital status are *nominal* (because we describe the categories with names) while age group is *ordered categorical* (or *ordinal*) because the age groups have a natural order. Another example of an ordered categorical variable would be disease stage. Categorical data with only two categories (e.g. dead/alive) are known as *binary*.

Numerical data can be either *discrete* or *continuous*. Discrete data take only integer values (e.g. number of visits an individual makes to the GP in a year) while continuous data are measured on a scale (e.g. height, weight, age). Often, variables such as these that are actually continuous get measured to the nearest integer for convenience, or because that is judged to give sufficient precision, but can still be treated as continuous for the purposes of analysis.

BOX 4.1 CATEGORICAL VERSUS CONTINUOUS DATA

We can manipulate the data type to a certain extent, to simplify the analysis. For example, we may have recorded exact year of age, but decide to categorise it (e.g. <18 years, 19–60 years, >60 years) for the purposes of analysis. Or we may have exact data on BMI, but categorise it into 'underweight', 'healthy weight', 'overweight' and 'obese' to describe the distribution of BMI in the sample. (The reverse is not true – we cannot turn a categorical variable into a continuous one.)

Though there may be strong arguments for categorising continuous data for the purposes of illustrating the data, it is usually better not to do this for further analyses, because by doing so, some information is lost (to know the category is not as informative as to know the actual number). This generally means that the statistical techniques applied lose *power* – in other words, the ability to detect a difference or an association if one exists.

Descriptive analysis

Techniques used in descriptive analysis

'Descriptive analysis' covers a range of techniques used to highlight patterns in the data – usually data on a health status or outcome (e.g. skin cancer incidence), or an important risk factor (e.g. exposure to sunshine) or both. Most often, we are interested in variations over *time*, by geographical area (*place*), or by other demographic factors such as age, gender or ethnicity (*person*). Though these analyses may point to an apparent association between risk factor and outcome, and this could in turn lead to a hypothesis to be tested in further analyses, that is not the purpose of descriptive analyses, where the focus is on simply describing what is observed. There are several approaches that are commonly used to do this – descriptive statistics, tables, graphs, and disease atlases. Of these, visual displays (graphs and atlases) are usually the most effective way to describe data, while tables present more precise numbers than graphs. We start with descriptive statistics, which can be divided into those used to summarise numerical variables, and those used to measure risk.

Summarising numerical variables

The most obvious and well-known summary statistic is the average. This is known as a measure of *location*, because it tells us where the centre or average of the data is located on a scale. There are three commonly used measures of location – the mean (add up all the values and divide by number of observations, denoted by n), median (order the observations and pick the middle one) and mode (the most commonly occurring value). For a small example data set of heights, in metres, of a sample of n=8 participants, they can be calculated as follows.

1.69, 1.78, 1.56, 1.89, 1.91, 1.55, 1.78, 2.08 (data set 1)

Mean = (1.69+1.78+1.56+1.89+1.91+1.55+1.78+2.08)/8 = 1.78 metres

*Median = middle value of 1.55, 1.56, 1.69, **1.78, 1.78**, 1.89, 1.91, 2.08 = 1.78 metres**

Mode = 1.78 metres (the only value that occurs more than once)

*If there are an even number of values, take the mean of the middle two

In this example, the mean, median and mode are the same. The mean is most often used, and has the advantage of taking into account every observation (rather than just the middle or most common one). However, if the data contain outliers (very high or low values) or is skewed (non-symmetrical) then the three measures of location will differ. In this situation, the mean is prone to be overly sensitive to extreme values, and therefore not a good representation of the entire data set; the median is then preferable.

An average is useful to concisely summarise a set of data, but it doesn't give us any idea about variation within the data. For example, the following set of height measurements would also result in a mean of 1.78 metres:

1.76, 1.77, 1.78, 1.78, 1.78, 1.78, 1.79, 1.80 (data set 2)

but there is much less variation in this second data set. So, to adequately describe a data set, it is necessary to have a measure of variation as well as a measure of location. If the mean has been used to describe location, then the *standard deviation* should be used to describe variation. If the median has been used to describe location, then the *inter-quartile range* should be used to describe variation. These measures are now explained with examples.

The standard deviation (SD) is a summary of how much, on average, the individual values in the data set vary from the mean. It is calculated by taking the difference between each value (x) and the mean, and squaring it $(x-mean)^2$, and adding up across all values in the data set, then dividing by the number of values less one (n-1), and finally taking the square root.

$$SD = sqrt\{sum(x-mean)^2/(n-1)\}$$

For a small data set, SD can be easily calculated by hand, which is helpful for the purposes of illustration, but in practice, n is much larger than 8, and SD is calculated by software such as Excel or a dedicated statistics package.

For data set 1,

$SD = sqrt\{[(1.69-1.78)^2 + (1.78-1.78)^2 + (1.56-1.78)^2 + (1.89-1.78)^2 + (1.91-1.78)^2 + (1.55-1.78)^2 + (1.78-1.78)^2 + (2.08-1.78)^2]/7\}$

$= sqrt\{[0.0081 + 0 + 0.0484 + 0.0121 + 0.0169 + 0.0529 + 0 + 0.090]/7\}$

$= sqrt\{0.2284/7\}$

$= 0.181$

The SD has the same units as the mean, so we can summarise the heights in data set 1 by the mean of 1.78 metres and SD of 0.18 metres.

There is less variation in data set 2, so we would expect the SD to be less. It can be calculated similarly:

$SD = sqrt\{[(1.76\text{-}1.78)^2 + (1.77\text{-}1.78)^2 + (1.78\text{-}1.78)^2 + (1.78\text{-}1.78)^2 + (1.78\text{-}1.78)^2 + (1.78\text{-}1.78)^2 + (1.79\text{-}1.78)^2 + (1.80\text{-}1.78)^2]/7\}$

$= sqrt\{[0.0004 + 0.0001 + 0 + 0 + 0 + 0 + 0 + 0.0001 + 0.0004]/7\}$

$= sqrt\{0.001/7\}$

$= 0.012$

We can summarise the heights in data set 2 by the mean of 1.78 metres and SD of 0.012 metres.

BOX 4.2   CONFIDENCE INTERVALS

Note that the mean of 1.78 metres for sample 1 is a *point estimate* – that is, our best estimate based on the available sample. Since this is unlikely to be the same as the actual mean in the whole population (which we are trying to describe using the sample), it is good practice to provide a *confidence interval* around the mean. A 95% confidence interval is usually calculated (though you may occasionally see others such as 90% or 99% confidence intervals) to provide a range within which we are 95% confident that the true value lies. The less confident we are about the estimate (either because of the small size of the sample, or the variability of the observed data) then the wider the confidence interval should be to reflect this.

Confidence intervals can be calculated by hand, but are not done so in practice. They are calculated using something called the *standard error*, which is based on the SD and the size of the sample. For sample 2, which has the same sample size but a smaller SD, the standard error will be smaller and the confidence interval for the mean will be narrower.

The inter-quartile range (IQR) comprises a *lower quartile* and an *upper quartile*. As with the calculation of the median above, the data need to be ranked before these can be picked out.

1.55, 1.56, │ 1.69, 1.78, │ 1.78, 1.88, │ 1.89, 2.08   *(data set 1, ranked)*

The median is the value that occurs midway through the ranked data, or divides it in half, as denoted by the solid line. Similarly, the lower quartile, median and upper quartile divide the data into quarters, and the lower and upper quartiles in this example are shown by a dotted line. Clearly, the number of data points in each quarter of the data set will depend on the number in the sample (n), and will usually be larger than 8! Since there are an even number of observations in this data set, the median line falls between two data points. To calculate the lower quartile, median and upper quartile in this case, we simply have to take the mean of the numbers either side of the line. In other words:

Lower quartile = (1.56+1.69)/2 = 1.63

Median = (1.78+1.78)/2 = 1.78 (as above)

Upper quartile = (1.88+1.89)/2 = 1.89 (rounding up from 1.885)

We can summarise the heights in data set 1 by the median of 1.78 metres and IQR of 1.63-1.89 metres.

To see how the IQR reflects the spread in the data, we can calculate the median and IQR for data set 2:

1.76, 1.77, 1.78, 1.78, 1.78, 1.78, 1.79, 1.80 (data set 2, ranked)

Lower quartile = (1.77+1.78)/2 = 1.78 (rounding up from 1.775)

Median = (1.78+1.78)/2 = 1.78

Upper quartile = (1.78+1.79)/2 = 1.79 (rounding up from 1.785)

We can summarise the heights in data set 2 by the median of 1.78 metres and IQR of 1.78-1.79 metres. It is clear from these summary statistics that there is less variation in data set 2 than data set 1, despite the medians being the same. As with the median as a measure of location, the IQR is a robust measure of spread that is not affected by outliers. To see this, consider data set 3 below, which differs from data set 1 by only the first observation:

0.92, 1.56, 1.69, 1.78, 1.78, 1.88, 1.89, 2.08   (data set 3, ranked)

If you calculated the median and IQR for this modified data set, they would be unaffected. If you were using the mean and SD to summarise the data set, they would compare with the original data set as follows.

Table 4.1 Mean and SD for data set 1 and data set 3

	Data set 1	Data set 3
Mean	1.78	1.70
SD	0.18	0.35

We see that the very low observation of 0.92 metres instead of the original value of 1.55 has reduced the mean considerably, and doubled the SD. Since this outlier could be a transcription error, or a true but unusual, and therefore unrepresentative, measurement (in this example, perhaps a child), it would be preferable to use the median and IQR to describe the data which, as already established, is not affected in the same way by outliers.

Measuring risk

There are various ways to measure risk, from simple percentages to rates, which can be used to compare the risk in different populations, or between different groups (e.g. by smoking status). Consider the categorical exposure variable 'smoking status' (measured as never smoked/ex-smoker/current smoker). We can summarise this for a sample by saying, for example, that 10% of the sample are current smokers. Percentages are also used to summarise the frequency of health outcomes. If the outcome of interest is lung cancer, then a summary statistic for the sample might be that 0.1% of the sample currently has lung cancer – this is known as *point prevalence* (how many people have a condition at one point in time). *Period prevalence* is a related measure, also expressed as a percentage, which takes into account all instances of the outcome within a fixed time period (say a week). If out of a sample of 100 people, 10 report having a cold at the moment I survey them, then the point prevalence of having a cold is 10%. If a further 10 report that they have suffered from a cold in the preceding week, then the period prevalence (for one week) is 20%. This is often a more useful measure than point prevalence when assessing infectious diseases or symptoms that fluctuate over time (such as back pain or depression). Statements such as *'In England, 1 in 6 people report experiencing a common mental health problem (such as anxiety and depression) in any given week'* (McManus et al., 2016) are measures of period prevalence.

Often, we are interested in the number of new cases in a certain time period, and this is called *incidence*. For example, in a cohort study following children through adolescence, we may wish to compare the incidence rate of diagnosed eating disorders for boys and girls between the ages of 10 and 17. Let's say that in this seven-year period, there were 100 new cases diagnosed among girls, and 25 among boys. To calculate the incidence rates, we need to know how many boys and girls were followed up to age 17 – 15,000 for girls and 10,000 for boys.

> *Incidence rate of eating disorders for girls = 100/15,000 over 7 years = 6.7 per 1,000 over 7 years, or 0.95 per 1,000 girls per year*
>
> *Incidence rate of eating disorders for boys = 25/10,000 over 7 years = 2.5 per 1,000 over 7 years, or 0.36 per 1,000 boys per year*

In other words, if we were following up 1,000 adolescent girls and 1,000 adolescent boys, we would expect to see approximately one new case of eating disorders a year among the girls, and one every three years for the boys.

Prevalence and incidence rates measure *morbidity* – that is how many people are developing a condition or are living with a condition. Another way of measuring the burden of disease due to a condition is *mortality* rates. Sticking to the above example, if in the seven-year period studied, 3 girls and 1 boy died due to an eating disorder, then

Mortality rate of eating disorders for girls = 3/15,000 over 7 years = 20 per 100,000 over 7 years, or 2.86 per 100,000 girls per year

Mortality rate of eating disorders for boys = 1/10,000 over 7 years = 10 per 100,000 over 7 years, or 1.43 per 100,000 boys per year

Note that, whichever measure of risk is used (prevalence, incidence or mortality), it should be presented with a confidence interval to communicate the level of precision of the estimate.

BOX 4.3 MORTALITY VERSUS MORBIDITY

Mortality rates are more useful when studying conditions that commonly lead to death (such as lung cancer) than those which are usually managed successfully (such as asthma). If we were to compare mortality rates from asthma in different countries, any differences observed are likely to reflect variations in care for asthma patients as much as differences in the prevalence of asthma, and it is important to bear in mind that mortality rates are a function of incidence and management (related to the availability of optimal health care services).

The other problem with using mortality rates as a measure of the burden of disease, is that it represents only the 'tip of the iceberg', as described by Bhopal (2016). If we use suicide rates to compare mental ill-health across different countries, then this tells us nothing about the burden of disease seen by primary and secondary care services; in other words, those people living with mental ill-health rather than dying from it. See Rudge and Gilchrest (2005) for a further example. There are, however, also good reasons why mortality rates are used for public health analyses – compared with other data sources they are generally accurate, complete and readily available.

Tables

A table of data is perhaps the most commonly used method to present descriptive data. The first table in a report or paper often describes the demographic characteristics of study participants. This allows comparison with the population from which the sample is drawn (to assess representativeness), and to compare the characteristics of different groups within the study (for example, to compare cases and controls, or to compare those exposed to a risk factor with those not exposed). Consider a hypothetical trial to test a new intervention – the age of participants in the two arms of the trial may be compared as in Table 4.2.

Table 4.2   Age of study participants (numbers and percentages)

Age group (yrs)	Intervention arm	Control arm
<18	5 (8%)	7 (10%)
18–25	9 (15%)	10 (14%)
25–35	14 (23%)	15 (21%)
35–45	13 (22%)	17 (24%)
45–55	10 (17%)	13 (19%)
55+	9 (15%)	8 (11%)
Total	60 (100%)	70 (100%)

As well as conveying the numbers for each age group, the percentages allow the reader to compare the age *distribution* in the two arms of the trial. It shows that, although there are more participants in the control arm (70) than the intervention arm (60), the age distribution is broadly similar in each arm of the trial. Any table such as this, which describes the sample according to two categorical variables (here 'trial arm' and 'age group'), is known as a *contingency table*. Further analyses of contingency tables are discussed below. Tables are also often used to present summary statistics for different samples, or measures of risk in different groups (e.g. exposed and unexposed).

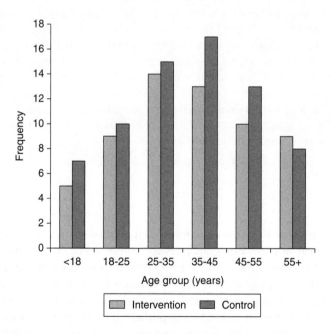

Figure 4.1   Number of study participants in each age group, by trial arm

Graphs

There are many different types of graph (Tufte, 1983; McCandless, 2012). More commonly used ones include the pie chart, bar chart, histogram, scatter plot and line graph. Of these, the first two can be used to illustrate data that fall into different categories (or 'categorical' data). If these categories have an order, as in the age groups in Table 4.2, then a bar chart is preferable. A bar chart could therefore be used to show the data, as in Figure 4.1.

This is a clustered bar chart, because for each age group represented, the data for the intervention and control arm is shown side by side. This enables comparison of the numbers in each age group for each arm, and the overall distribution by age. Arguably, this visual representation is a more effective way of conveying the information than Table 4.2.

If participants' exact age, rather than age group, had been recorded, then we can treat age as a continuous variable rather than a categorical variable, and represent it using two separate histograms instead of a bar chart. As you will see below, the shape of the distribution is similar to that shown by the bar chart, but there are no gaps between the bars (reflecting the continuous nature of the data).

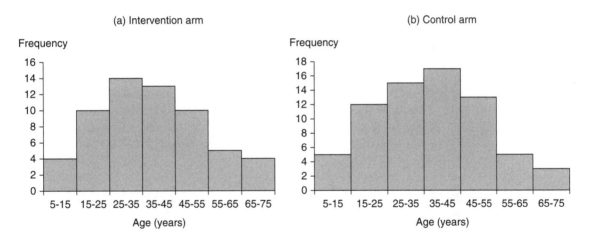

Figure 4.2   Age distribution of participants in each arm of the trial

Scatter plots are used to illustrate the relationship between two continuous variables, where each observation is marked by a dot (or some other symbol). The scatter of the dots allows any association between the variables to be seen visually. In Figure 4.3, each dot represents one of 35 electoral wards in South Gloucestershire (England). The two variables presented for each ward are an indicator of deprivation on the horizontal axis, known as the Index of Multiple Deprivation (IMD, 2010), and the number of fast food outlets per 1,000 population on the vertical axis. The scatter plot suggests a positive correlation between these two variables (summarised here by the dotted line of best fit).

The correlation coefficient between fast food outlets per 1,000 population and deprivation in Figure 4.3 was 0.71, confirming a strong positive correlation (Pearce et al., 2017).

BOX 4.4 INTERPRETING THE CORRELATION COEFFICIENT

The degree of correlation can be summarised by the correlation coefficient (r). r is on a scale from -1 to +1, where -1 is perfect negative correlation (as one variable increases the other decreases, with the points in a perfectly straight line), 0 is no correlation and +1 is perfect positive correlation (as one variable increases so does the other, with the points in a perfectly straight line). While perfect correlations are unlikely to arise in practice, values near zero suggest little or no correlation, while values closer to -1 and +1 indicate increasingly strong negative and positive correlations, respectively. It is important to remember that correlation is measuring linear association, and therefore lack of correlation does not mean that there is no association between the two variables. Non-linear associations can be described by other functions (e.g. exponential) but are beyond the scope of this book.

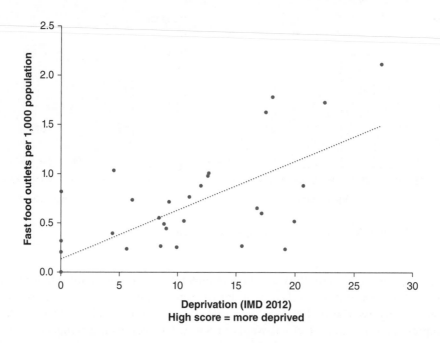

Figure 4.3 Scatter plot showing the association between density of fast food outlets and deprivation for each ward in South Gloucestershire, England

Source: Pearce, M., Bray, I. and Horswell, M. (2017)

Figure 4.4a shows a quite different looking scatter plot, of statutory notifications of food poisoning in England and Wales over a five-week period (note that short-term changes in infectious diseases rates are of interest for identifying outbreaks). There are only five data points, representing the number of notifications during each of five weeks. Since one of the axes represents time, the convention is to represent this information as a line graph (Figure 4.4b). This is a special case of a scatter plot, used when one of the continuous variables is time, in which the trend over time is shown by a line (with or without symbols marking the observed value at each time point, but here, with). Trends over time are important in public health – from showing long-term changes in mortality rates (e.g. over decades), to fluctuations in road traffic collisions at different hours of the day (e.g. within a 24-hour period) – and are easier to detect visually than in a table.

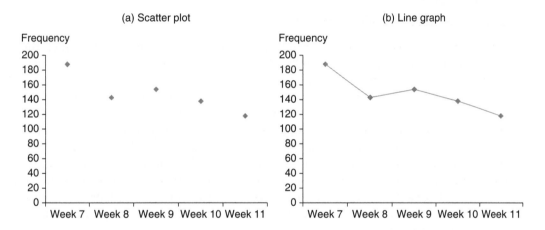

Figure 4.4 **Statutory notifications of food poisoning from week 7 to week 11 of 2018, England and Wales**

Source: Public Health England (2018). Statutory Notifications of Infectious Diseases, Week 2018/12 www.gov.uk/government/uploads/system/uploads/attachment_data/file/694900/NOIDS-weekly-report-week12-2018.pdf

Disease atlases

Descriptive epidemiology is concerned with describing patterns in terms of time, place and person. We have established that time trends in health outcomes are effectively communicated by line graphs, and demographic characteristics can also be summarised by graphs, such as bar charts. There is no reason why this information cannot be shown in a table, except that it is somewhat harder to digest (although when precision is important then actual numbers in a table may be preferable to a graph). When it comes to describing differences in health outcomes by place, then a map is an obvious choice. 'Disease atlases' are widely used to show differences in disease incidence or mortality across geographical areas (such as countries or administrative areas), or differences in exposure to risk factors, via gradated shading. Clearly, if the outcome of interest is a rate, then the size of the population in each area must be taken into account. Figure 4.5 shows global variation in the proportion of total disease burden that is due to mental and substance use disorders. As well as being commonly used to describe geographic variations in non-communicable diseases, and their risk factors (for another example, see Barnett et al., 2001), they are a useful tool in illustrating the spread of communicable diseases (see, for example, Hempel, 2018), and can be used for surveillance purposes (Rolfhamre et al., 2004).

Aetiological analysis

Techniques used in aetiological analysis

What can be inferred from data depends in part on the study design from which the data arose. For example, data from an RCT is more useful in inferring causality than data from a case-control study (as explained in Chapter 1). And data from a cross-sectional study should not be used to infer causality at all, because it is not clear whether the exposure or outcome occurred first (as both are measured at the same time). Nevertheless, the techniques used to analyse quantitative data in public health projects depend as much on the type of data as the study design used to generate the data. For this reason, the rest of this chapter is organised into sections on the basis of data type. First, we consider the association between two categorical variables, then the association between a categorical variable and a continuous variable, and finally the relationship between two continuous variables. We then introduce methods that can be used to control for confounding variables.

BOX 4.5   STATISTICAL TESTS AND P-VALUES

Note that the techniques described in this section generally involve the calculation of a *test statistic*, the comparison of this statistic with a standard *distribution* to determine a *p-value*, and interpretation of this p-value. While this process is explained in some detail for the first of these tests (the chi-square test), the reality is that such calculations are carried out in packages such as Excel or SPSS rather than by hand, so space is not devoted to describing the formulae and calculations for other tests. The reader is referred to other software-specific texts (e.g. Pallant, 2016) for guidance on performing the tests described here.

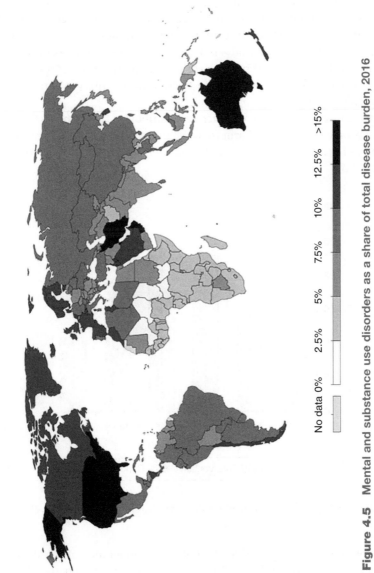

Figure 4.5 Mental and substance use disorders as a share of total disease burden, 2016

No data 0% 2.5% 5% 7.5% 10% 12.5% >15%

Source: Global Burden of Disease Collaborative Network. Global Burden of Disease Study 2016 (GBD 2016) Results. Seattle, United States: Institute for Health Metrics and Evaluation (IHME), 2017

The association between two categorical variables

Chi-squared tests are used to assess the relationship between two categorical variables. Table 4.2 above shows the number of participants in a study by trial arm and age group. Any such table, which gives the number of observations for two categorical variables, is known as a contingency table. Although the age categories are ordered, these are both categorical variables. Let's say we want to know whether the age distribution in the sample is different in the two arms of the trial – that is, whether there is an association between age and trial arm. This is important because age is a common confounder (in other words, it is likely to be associated with both the effectiveness of the intervention and the health outcome of interest).

It is hard to tell from Figure 4.1 whether age distribution differs by trial arm, because there are more people in the control arm than the intervention arm. So, instead, we could draw a bar chart of the *percentage* of the sample in each age group, for the two arms of the trial (see Figure 4.6).

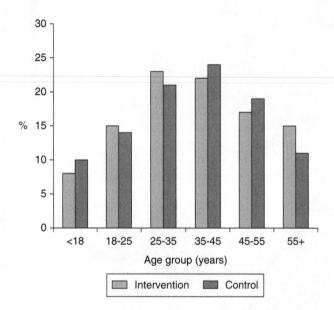

Figure 4.6 Percentage of study participants in each age group, by trial arm

Based on Figure 4.6, it appears that there is a preponderance of middle-age participants (35–55 years) in the control arm. But the total numbers of each are relatively small (60 in the intervention arm and 70 in the control arm), so how do we know whether this is an important difference in age distributions e.g. greater than we would expect by chance?

To test the hypothesis that the age distribution is different for the two arms of the trial, we need to compare the *observed* age distributions with those that would be *expected*, if there were no association between trial arm and age (in other words, there was exactly the same age distribution for the two arms of the trial).

Expected values, shown in Table 4.3 below, can be calculated for each observation (cell) in the table by multiplying the row total and column total, then dividing by the overall total. For example:

expected number <18 years in the intervention arm = (12 × 60)/130 = 5.54

Table 4.3 Observed and expected numbers of study participants, by age group and trial arm

Age group (yrs)	Intervention arm Observed (Expected)	Control arm Observed (Expected)	Row total
<18	5 (5.54)	7 (6.46)	12
18-25	9 (8.77)	10 (10.23)	19
25-35	14 (13.38)	15 (15.62)	29
35-45	13 (13.85)	17 (16.15)	30
45-55	10 (10.62)	13 (12.38)	23
55+	9 (7.85)	8 (9.15)	17
Column total	60	70	130

The chi-square (x^2) statistic can then be calculated to summarise the differences between the observed and the expected values:

x^2 = sum {(observed − expected)^2 / expected}

For the observed and expected values in Table 4.3, the chi-square statistic is 0.64.

The value of this statistic is then compared with the chi-square distribution, for the given *degrees of freedom* (d.f.), which depends on the size of the contingency table as follows (excluding total rows and columns):

Degrees of freedom = (the number of rows -1) x (the number of columns -1)

In this case, d.f. = (6-1) x (2-1) = 5

Comparison with the chi-square distribution with 5 d.f. (x^2_5) can be used to generate the probability that the data observed could have occurred by chance alone, if there really is no association between the two variables (in this case, age and trial arm). This probability is known as a *p-value*, and was introduced in Chapter 1. If it is small, typically less than 0.05, which corresponds to 5%, then it is unlikely that the observed data would have arisen if there were no association between the two variables. It is therefore likely that an association exists between the two variables. However, in this case, the $x^2{}_5$ statistic yields a p-value of 0.99, so does not support an association between age group and trial arm. We can conclude that any differences observed in the sample are most likely due to chance.

Contingency tables are commonly used to represent two binary categorical variables – these are known as *two-by-two* tables. Note that for two-by-two tables, d.f. = (2-1)x(2-1) = 1. The age categories in Table 4.3 above could be collapsed to generate a two-by-two table, as in Table 4.4.

Table 4.4 Number (and percentage) of study participants by age group (<45, >45 years) and trial arm

Age group (yrs)	Intervention arm	Control arm	Row total
<45	41 (68%)	49 (70%)	90
>45	19 (32%)	21 (30%)	40
Column total	60 (100%)	70 (100%)	130

Two-by-two tables are often used to summarise the outcomes for exposed and unexposed groups (in a cohort study) or intervention and control arms (in a trial). These tables are used to calculate and compare risk in the two groups.

Referring back to the eating disorder example used earlier, the data arose from a cohort study and the sample for analysis comprised 15,000 girls and 10,000 boys. In this case, the demographic variable 'gender' can be thought of as an exposure variable or risk factor. The results are presented as in Table 4.5.

Table 4.5 Eating disorder incidence during 7-year follow-up among girls and boys in a cohort study

Outcome	Girls	Boys	Total
Eating disorder	100	25	125
No eating disorder	14,900	9,975	24,875
Total	15,000	10,000	25,000

From this table, we can calculate the incidence rates (over 7 years) as 6.7 per 1,000 for girls, and 2.5 per 1,000 for boys, as above. These are known as *absolute* risks. If we want to compare these two different risks there are two options. One is to look at the *difference* between them.

Risk difference[1] $= risk_{group1} - risk_{group2}$

$risk_{girls} - risk_{boys} = 6.7 - 2.5 = 4.2$ *per 1,000*

The other is to calculate consider *relative* risk, and calculate the risk ratio.

Risk ratio $= risk_{group1} / risk_{group2}$

$risk_{girls} / risk_{boys} = 6.7/2.5 = 2.7$

As explained in Chapter 1, data from a case-control study cannot be used to calculate incidence rates or relative risks. The results from a case-control study can, however, be presented in a two-by-two table, and used to calculate an *odds ratio,* which is a good approximation to the risk ratio, when the outcome is rare. Table 4.6 presents an example in which cases and controls were individually matched, so there is an equal number of each. The outcome is children who have died from anorexia nervosa and the exposure of interest is having a mother who was ever diagnosed with any eating disorder.

Table 4.6 A case-control study comparing maternal diagnosis of eating disorder with cases of child mortality due to anorexia nervosa

Exposure	Cases	Controls	Total
Maternal diagnosis	10	5	15
No maternal diagnosis	65	70	135
Total	75	75	150

The odds of exposure for the cases is the number of cases who were exposed divided by the number of cases who were not exposed (10/65 = 0.154). This can be compared with the odds of exposure for the controls (5/70 = 0.071) using the odds ratio.

Odds ratio $= odds_{group1} / odds_{group2}$

$odds_{cases} / odds_{controls} = 0.154/0.071 = 2.2$

Note that this is equivalent to the odds ratio comparing the odds of having the outcome (being a case) for those exposed (10/5 = 2) and those not exposed (65/70 = 0.929):

Odds ratio $= odds_{group1} / odds_{group2}$

$odds_{exposed} / odds_{not\ exposed} = 2.000/0.929 = 2.2$

---

[1]also known as attributable risk

BOX 4.6   INTERPRETATION OF THE RISK RATIO, ODDS RATIO AND RISK DIFFERENCE

The risk ratio (RR) is commonly used in public health research, and tells us how much more (or less) likely the outcome is to occur in one group compared to another. A RR of 2.7 would suggest that eating disorders are nearly 3 times more likely to be diagnosed in girls than boys in this age group. The interpretation of RRs is not totally intuitive, so a range of examples are given:

RR=10 There is a 10-fold increase risk (of having the outcome) for those exposed*

RR=2 There is a doubling of risk for those exposed*

RR=1.7 There is a 70% increase in risk for those exposed*

RR=1.3 There is a 30% increase in risk for those exposed*

RR=1 There is no association between the exposure and the outcome

RR=0.75 There is a 25% reduction in risk for those exposed*

RR=0.50 There is a 50% reduction in risk for those exposed*

RR=0.25 There is a 75% reduction in risk for those exposed*

* compared with those unexposed

The odds ratio (OR) is, if anything, even more commonly used in research. Even though it is less straightforward to interpret it arises for two main reasons. The first is that, as already discussed, case-control studies can only be used to estimate ORs (not RRs). The second is that the statistical models used to analyse data from epidemiological study designs (such as case-control studies, cohort studies and trials) often estimate ORs rather than RRs. To interpret the OR, simply replace 'risk' with 'odds' in the above statements, and remember that the OR is approximately equivalent to the RR for rare outcomes.

The risk difference is used less, but is arguably more important when communicating research findings. Consider an exposure that is associated with a 5–fold increase in risk, but the risks for both exposed and unexposed are very low (say 5 per 100,000 and 1 per 100,000 respectively, per annum). Presenting an RR or OR of 5 gives a very different message (exposure is associated with a 5-fold increase in risk/odds) than presenting a risk difference of 5-1 = 4 per 100,000 per annum. This is the number of new cases per year that are due to the risk factor in question, and therefore the number that could be avoided per year if the risk factor were eliminated.

Confidence intervals and/or p-values can be calculated for the risk difference, RR and OR, and should always be considered when interpreting these statistics. For further information about these measures of association, and others, see Tripepi et al., (2007).

The association between a categorical variable and a continuous variable

To test for an association between a categorical variable and a continuous variable, different methods are used. Figure 4.2 presented data on continuous year of age and trial arm. Again, although the age distribution in the two histograms looks similar, it is difficult to tell by eye whether the differences observed are important. If we know the exact age of participants in each arm of the trial, then we can test whether there is a difference in the ages of participants in each group using an independent samples t-test. This compares the means in the two independent groups, as we have here. It is only appropriate to use this test if the distributions are approximately Normally distributed (or bell-shaped), which we can see from Figure 4.2 holds in this case. Otherwise, a non-parametric test known as the Wilcoxen rank sum test is used instead. This test statistic is based on the ranks of the recorded ages in the two groups of participants, rather than the actual ages. For a simplified example of what this means, see Table 4.7 below.

Table 4.7 Example of actual ages and rank ages in two groups of five participants

	Group 1					Group 2				
Actual age	16	80	45	57	22	18	60	46	33	52
Rank age	1	10	5	8	3	2	9	6	4	7

The independent sample t-test compares the mean age for group 1 (44.0 years) with the mean age for group 2 (41.8 years) while the Wilcoxen rank sum test compares the ranks for group 1 (1, 3, 5, 8 and 10) with the ranks for group 2 (2, 4, 6, 7, 9). Both are testing for a difference in ages between the two groups, and both generate a test statistic and corresponding p-value, which can be interpreted in the usual way.

It is also possible to test for a difference in a continuous variable in more than two groups. This extension to the independent sample t-test is known as Analysis of Variance (ANOVA), while the non-parametric alternative (extension of Wilcoxen test) is known as Kruskal-Wallis test. Although the names are different, the explanation given above about testing for differences in means or ranks still holds, but comparing more than two groups. However, if the ANOVA or Kruskal-Wallis test provides evidence of an association between the two variables, in other words a difference in the continuous outcome between groups, it does not tell you between which particular groups these differences lie. For example, groups 1 and 2 may be similar to each other but dissimilar from group 3 but you will only know this from looking at the means or medians in each group, and confirming differences with pairwise t-tests or Wilcoxen tests.

BOX 4.7   PARAMETRIC VERSUS NON-PARAMETRIC

Note that the use of ranks rather than actual values results in a loss of information, therefore a loss of statistical power (meaning that if there is a difference in ages between the two groups, then the test comparing means is more likely to detect this difference than the test based on ranks). Therefore, the non-parametric tests are not usually used unless dictated by a skewed (non-Normal) distribution.

A final situation to consider is that in which you are comparing two sets of continuous data but they are paired. For example, this might arise when analysing a before-and-after study – you could have blood pressure readings on the same people before and after an intervention. In this case, the test to use is a *paired t-test*.

The association between two continuous variables

The relationship between two continuous variables should first be explored by a scatter plot, as described above. We have already seen how a linear association can be described by the correlation coefficient, r. A confidence interval can be calculated for this statistic, and the association described by the scatter plot and correlation coefficient can be formally assessed with a p-value for r. This is a parametric test which relies on the variables being approximately Normally distributed. As with the tests introduced above, there is a non-parametric alternative called Spearman rank correlation (r_s). This is also based on ranks rather than actual values.

So, correlation can be used to tell us whether there is evidence of a linear association between two variables (p-value), and the strength of the association (r or r_s with confidence interval). Simple linear regression uses the same line of best fit as correlation but goes a step further in explaining the relationship between exposure (horizontal axis) and outcome (vertical axis). A regression line is described by the following formula:

Outcome = intercept + (gradient x exposure)

The *intercept* is where the line of best fit crosses the vertical axis and the *gradient* measures the steepness of the slope (change in outcome for a unit change in exposure). In Figure 4.3, the intercept is 0.13. The slope can be estimated by observing that the outcome increases from 0.13 to 1.40 (a difference of 1.27) while the exposure increases from 0 to 25. The difference in outcome for a unit increase in exposure can be estimated as 1.27/25 = 0.05. So, the regression line in Figure 4.3 can be summarised as

Fast food outlets per 1,000 population = 0.13 + (0.05 x IMD score)

We can use this to estimate the number of fast food outlets per 1,000 population for any IMD score, given that it is within the range of the original sample (i.e. IMD is between 0 and 30).

For a ward with an IMD score of 5 (less deprived), we estimate that the number of fast food outlets per 100,000 to be $0.13 + (0.05 \times 5) = 0.38$.

For a ward with an IMD score of 20 (more deprived), we estimate that the number of fast food outlets per 100,000 to be $0.13 + (0.05 \times 20) = 1.13$

In practice, the model would be fitted with the help of statistical software, which produces precise estimates of the intercept and gradient, with confidence intervals and p-values. It is the gradient that is of interest for drawing conclusions about the relationship between the exposure and the outcome.

Controlling for confounding

The problem of confounding in epidemiological studies was discussed in Chapter 1. Approaches for controlling confounding in the design of studies were dealt with in that chapter. Here, we introduce briefly two statistical techniques often used to control for confounding at the analysis stage. The first is standardisation. This is usually only used to control for the very common confounder of age group (and sometimes gender too) when comparing rates between different populations with different age (and gender) structures. To see why this is necessary, consider a crude analysis of lung cancer mortality rates in a retirement town and a capital city dominated by working-age people – clearly, the rates will be higher in the retirement town and if you did not take into account the different age structures of the two populations then you might conclude that the observed difference was due to something else (such as deprivation or health service provision).

There are two alternative methods (called *direct standardisation* and *indirect standardisation*) and the choice will depend in part on the data available. However, both use a *standard population* (standard in terms of age and gender) to allow comparisons between rates that are not affected by the different demographics. For example, Stefan et al. (2017) compared rates of childhood cancers across 18 African populations and 4 US/European populations by standardising to the 'standard world population', to take into account the different age structures in these countries.

The second and more flexible approach is an extension of the simple linear regression. By including more variables in the model, we can estimate the effect on the outcome of any potential confounder for which we have data, as well as additional risk factors. A gradient (also known as the *slope* or *regression coefficient*) is estimated for each confounder and exposure – in fact, there is no need to differentiate between potential confounders and risk factors. Here is a possible model for the prevalence of obesity by ward (note that we are now considering fast food outlet density as a risk factor):

$$\text{Obesity prevalence} = \text{intercept} + (\text{gradient}_1 \text{ x fast food outlet density})$$
$$+ (\text{gradient}_2 \text{ x median age of population})$$
$$+ (\text{gradient}_3 \text{ x deprivation score})$$

Three separate coefficients now describe the influence of three separate variables on obesity prevalence (but taking the other variables into account). This model will allow obesity prevalence to be estimated for any ward based on fast food outlet density, the median age of the population and the deprivation score. But it will also allow the relationship between fast food outlet density and obesity prevalence to be estimated, taking into account the potential confounders of population age and deprivation.

While simple linear regression is used for a continuous outcome, logistic regression is used when the outcome is binary. It is commonly used in public health research, for example, to analyse survival, relapse, or other changes in status (e.g. smoking cessation). The regression coefficients estimated for each variable in the model when using logistic regression can be used to provide estimates of ORs (with confidence intervals and p-values for each). As an example, Di Gregori et al. (2014) used logistic regression to determine the most important factors associated with uptake of influenza vaccine among medical students in Italy. For students wishing to undertake regression modelling, further information can be found in software specific texts, such as Pallant (2016) for SPSS, or a more comprehensive textbook dedicated to regression techniques, such as Pardoe (2012).

Conclusion

This chapter has introduced a number of tools used for descriptive epidemiology (tables, graphs, disease atlases) and analytical epidemiology (statistical tests of hypotheses and methods of dealing with confounding). The importance of using non-parametric methods when appropriate has been highlighted. Various measures of risk have been described, including risk difference, risk ratio and odds ratio, and their utility in public health discussed. Although this chapter provides a basic introduction to regression, with an emphasis on interpretation, further reading will be necessary before undertaking a regression analysis.

Further reading

Altman, D. (1991) *Practical Statistics for Medical Research*. London: Chapman and Hall.
Campbell, M.J. and Machin, D. (1999) *Medical Statistics: A commonsense approach* (Third edition). Chichester: Wiley.
Pallant, J. (2016) *SPSS Survival Guide* (Sixth edition). Oxford: Oxford University Press.
Rowntree, D. (2018) *Statistics without Tears: An introduction for non-mathematicians*. London: Penguin.

5 QUALITY AND RIGOUR IN QUANTITATIVE RESEARCH

=========== CHAPTER SUMMARY ===========

The collection of **primary data** was discussed in Chapter 3. Whether you are using primary data collected for the purposes of your study, or **secondary data** that can be re-used to help answer your research question, it is important to consider the quality of the data and whether it is 'fit for purpose'. The following discussion about assessing the **validity and reliability of primary data** aims to be pragmatic and relevant to public health practice, rather than theoretical and academic. The quality of secondary data is then considered, with reference to some common sources of secondary data. Finally, methods to assess the quality of published research are introduced in the section on 'Critical Appraisal'.

Validity

Testing validity means asking yourself whether the data is measuring what you think it is, or what it should be measuring. For example, if you are using a tool (in this case, a questionnaire) to measure mental health, but the questions are constructed in such a way that respondents give 'socially desirable' answers, then the data you have collected will not allow you to accurately identify those with poor mental health. In other words, it is not a valid measure of mental health. Very often we use a tool (sometimes also known as an 'instrument') that has already been validated, because there exists a particular set of questions or way of measuring an exposure or outcome (such as a technique for measuring percentage body fat or other anthropometric measure), which has been shown elsewhere to be a good (valid) measure. In this case, it is important to reference evidence (usually a peer-reviewed journal article) that the measure you are using is validated. If it is not possible to use a measure that is validated, you may be able to adapt an existing measure.

BOX 5.1 VALIDITY TOOL EXAMPLE (BRAY ET AL., 2016)

We wanted to measure student nurses' self-confidence and attitudes towards family-witnessed resuscitation. Such a tool already existed for qualified nurses (Twibell et al., 2008), but not all the questions were relevant to student nurses. So, we adapted the tool, and validated the new version, to ensure that it was appropriate for use with student nurses (Bray et al., 2016).

Sometimes, however, it is not possible to use or adapt an existing tool. If you are using a novel method of measurement, then you should consider the validity of this method, ideally at the piloting phase before you invest in data collection on a larger scale. There are various ways this can be done, some more formal than others. It is worth noting here that much of the standard teaching on assessing validity and reliability stems from the psychology literature, and is therefore suitable for the situation where you are using a tool to measure a construct (such as 'happiness' or 'body dissatisfaction'). In this situation, it is necessary to use statistical techniques to assess the validity and reliability of the scale, and these are described below. However, if your data collection does not fall into this category (maybe you are collecting purely factual information, such as parity or height, rather than measuring a construct), then these more formal methods of assessing validity will not be necessary.

Face validity

This is the simplest type of validity, meaning whether 'on the face of it' a tool seems to measure what it claims to. For example, a relatively superficial and subjective assessment of the relevance of a questionnaire can be carried out by asking whether the questions appear relevant, reasonable, unambiguous and clear. As a minimum, this type of validity should be assessed. Depending on the situation, this may be all that is possible (if time or resources are very limited) but more usually this will be just the first step in assessing validity.

Content validity

This refers to the extent to which the content of the tool appears to examine the full scope of the characteristic or domain it is intended to measure. Although this sounds similar to face validity, it takes a more systematic approach to answering the same question. Content validity is usually judged by a panel of experts and therefore can quite easily be achieved, so should be considered wherever possible. Experts may be practice-based or academic (ideally include both), and depending on the topic and your contacts, the experts may be people you know locally, or you might need to turn to nationally recognised experts.

Criterion validity

This concept measures how closely the tool or method being used mirrors the best-known measure, or 'gold standard'. This can be formally assessed using the correlation between the tool being used and the 'gold standard'. For example, a set of questions designed to detect clinical depression could be compared against clinical assessment of the participants, if both measures are applied to a sample for validation purposes. If no such 'gold standard' exists, there may be an acceptable proxy measure that can be used instead. The main issue is in deciding what other measure or proxy measure is appropriate (if one exists). As an example, imagine that you are developing a new tool to measure quality of life among children with a long-term illness. If there is no established tool for measuring quality of life for these children based on their own responses, but a validated questionnaire tool does exist to measure parent-reported quality of life, then this could be used as a proxy for the purposes of validating the new questionnaire to be delivered to children. Statistical analyses are required to quantify the correlation, as described in Box 5.2 below.

BOX 5.2 STATISTICAL MEASURES OF AGREEMENT

Kappa quantifies agreement between measures on a categorical scale. It is therefore widely used to assess criterion validity for tools that are measured using categories (e.g. 'has disease' versus 'disease-free') or ordered categories (e.g. stage of disease). The Kappa statistic is a number from -1 to +1. Zero suggests the agreement is not better than that expected by chance. (Negative values are worse than you would expect by chance.) '1' corresponds to perfect agreement, which is unlikely, but when you are validating a tool you are aiming for a Kappa statistic close to 1. Results can be classified as follows: 0.40–0.59 is fair agreement, 0.60–0.74 is good agreement, 0.75–1.00 is excellent agreement. However, other classifications are possible; see for example, www.medcalc.org/manual/kappa.php. The following example illustrates the application of Kappa. To test whether a self-completed questionnaire is a valid measure of depression among adults, the classifications ('depressed' versus 'not depressed') according to both this questionnaire and clinical assessment are compared by calculating the Kappa statistic, which is 0.70. This suggests that there is a good agreement and the questionnaire is a valid measure of depression. Finally, note that if

(Continued)

(Continued)

the data are ordered categorical (e.g. four stages of disease rather than 'has disease' versus 'disease-free'), then the Kappa statistic should be weighted to take account of this.

Pearson correlation is used to assess agreement between two continuous measurements (e.g. two methods of measuring a person's height). The measurements should be approximately Normally distributed (otherwise a Spearman rank correlation coefficient is more appropriate). The coefficient lies between -1 (perfect negative correlation) and +1 (perfect positive correlation). Zero denotes no correlation. Results can be classified e.g. <0.5 is unacceptable reliability, 0.5–0.6 is poor reliability, 0.6–0.7 is questionable reliability, 0.7–0.8 is acceptable reliability, 0.8–0.9 is good reliability and >0.9 is excellent reliability. Since height is approximately Normally distributed, Pearson correlation would be appropriate to assess the agreement between two alternative methods of measuring height.

Spearman correlation is based on the ranks of the measurements rather than the actual values of the measurements. It is therefore more appropriate than the Pearson correlation coefficient for non-Normal data or small samples. Consider the situation where you are assessing the agreement between two alternative methods of measuring weight. Since this variable is not Normally distributed, Spearman correlation would be more appropriate than Pearson correlation.

Construct validity

Construct validity is the extent to which a measure based on a questionnaire tests the hypothesis or theory it is intended to measure. This is usually assumed to mean it correlates well with related variables (convergent validity) or does not correlate with unrelated variables (discriminant validity). This then involves deciding what are the related (or unrelated) variables, and locating suitable ways to measure them. Returning to the example of a questionnaire tool to measure depression, we could test convergent validity by comparing the results of this new tool with existing tools for anxiety (which we would expect to be related to depression). Discriminant validity could be assessed by checking that it doesn't also correlate positively with a measure of 'happiness'. As with criterion validity, the statistical methods used will be Kappa or a correlation coefficient, depending on whether the variable is categorical or numerical.

External validity

More generally, the term *validity* can be used to refer to the overall rigour of a study. *External validity* is the extent to which research findings can be generalised to the wider population of interest, and applied to other settings (Bowling and Ebrahim, 2005). This is influenced by sampling (see Chapter 2) but also by other processes that seek to eliminate bias from the study. These are discussed below in the section on critical appraisal. Note that a tool is unlikely to be valid if it is not *reliable*, a concept we deal with next.

Reliability

Reliability refers to the extent to which a tool or measure performs consistently over time or across different researchers. There are several different types of reliability that you may need to consider, depending on the nature of your research.

Inter-rater reliability

This is the extent to which the results obtained by two or more 'raters' or researchers apply-ing the same method of measurement, or tool, are in agreement for similar or the same populations. The following example illustrates why this should be considered. A cohort study investigating predictors of breast cancer, the Guernsey IV cohort, included anthropo-metric measurements such as height, weight, and other measures of adiposity such as waist and hip circumference and skin-fold thickness. The cohort is described by Fentiman et al. (1994). Several research nurses were employed to record these measurements for the cohort. Analysis of data revealed significant differences in all anthropometric indices apart from height and weight, depending on who had taken the measurement, thereby yielding these measures unreliable. In this case the raters were not taking measurements on the same sam-ples, but each sample would have been similar in that it was drawn from the same population of women. The best way to test inter-rater reliability is for all the raters to assess a sample of participants (ideally at the same time point), and assess levels of agreement between raters using the same methods as those introduced above for assessing validity – that is, Kappa, Pearson correlation or Spearman correlation, depending on the type of data. Note that inter-rater reliability can also be an issue with interviewer-completed questionnaires, as individual interviewers may illicit different responses through their style of interviewing. One advan-tage of using self-completed questionnaires is that it eradicates any such interviewer bias.

Intra-rater reliability

This is assessing whether the same rater applying the same tool to the same participant (within a relatively short time period) will get a consistent result. This could be important for a variety of outcomes, e.g. a research nurse using callipers to measure skin-fold thick-ness, or a researcher using an interviewer-led questionnaire to gather information from participants. Before assessing intra-rater reliability, first consider how much the outcome fluctuates over time, and decide over what interval it would be reasonable to expect the outcome to be stable. You can then assess agreement between two sets of measurements taken on a sample of participants by the same person (using Kappa, Pearson correlation or

Spearman correlation). A good measure or tool will be reliable when used on different occasions by the same person.

Test-retest reliability

This is a test of the stability of a measure itself over time. In contrast to inter-rater reliability and intra-rater reliability, this is not about the person using the tool. To exclude the possible effects of the person administering the measure, let's consider a self-completed question-naire. Test-retest reliability of the tool is assessed by asking a sample of participants to complete the questionnaire on two different occasions and then assessing agreement of scores obtained at the different time points, using Kappa, Pearson correlation or Spearman correlation. As with intra-rater reliability, it is important to be comparing repeat measures over a time period in which we would not reasonably expect the outcome being assessed to have changed. This is obviously more of an issue for some variables than others. An adult's height should not change from one week to the next, so a good method of measuring height should yield high levels of test-retest reliability over this time period. A questionnaire tool to measure mood, on the other hand, may lead to quite different responses from one week to the next, as mood is something that fluctuates over time, and therefore a high level of test-retest reliability would not necessarily be expected for this measure.

Internal consistency

A questionnaire often comprises several sets of questions (tools or instruments) that relate to a particular domain (e.g. physical ability) or together can be used to measure a particu-lar construct (e.g. socio-economic status). If these tools are not previously validated, then it is important to assess the extent to which the individual questions *belong* in that domain. In other words, do all the questions contribute usefully to the measurement of that domain or construct? If they do not, then they should be removed as part of a testing and validation stage, to ensure that the questionnaire is as concise and relevant as pos-sible. Internal consistency can be formally assessed using item-total correlations and Cronbach's alpha.

BOX 5.3   STATISTICAL MEASURES OF INTERNAL CONSISTENCY

Item-total correlation measures the association between each item (question) and the total score (for that set of questions). A low score suggests that the item is not measuring the underlying concept that the tool is designed to measure. Item-total correlations <0.2 usually suggest that the item should be removed from the tool (Everitt, 2002).

Cronbach's alpha is a measure of correlation between all the items in the tool or instrument (an average correlation among the items). It will take a value between 0 and 1. A low value suggests that the items do not belong to the same conceptual domain. It is generally accepted that Cronbach's alpha should be at least 0.7 but different cut-offs are used (Nunnaly, 1978).

BOX 5.4   INTERNAL CONSISTENCY (BRAY ET AL., 2016)

The following example, introduced in Box 5.1 above, demonstrates how item-total correlations and Cronbach's alpha are applied to test the internal consistency of a set of questions. In this case, there were two measures to be assessed by self-completed questionnaire, one to measure perceived risks and benefits, and one to measure self-confidence, both relating to student nurses' views on family-witnessed resuscitation.

Background: There is increasing debate about the advantages and disadvantages of family-witnessed resuscitation. Research about the views of healthcare providers depends upon reliable tools to measure their perceptions. Two tools have been developed for use with nurses – a 26-item risk-benefit (RB) tool and a 17-item self-confidence (SC) tool.

Objective: To validate these tools for use with student nurses in the UK.

Methods: A sample of 79 student nurses were invited to complete the tools. Item-total correlations and Cronbach's α were used to determine internal consistency.

Results: Item-total correlations suggested that some of the questions in the RB scale were discriminating less well (item-test correlation<0.2 for questions 4, 7, 8, 10), so these questions were removed from the scale. The Cronbach's α reliability of the 22-item scale was 0.86. All the items in the SC scale were found to offer very good discrimination (item-test correlation ranged from 0.53 to 0.81) so none were removed. The Cronbach's α reliability of the 17-item scale was 0.93.

Conclusions: There is first evidence that these tools are valid and reliable for measuring student nurses' perceptions about family-witnessed resuscitation.

In summary, initial testing at a pilot phase should be used to ensure adequate reliability and validity before the measurement tool is used. If measures of reliability and validity have been calculated, it is also important to present these as part of your research findings. Most of these statistics will only be available for the pilot sample but statistics demonstrating internal consistency should be presented for the final sample, as in the example above.

Assessing the quality of secondary data

The use of secondary data, which has already been collected for another purpose but which can be reused to help answer your research question, for public health research has been described in Chapter 3. Such data may arise from previous research, or from routinely collected data. There are many good reasons for using secondary data, not least because it is cheaper and faster than collecting new data, and because if relevant data already exist, then it is not ethical to spend resources and participants' time to collect more data. For this reason, those funding large research studies often stipulate that the data be made available to other researchers, and researchers are encouraged to make use of secondary data (see, for example, the *ESRC Secondary Data Analysis Initiative* (ESRC, 2018)). Data archives are now commonly used to store research data for reuse. Of course, there are also ethical issues with reusing data that have been collected for a different purpose (for example, see Malin et al., 2010), and these will be covered in more detail in Chapter 14 on ethics.

On the other hand, the downside of using secondary data is that you cannot control what is collected or how questions are asked. For example, the Avon Longitudinal Study of Parents and Children (ALSPAC) has been used to investigate the longitudinal relationship between body dissatisfaction in adolescence and later risky behaviours. This study started in 1990, and the method used to quantify body dissatisfaction (a five-point figure rating scale, Dowdney et al., 1995) is now considered quite out of date, and has been surpassed by other, more valid measures (many alternatives are discussed by Menzel et al., 2011). So researchers have to decide between using this secondary data, with its limitations, or using a data set that includes current measures of body dissatisfaction and waiting for follow-up data on risky behaviours to be collected. As well as the validity of the measures used, the frequency and timing of data collection points may not be optimal for the purposes of answering your research question, leading to many compromises in your analysis.

A further disadvantage of using routinely collected data is that it is generally collected for administrative purposes, and therefore not of the quality usually used for research. A key problem is often that much of the data is missing or inaccurate. A framework that is useful for assessing the quality of secondary data sources is CART:

Completeness

Accuracy

Relevance/**R**epresentativeness

Timeliness

Completeness

This usually relates to 'coverage' – the proportion of the sample or population of interest for whom we have data. For example, the UK census tends to be fairly complete and gives good coverage of the population. But it can also refer to the completeness of the data – questionnaires which are returned by 100% of the sample but which are only partially completed are of limited use. Data collected for administrative purposes is likely to be incomplete, particularly if only some fields are mandatory. For example, addresses are often only partially completed, and if postcodes are missing then this has serious implications for research that intended to use postcode to infer a measure of socio-economic status (e.g. Index of Multiple Deprivation). Turning to another example, completeness of reporting for notifiable diseases in England (Public Health England, 2010) will be much higher than for other infectious diseases that are not notifiable.

Accuracy

Accuracy of data collection will depend on many things, but it is clear that some sources of data can be expected to be more accurate than others. Self-reported data is prone to bias (e.g. social desirability bias) and is likely to be less accurate than clinical measurements, such as height and weight. Aside from the problem of social desirability bias, some variables are more likely to be reported accurately than others – 'age in years' or 'parity' should be fairly accurate compared with 'date of last tetanus vaccination' (which may be guestimated). Accuracy of routine data will vary with context – in many countries we take it for granted that death certification is generally accurate (although even in the UK there are concerns about accuracy, particularly in deaths of older people), whereas in other countries it is less so. Social and political influences may affect the accuracy of routinely collected data – attitudes towards suicide, for example, will result in under-reporting of this as the primary cause of death in certain countries, while political interference in the collection or reporting of official statistics may mean that researchers have less confidence in it under certain less democratic regimes.

Relevance/representativeness

We should consider whether data that are collected routinely are sufficiently relevant to our research question. For example, if we are investigating trends over time in the prevalence of asthma among children, one strategy would be to analyse asthma-related prescription data that is routinely collected by primary care providers (NHS Digital, 2018). The most common prescriptions for asthma would be identified, and records of such prescriptions to children extracted for analysis. This is an acceptable approach, but the researcher should question how relevant all these prescription records are to asthma – is it possible that some of the medicines prescribed could also have been given for a different condition, and therefore not relate to asthma at all? Bear in mind also that not all medicines prescribed are used by the patient, so it may be that some records reflect a doctor prescribing what they thought was appropriate (or might be necessary as a precaution) at the time the patient presented, but in fact the medicine was not needed or used. Routine data will not always be representative of the population that the researcher is interested in. For some conditions – we could take depression as an example – only the more serious cases present to healthcare providers, and therefore an analysis of primary data will exclude those who have not sought treatment, perhaps because their symptoms are milder or because they do not recognise that they need help. In some countries, individuals with a condition may not present to primary care because they cannot afford treatment (depending on the model of healthcare provision). So, if the objective was to measure the prevalence of depression in a population, then routinely collected from primary care would not be representative of all people with depression.

Timeliness

There can be delays in routinely collected data becoming available. Population estimates and key statistics by Local Authority and ward from the 2011 UK census were available in the following year, but detailed UK migration statistics were not available until 2015 (ONS, 2015). As an aside, there is a non-statutory 100-year rule in the UK, such that the Government intends to fully publish the 1921 Census in 2022. But even if researchers don't have to wait 100 years to access anonymised census data, the time delays in accessing such routine data can mean that it is somewhat out of date and therefore of limited use by the time it is available. In contrast, routinely collected data on infectious diseases is by necessity timely, since the aim is to detect outbreaks in time to take action. Weekly reports are published for England and Wales (Public Health England, 2018). Most routinely collected data will sit on a scale somewhere between these two examples in terms of timeliness. Researchers should consider the delays in accessing routine data, and whether this compromises its usefulness to answer the research question.

Critical appraisal

In this section we consider the quality assessment of published research evidence. The process is generally known as 'critical appraisal', but whatever we choose to call it, it is important that we consider the extent to which we trust the available evidence, and its relevance to the current context. This has important implications for how we use evidence (e.g. should it be used to change policy?). Critical appraisal is also a key step in the process of carrying out a systematic review (see Chapter 12).

Why is critical appraisal important?

Evidence-based practice demands that decisions made by policy-makers and practitioners are based on the best available evidence. This is important, because if they are not, then this leads to suboptimal use of resources and outcomes for both individual patients and the wider population. The problem is that, very often, high-quality evidence to support a particular decision or policy is not available, so we have to consider all the evidence that is available, bearing in mind its limitations. The key thing is to not take evidence on face value, and to question and be honest about the quality of the evidence.

Approaches to critical appraisal for standard epidemiological study designs

There are different approaches that can be taken to carrying out a critical appraisal. The choice will depend in part on the time available and the purpose of the appraisal.

Compared with the more detailed checklists described below, this exercise might seem rather cursory. However, it is important to recognise that in the real world, practitioners may sometimes only have the time to read the abstract rather than the full article – in this context a rapid appraisal of that information is better than none.

BOX 5.5 A RAPID APPRAISAL

A very quick appraisal can consist of asking yourself three questions:

1. What are the results?
2. Are the results valid (do you trust the results)?
3. Are the results relevant to your research question and setting?

If the appraisal is part of a systematic review, then a checklist that includes a scoring system is sometimes preferred. The overall score can then be used to make decisions about which studies are of sufficiently high quality to be included in the final synthesis of findings, to perform sensitivity analyses excluding lower quality studies, or even included as an explanatory variable in a meta-regression. The GRADE and Cochrane risk of bias tools, both designed for use in systematic reviews, are described in Chapter 12. Note, however, that the tool used can yield quite different results, leading some researchers to recommend that overall scores are not used in this way (da Costa and Jüni, 2014).

More generally, the purpose of a critical appraisal is to explore the strengths and weaknesses of a study and to document these so that those using the evidence are aware of the limitations. The key thing is that this is done in a systematic way, to reduce *reader bias* (Owen, 1982). The most well-known and commonly used checklists for carrying out critical appraisals are those produced by the Critical Appraisal Skills Programme (CASP, 2018). These are structured in sections around the three broad questions given above, and comprise more detailed questions, which are specific to each study design. Checklists are freely available from the CASP website to print or complete electronically. All the major epidemiological studies introduced in Chapter 1 are covered – case-control and cohort studies, randomised controlled trials (RCTs) – as well as qualitative studies (see Chapter 10) and systematic reviews, which will be covered in Chapter 12. These checklists were designed for use in an educational setting, and come with hints to help with answering each of the questions. Common themes include consideration of bias and confounding (key epidemiological issues introduced in Chapter 1), and the generalisability of the findings to the local population.

BOX 5.6   THE CASP CHECKLIST FOR COHORT STUDIES

Section A: Are the results of the study valid?

1. Did the study address a clearly focused issue?
2. Was the cohort recruited in an acceptable way?
3. Was the exposure accurately measured to minimise bias?
4 Was the outcome accurately measured to minimise bias?
5. (a) Have the authors identified all important confounding factors?
   (b) Have they taken account of the confounding factors in the design and/or analysis?
6. (a) Was the follow up of subjects complete enough?
   (b) Was the follow up of subjects long enough?

Section B: What are the results?

7. What are the results of this study?
8. How precise are the results?
9. Do you believe the results?

Section C: Will the results help locally?

10. Can the results be applied to the local population?
11. Do the results of this study fit with other available evidence?
12. What are the implications of this study for practice?

Study-specific questions include, for example, careful scrutiny of the randomisation process for RCTs. Each question (e.g. *'Was the assignment of patients to treatments randomised?'*) asks the researcher to select either *'Yes'*, *'No'*, or *'Can't tell'* – if these questions are completed they can be used to generate a crude scoring system, but generally the usefulness of these checklists lies in the observations that are made in response to these questions (e.g. *'Patients were randomly allocated to treatment arm using a computer-generated random number sequence'* or *'The method of randomisation was not described'*).

For case-control studies, cohort studies and RCTs an alternative study-specific checklist is available from the Scottish Intercollegiate Guidelines Network (SIGN, 2018). The purpose of these checklists is to generate evidence-based clinical guidelines, and they have been developed to provide a balance between methodological rigour and practicality. As with the CASP guidelines, there is the opportunity to treat these as closed questions, by completing closed *'Yes'* and *'No'* tickboxes, and to add further observations in response to these questions. Guidance notes are available to help with completing the checklists. Similarly, checklists for these key study designs have been developed by the US National Institutes of Health (NIH). These are based on consultation with a variety of organisations including SIGN, and are therefore not dissimilar to those already mentioned.

Other guidelines have been developed for specific disciplines rather than specific study designs. The 'Quality Assessment Tool for Quantitative Studies' was developed by the Effective Public Health Practice Project, funded by the Ontario Ministry of Health and Long-Term Care (Canada) (Effective Public Health Practice Project, 1998a). It is especially aimed at those designing, implementing and evaluating public health programmes and policy. It leads to an overall methodological rating of 'strong', 'moderate' or 'weak' in eight sections – selection bias, study design, confounders, blinding, data collection methods, withdrawals and dropouts, intervention integrity, and analysis. A companion 'dictionary' is provided to assist with completion (Effective Public Health Practice Project, 1998b). This checklist is a good one to consider as an alternative to CASP or SIGN because it takes quite a different approach, comprising of more closed questions with a range of options.

BOX 5.7   A QUESTION FROM THE QUALITY ASSESSMENT TOOL FOR QUANTITATIVE STUDIES

What percentage of selected individuals agreed to participate?

1. 80–100% agreement
2. 60–79% agreement
3. less than 60% agreement
4. Not applicable
5. Can't tell

Many of the tools mentioned in this section are included in the compendium of critical appraisal tools compiled by Ciliska et al. (2012).

Approaches to critical appraisal for other study designs

Consider a proposal to place GPs in emergency departments – this idea has been put forward to relieve pressures and reduce waiting times. The ideal study design to test such an intervention would be a randomised controlled trial, but in practice it is difficult to conduct such a trial (e.g. it would require a large number of emergency departments to take part, which would be difficult to organise and resource). If you searched for the available evidence on the topic, one of the studies you would find would be a 'before-and-after' study (see Chapter 1) by Boecke et al. (2010). This illustrates nicely the problems with assessing evidence for 'real-life' public health issues, because it doesn't fit neatly into one of the main epidemiological study designs described in Chapter 1, for which we have standard critical appraisal tools (described earlier in this chapter).

The US National Institutes of Health has produced a number of critical appraisal tools for some of these more pragmatic study designs, including cross-sectional studies and before-and-after studies (NIH, no date given). Application of this tool to the Boecke et al. (2010) paper highlights a particular problem with loss to follow-up – it was not possible to collect outcome data for many of the participants. Only through careful scrutiny of the numbers in each of the tables of results, prompted by a question on the checklist, does this issue become clear. Some of these tables do not include totals, which is why the issue is not obvious on first reading.

BOX 5.8   APPLICATION OF THE US NATIONAL INSTITUTES OF HEALTH CHECKLIST FOR BEFORE-AND-AFTER STUDIES TO BOECKE ET AL. (2010)

Question 9. Was the loss to follow-up after baseline 20% or less? Were those lost to follow-up accounted for in the analysis?

After applying exclusion criteria, and enrolling those willing to take part, no loss to follow-up is described by the flow diagram in Figure 1. However, the number of patients for whom demographic data is available is considerably lower (Table 1). It is not clear from Table 2 how many patients returned a patient satisfaction questionnaire – this was the main outcome measure. The totals in Table 3 show that data on the number of additional tests requested was available for all 832 in the usual care group and all 695 in the new care group. Adding up the treatment times in Table 6 suggests that this data was available for 742 in the usual care group (89%) and 652 in the new care group (94%). Data on quality of diagnosis was only available for 1105 patients, representing a loss of 28% of the original sample. These losses to follow-up are not explicitly acknowledged and it is not clear how they were accounted for in the analysis.

Another set of critical appraisal tools is available from the Joanna Briggs Institute in Australia (Joanna Briggs Institute, 2018), which has a focus on improving global health problems. Included here are checklists for prevalence studies, for non-randomised experimental (intervention) studies and for analytical cross-sectional studies. There may be other types of evidence that are not addressed by any of the critical appraisal tools mentioned so far in this section. Many of these are likely to be found in the *grey literature*, which is not peer-reviewed. The AACODS checklist (Tyndall, 2010), developed at Flinders University (Australia), can be used to critically appraise grey literature. The acronym stands for the main headings of the checklist – **A**uthority, **A**ccuracy, **C**overage, **O**bjectivity, **D**ate and **S**ignificance.

BOX 5.9   BESPOKE CRITICAL APPRAISAL TOOL (MCLAUGHLIN ET AL., 2017)

1. Year of publication
2. Appropriate study design?
3. Baseline demographics of subjects given?
4. Population choice, representative of:

   UK primary care patients nationally
   UK primary care patients in a local area
   A specific group
   Not specified

5. Predefined sampling frame?
6. Sampling type:

   Census/100% sample
   Random
   Systematic
   Convenience
   Not specified

7. Setting and location of recruitment identified?
8. Applied equally to all subjects?
9. Validated/standardised extraction technique?
10. Data from quality-controlled database of secure records?
11. Time period included clear (post-QOF data identified)?
12. Clearly defined outcome measures, for example, BMI-defined obesity
13. Primary outcome was BMI or calculable BMI record

Despite the wide range of critical appraisal tools available, it is sometimes the case that an appropriate one cannot be identified, in which case one option is to design a bespoke tool for the task. This can arise when carrying out a systematic review because a variety of different study designs are included – an example of this is found in McLaughlin et al. (2017). This was a systematic review of the recording and management of adult over-weight by UK GPs. A bespoke critical appraisal tool that incorporated important aspects of study quality, irrespective of the mix of study designs to allow improved comparability between studies, was developed and tested through piloting.

Conclusion

In conclusion, this chapter has stressed the importance of considering the quality of data used for public health research, whether that be primary data, secondary data or existing research evidence. In each case there are tools and frameworks that help us to assess the quality of the data or evidence. Whatever the context, the important thing is to question and be honest about the quality, and to acknowledge the likely implications of any limitations.

Further reading

Ajetunmobi, O. (2019) *Making Sense of Critical Appraisal* (Second edition). London: Hodder Arnold.

Bowling, A. and Ebrahim, S. (eds) (2005) *Handbook of Health Research Methods: Investigation, measurement and analysis*. Maidenhead: Open University Press.

Dawes, M., Davies, P., Gray, A., Mant, J., Seers, K. and Snowball, R. (2004) *Evidence-Based Practice* (Second edition). Edinburgh: Churchill Livingstone.

Greenhalgh, T. (2014) *How to Read a Paper: The basics of evidence-based medicine*. Chichester: Wiley.

PART 2
QUALITATIVE METHODS FOR PUBLIC HEALTH

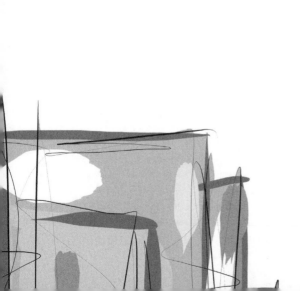
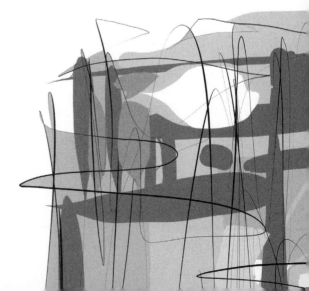

PART 2

QUALITATIVE METHODS FOR PUBLIC HEALTH

6 METHODOLOGICAL APPROACHES AND BASIC PRINCIPLES

=== CHAPTER SUMMARY ===

In this chapter we introduce the **methodological approaches** used most commonly in qualitative research, such as **ethnography, grounded theory** and **phenomenology**. Attention is paid to the traditions of **qualitative research**, the social science underpinning, and the philosophical considerations that help us to see the value of qualitative research for public health. The key qualitative study designs are described using a wide range of examples, relevant to our intended public health audience. Throughout the chapter we focus on the specific strengths and limitations of each methodological approach, and how they can enhance public health knowledge.

The philosophy of social science (and qualitative) research

Qualitative research, to put it simply, is a term used to describe research methods that seek to explore and understand individuals' experiences, lifeworld and the 'collective' social meanings that underpin that lifeworld. Contrasting with epidemiological science and some quantitative methods, it is fair to say that qualitative research is influenced by a more diverse set of traditions, many of which stem from the social sciences, in subjects like social anthropology, sociology, economics, psychology and geography. To the student it can seem like there is a confusing number of choices in carrying out qualitative studies. The history of these methods in terms of the study of public health, and health and well-being more generally, is well established and arose out of both public health medical schools in the middle of the twentieth century, and within academic social science departments. As such, qualitative approaches to public health issues are informed by two distinct traditions, one of which stems from the social sciences, the other of which stems largely from applied health science and health services research. Arguably, public health research can learn from both traditions.

Here, we discuss the main features of qualitative research, sometimes compared to quantitative research, with the aim to try and break down the barriers between them and view them as part of the same central issue, which is about how to investigate the human and social world. In qualitative research varied methodological approaches exist, each with their attendant ways of asking the same questions and investigating the same issue, but fundamentally they all come under the banner of qualitative research. To use quantitative or qualitative research is not a question of having a fixed viewpoint on what is better (or even a judgement of the 'value' of the research), but about using the best available approach to what you are wanting to find out. Qualitative methods are not the best approach for answering certain questions (an issue we explored in the main Introduction to our book). Taking this pragmatic approach will help you to discover whether quantitative or qualitative research is the most appropriate research design, or whether using both (in mixed methods as we will see in Chapter 11) will enhance our understanding even more.

To fundamentally understand why qualitative research is used in human and social research we need to take a step back to help us understand a number of key issues: namely, why researchers investigate different phenomena in fundamentally different (sometimes opposing) ways, and why they may not always understand each other. This issue has been called the 'commensurability' problem – that is, how can researchers from two different ways of thinking about the social world come together to understand each other's viewpoint and work collaboratively. This issue is also known as the fundamental problem of ontology, epistemology and methodology, or what Moses and Knutsen (2008) creatively refer to as the 'three musketeers of speculative philosophy'.

BOX 6.1 WAYS OF KNOWING (MOSES AND KNUTSEN, 2012)

1. Implicit in a research design is an understanding of the nature of the world and *how* it should be studied.
2. Researchers rarely pay attention to these philosophical and methodological issues as more attention is given to innovating methods.
3. The two main philosophical camps are *naturalism* and *constructivism*: they draw on different understandings of the social world.
4. Students engaging in research should be aware of their own methodological assumptions.

Naturalistic and social constructionist approaches within public health research

First of all, basic principles should apply about how researchers, including public health researchers, see the human and social world and what they think they can understand from it. In other words, how far they can relay back (i.e. represent) the social reality that is presented before them. Can researchers provide an objective account of social reality or will their view and 'picture' of the social world always be mediated in ways that distort or provide a more or less subjective and one-sided account?

In the philosophy of social research, which it is important we also apply to public health research (for the fundamentals are essentially the same), the first basic principle is about asking questions about what knowledge can be gained from the social domain and what is known to exist. So, for example, we can think about public health concepts like 'risk' and 'prevention', which are abstract in many ways and can to some extent be only known to exist through the mediated language that we use to understand the social world. Yet, in more orthodox public health they are directly seen to be 'social facts', that is, as solid and immutable as the atoms and quarks that 'hard' scientists have identified. These are important issues, and because of this qualitative researchers can be placed on a continuum between a *positivist* orientation (viewing them as social facts) on the one hand and a *social constructionist* (the mediated idea about social reality) viewpoint on the other, but as we will see the majority of researchers are not on opposite ends of a continuum.

BOX 6.2   NATURALISM (POSITIVISM) VS SOCIAL CONSTRUCTIONISM (MOSES AND KNUTSEN, 2012)

Naturalism:

- A forensic natural science approach
- The experimental method
- Focus on empiricism evidence
- Establishing the facts from the case (one truth)
- The correspondence theory of truth
- The high (or expert) view, and removed from the community perspective

Social constructionism:

- Tends to see many truths
- A different notion of what constitutes a fact
- Less reliance on the formal rules of method – imagination and other forms of reasoning
- Intimate knowledge of people and the community

Ontological issues concern, then, the ideas about what we agree exists out there in the world (e.g. obesity or community mental health) and then seeking to try to understand it. For those of a more *positivist* persuasion there is a view that the problem is relatively straightforward – that is to say, obesity exists, such social phenomena can be measured using the deductive principles of the scientific method (Bowling, 2014), we can see who is more likely to have it (or suffer from it), and how it can be treated. Public health research from a qualitative perspective that uses a more positivist orientation may then seek to find out how to understand people's perceptions of obesity in order so that it may be better prevented, or it may be to establish what interventions might work better from the perspective of the individuals – what is more acceptable, can use, and so on. But the fundamentals about what exists – in this case, obesity – is not in doubt.

Let us now take a more *social constructionist* approach. Here, we see that some additional critical questions are thrown into the research problem, to interrogate what it is that we think we know, therefore establishing some doubt into our fundamental public health issue. What this means, then, is taking a more critical perspective on the ontological principles. Our researcher that is more influenced by social constructionism will ask two additional questions. First, how can we understand this public health issue – obesity – in historical time? That is to say, what does it mean to say that there may be different constructions of what obesity is and how it is perceived in society across time? Second, they would also ask the question about social and cultural space – that is, how is obesity understood in different societies and cultures and what impact does that have on the way we might research it as well as the taken-for-granted perspectives we may take? Both of those questions help the social constructionist researcher to 'problematise' the issue and ground it in a social (as well as clinical/physiological) reality.

BOX 6.3 POSITIVIST VS. SOCIAL CONSTRUCTIONIST 'FRAMING' OF A PUBLIC HEALTH ISSUE

Let us assume that a public health researcher is interested in how and why young people (aged 18–25) consume 'designer' alcoholic drinks (in the UK this would include drinks like 'Bacardi Breezer' and 'Smirnoff Ice'). In the positivist approach, the researcher would look at the issue in the following way:

- There is a public health 'crisis' surrounding alcohol use/misuse.
- We have 'hard' data on this to tell us what the reality is.
- It is a 'problem'.
- We can provide solutions.

For the social constructionist public health researcher, the issue is 'framed' in a different way, taking into account:

- How is this issue constructed? – e.g. what system of talk (discourse) does it invoke when people mention it?
- 'Young people' may frame this differently – e.g. gender, ethnicity, other characteristics.
- Highlighting – a) historical and b) cultural variation.
- We can understand how and why it is constructed as a 'problem'.

These contrasting approaches (or paradigms) therefore offer a framework (and corresponding rules) comprising an accepted set of theories, methods and ways of defining the problem as well as the data that is produced. They are different in terms of their different assumptions about *social reality* (what it is, and what is knowable); different assumptions about *how to know social reality and the questions we ask*; and different assumptions about the *data we 'collect', how we collect it, and how we interpret it*. Thus, leading to different assumptions about the *conclusions we can draw*. This leads us to two different ways to think about the public health problem (though as we have said, most qualitative researchers tend to sit on a continuum and do not usually take extreme views), and may then have an impact on the kind of qualitative research they carry out as well as the methods that are used.

Using qualitative methods in public health research

In the philosophy of social research, ontological questions and fundamentals lead on to epistemological ones, where epistemology is taken to mean 'how do we know what we know?' In other words, what broad approaches to making sense of something and investigating it can we use, and how far can we use this to answer our research questions. Epistemology is usually taken to mean 'theory of knowledge' in a rather basic sense. The epistemological foundation for research is fundamental, and researchers in many traditions (particularly 'hard' sciences) do not 'navel gaze' about this issue, and that is largely because it is taken-for-granted knowledge. In understanding people, sociality, communities, and the public at large, those taken-for-granted principles are not there in the same way, and so there is room for doubt as well as different perspectives on what it is that we think we know and how we might know it.

BOX 6.4   QUALITATIVE RESEARCH AS ENHANCEMENT IN PUBLIC HEALTH TRIAL-BASED METHODS (RESALAND ET AL., 2015)

This study, based in Norway, sought to understand the possible impact of physical activity (PA) on children's academic performance at school (for which some evidence is emerging). In order to assess the relationship between PA and school performance the researchers employed a cluster randomised controlled trial methodology (see Chapter 1) to identify the key variables and to assess, at different time points/stages, the effect of PA on the school children's performance.

Qualitative methods (mostly interviews and some video recorded observation) were used to obtain an in-depth understanding of children's own 'embodied experiences' and

(Continued)

(Continued)

pedagogical processes taking place. Teachers were also interviewed and observed individually and in groups.

This paper focuses on the importance of and value gained from employing mixed methods in research with children, which the authors felt achieved 'a deeper understanding of children's, teachers', and parents'/guardians' perspectives enriched and gave a nuanced picture of processes leading to certain outcomes from the main trial' (Resaland et al., 2015: 15). The qualitative data helped to shed light on what was happening in the schools during the intervention period and what it is like to be a child in a school where such interventions are happening, therefore providing some enhancement to what is primarily an RCT study.

In public health research (as in other applied health research) there tend to be two ways of thinking about and researching public health problems. The first is to take an approach to the research that considers how qualitative studies can *enhance* quantitative findings, or enhance ways that we already understand the issue. For example, in a lot of trial-based research for public health and other health services research (and also largely mixed methods), qualitative research is starting to play a key role. However, its role is often a somewhat limited one, which is to help clarify or answer key issues that have arisen during the main part of the trial (which will mostly be about measuring the effectiveness of x intervention for a public health issue). This way of thinking about qualitative research also fits most appropriately with an evidence-based viewpoint, with fixed views and guidelines about qualitative research (and its place within the evidence-based hierarchy – see the main Introduction for a critique of this).

An alternative to this is to use qualitative methods in a way that employs more of a 'critical' approach – that is to say, one based more in the social sciences, one that uses a variety of methodological approaches (which we will come on to), and one that concerns itself more with qualitative paradigms that have some influence over the researcher's perspective and world-view. Unsurprisingly, this way of using qualitative research tends to be used more as a stand-alone approach, as opposed to being used alongside quantitative methods. Indeed, many qualitative researchers of this persuasion (and not the authors of this text) would suggest that quantitative and qualitative methods cannot be combined in any meaningful way due to key differences in their ontological and epistemological viewpoints (see Lincoln et al., 2013).

Thinking about qualitative research in terms of how it can enhance scientific studies of effectiveness is extremely useful, and probably accounts for the majority of funded public health research, as it is a fundamentally pragmatic or 'what works' approach. But, there are important areas where it falls down and there are research questions that it really cannot answer.

One of the key issues here is about the ways that researchers think about social reality. In the majority of public health research today where qualitative methods are used, it is used to ask people questions (in qualitative interviews) about what they think about something, what their experiences of that are, and so on. Atkinson (2017), for example, is rather critical of this way of using qualitative research, arguing that one of the problems is that it does not provide a theoretically informed study of social phenomena; such theories and conceptual architecture are provided by the social sciences. This more simplistic approach relies on some conventional approaches in qualitative research as the main aim is just to understand what people say they think, how they act, and how they feel about it. So, what does it not help us to understand?

People in social worlds deal in social meanings

One of the key issues that remains is about how well some qualitative research helps us to understand the complex social realities in which people live out their lives, and how important it is to make sense of this in order to understand key social, or public health, issues. Let us take an example – in this case, outbreaks of measles in different communities. Measles outbreaks are relatively rare, but when they do occur public health professionals are keen to establish the reasons for the outbreak and how best to address it, and one of the ways they might do this is to use qualitative research to ask people within the communities, and other key stakeholders, questions about their understanding of vaccinations and risk as well as health beliefs. On the one hand, this approach can work well, but there are limitations to really getting to the heart of the issue and it can fundamentally miss some critical issues that do not just take a knowledge deficit approach to lay people's understanding of health issues. If qualitative research exclusively involves interviews with people in the community then many of those people may not want to disclose important information or they may seek to deliberately deceive the interviewer. More importantly, wider social, economic and cultural issues can be relatively ignored at the expense of getting the participant's perspective.

Researchers such as Kitta and Goldberg (2016), for example, describe the problems with conventional ways of understanding vaccination refusal, saying that the root causes include understanding the entrenched medical folklore of lay beliefs and that research should seek to highlight the structural determinants of health behaviours. Some qualitative methodological research designs (e.g. ethnography) take into account more of the wider social reality and context so that it can investigate in more depth the key issues of local people. For example, in Closser et al. (2016) we see comparative ethnographic studies being used in eight countries to understand the underlying reasons behind polio vaccine acceptance, and a methodology grounded in some nuanced understanding of local contexts (as well as paying attention to global trends).

There are a few other key aspects to this more critical qualitative approach. First, that it takes a largely social actors' approach to social and public health problems, where people live out complex lives with multiple social roles and they perform versions of their self in different contexts (see sociologist Erving Goffman's 1956, *The Presentation of Self in Everyday Life*). Hence, interviewing only really captures a 'version' of that multiple self. Second, it highlights the importance of both the wider – global and upstream – social context as well as the local social-cultural context – that is, what else is going on in their lives that is important to understand and help 'frame' the issue. Third, such an approach stresses the importance of a 'holistic' understanding of that social reality; how can we properly understand complex public health issues without understanding the whole social context of people's/community lives? The issue needs to be framed within a larger context.

Qualitative methodologies

Qualitative researchers use different methodological approaches, but we need to think about the most useful approaches for public health researchers and students understanding public health problems. Creswell and Poth (2018), for example, talk about five 'traditions' in their book on qualitative research, focusing on ethnography, case study, phenomenology, narrative and grounded theory, but one could also include action (and co-production) research, auto-ethnography and ethnomethodology. Also, some of these approaches (e.g. narrative and case study) are more about methodological techniques and approaches to the data than rounded methodological approaches that could be called traditions. Knowledge always moves forward and rejects approaches that are weaker and lack utility. Grounded theory equally is often perceived as an approach to data analysis, as the original proponents of the approach, Barney Glaser and Anselm Strauss (Glaser and Strauss, 1967) wanted to provide more of a systematised blueprint for analysing qualitative data in the social sciences. To make this useful for public health research, therefore, we will discuss some of the methodologies that, for us, either have to date (or could in the future) provide the most interesting and useful inspiration for public health research.

Ethnography

Ethnography literally means 'folk writing' or what we can understand as writing about other societies and cultures, but it is not associated with a single method, though participant observation has become the *sine qua non* of ethnographic endeavours. It has its roots fundamentally in two key traditions: the first of which is in the anthropological fieldwork of the twentieth century. At the turn of the twentieth century, anthropologists were often employed *ad hoc* in the local colonial administrations in countries like Nigeria (Kuper, 1996) to help supplement some of the census data, though more sophisticated ethnographic detail was not particularly encouraged. What we now understand as the ethnographic method was symbolised most distinctively in the work of the anthropologist Bronislaw Malinowski where his 1922 classic work on the Trobriand Islands – *Argonauts of the Western Pacific* – is particularly well known and seen as an early example of lengthy and detailed ethnographic fieldwork. Other notable anthropologists producing similar lengthy fieldwork accounts included Margaret Mead, E.E. Evans-Pritchard and Pitt-Rivers, where the distinctive feature was on intensive work with a particular culture/society, living for a year or more with the people, and making an account that could vary from descriptive to more analytical and theoretical considerations in the work of Radcliffe-Brown and other British functionalist social scientists. Much of this work has received considerable criticism as a reflection of social anthropology as a colonial science (Asad 1973; Pels and Salemink, 1999), which has both led to attempts at de-colonisation of methodologies (Tuhiwai Smith 1999), as well as some self-reflection in anthropology as researchers sought to address how they represented 'other cultures' as well as their own (Clifford, 1986).

The second key tradition was in the emerging professional sociology in the USA and specifically what was known as the Chicago School of the 1930s (Bulmer, 1986; Deegan, 2001). Much of that work was characterised as ethnography and was concerned to understand the new quality of urban community life in American cities as they diversified and inequalities grew in urban areas. Key ethnographic work during this period included the work of William Foote Whyte (1943, *Street Corner Society*), and W.I. Thomas and Znaniecki (1918, *The Polish Peasant in Europe and America*), among others. Looking back on some of this work can provide some inspiration for modern-day public health, as many of the issues social scientists focused on in the growth of American cities have similarities with the concerns and challenges of public health.

So, what do these approaches have in common, and what are some of the key characteristics of ethnographic research? The first is that ethnography is research based on long-term and intensive immersion in a setting (e.g. a community, school, local organisation) where the ethnographer spends as much time as possible in that setting. It can be, therefore, a very demanding form of research activity, perhaps not necessarily practical for a small-scale student project. Another key feature is that the ethnographer seeks to grasp a more holistic understanding of the issue they are seeking to understand, so they do not necessarily predetermine the issues of interest in advance – this might be important as the ethnographer is seeking to grasp an understanding of the interrelated aspects of social life – e.g. as we have highlighted, if we were seeking to understand why some individuals choose not to immunise their children against diseases like measles it might be important to understand more fully the social context in which those decisions are made – it is not that all people who decide not to immunise their child make the same decision for the same reasons.

BOX 6.5   US–MEXICO BORDER TRANSNATIONAL MIGRATION AND PUBLIC HEALTH (HOLMES, 2013A)

As a public health doctor and medical anthropologist, Holmes' work has been focused on social hierarchies and health inequalities in the context of US–Mexico migration. This

(Continued)

(Continued)

work has drawn upon 18 months of full-time participant observation, during which time Holmes has migrated with undocumented indigenous Mexicans in the United States and Mexico, picked berries and lived in a labour camp in Washington State, pruned vineyards in central California, harvested corn in the mountains of Oaxaca, accompanied migrant labourers on clinic visits, and trekked across the border desert into Arizona.

His work is documented in detail in his award-winning book *Fresh Fruit, Broken Bodies: Migrant Farmworkers in the United States* (2013b), though in one of his more illuminating articles he documents his accompanied border crossing from Mexico to the US and details the participant observation and what that involved: ...

'Before, during, and immediately after the border crossing in which I participated, I wrote hundreds of pages of field notes involving observations, conversations, and my own embodied experiences. In addition, I took photos and tape-recorded conversations and interviews. The field notes in this article were taken during this in-depth, extended case study of a border crossing beginning with preparations in the mountains of Oaxaca and culminating in the borderlands of Arizona. The field notes are analyzed in the context of the 18 months of full-time migratory participant observation in Mexico and the US with extended indigenous Triqui families.' (Holmes, 2013a: 154).

Ethnographic research allows one to witness decision making and actions in context, as well as the relationship between micro-level actions and decisions and the macro-level socio-cultural and economic context in which people live their lives. As Holmes says, 'the thick description of ethnography provides complex and powerful narratives of the every-day lives of real people that have the potential to influence public opinion and policy' (2013a: 154). It traces the grain of everyday life. Ethnography has a duty to report back on the way in which social life is ordered and conducted; in other words, how is social life accomplished. It is not just about empathetic commentary or celebrating distinctive ways of life. What we see primarily in the ethnographic tradition then is the use of participant observation (see Chapter 8 for a further discussion of this approach), the stock-in-trade of social anthropology. In participant observation the researcher immerses themselves into the socio-cultural sphere of the participants, which poses practical as well as ethical challenges in the context of public health research.

Why ethnography for public health research?

There are clear reasons for the advantage of this approach to public health research, but the one that sticks out is the problematisation of one of the main public health paradigms, which is about individual behaviour and choice. As Holmes (2013a) says in his paper, one of the core public health perspectives sees individuals as rational actors, weighing up the pros and cons of actions and maximising self-interest. Clearly, in Holmes' research on

Mexican migrants crossing the US border, the social actors crossing the border do not do this and ethnography allows one to see things more clearly from an 'emic' (or insider perspective). It enables us to get under the representational problem of much qualitative research – given that other qualitative studies involving interviews exclusively will perhaps only address an issue at a surface level and not be able to see, over time, patterns in the data.

BOX 6.6   COMPLEMENTARY HEALTH PRACTITIONERS AND WELLBEING (MCCLEAN, 2006)

Wellbeing practices, such as complementary and alternative health, are playing a key part in people's strategies for keeping well and preventing ill-health. McClean (2006 to conducted an ethnographic study into a local group of people who both used and practised what might be considered more 'fringe' and esoteric wellbeing therapeutic practices, like crystal and spiritual healing.

The study provides insight into why people would use and practise something that is on the margins. The study provides theoretically informed findings about how these practices become normal for the participants (as opposed to being perceived as irrational or not evidence-based), and at the same time shows us how societal trends, such as personalisation, are changing the way people think about their wellbeing beyond traditional solutions. It explored the nature of victim blaming and stigma, personal responsibility and ideologies of health and wellbeing.

Through long-term immersion (two years of fieldwork) in the community of healers and users, this ethnographic study has contributed to how we think about wellbeing and culture.

Ethnographic methods are also gaining traction in co-production/co-creation methodologies. In applied areas of research, and in public health studies, co-production (variably described also as co-creation) has emerged as a way of addressing a criticism of research that is done to people, as opposed to thinking about research that is carried out *with* people and communities (Wherton et al., 2015). Within a 'positivist' way of framing research, research conducted in communities neglects to use communities in the whole research process, from the ideation stage through to undertaking. Co-production is now also perceived as a solution to how to make research more relevant to communities and improve 'impact'. It offers work with communities, providing citizens with greater control over the research process. Ethnographic methods such as participant observation, immersion in the social and cultural context and lifeworld of the people, and the principles of giving voice to hard-to-reach communities, are methods that are increasingly a part of co-production design as users of research become co-producers and not passive consumers of academic research.

Grounded theory

Grounded theory is a commonly used approach in qualitative research, for the simple reason that it mostly uses a clear step-by-step approach to data analysis procedures and appeals to applied researchers, and also researchers that come from a more quantitative tradition. Originally expounded by the American sociologists Barney Glaser and Anselm Strauss in their *Discovery of Grounded Theory* (1967), the key principles of grounded theory have changed and fluctuated as Glaser and Strauss went their separate ways having disagreed on some fundamental approaches, and the method broadened in terms of its appeal with the publication of Strauss and Juliet Corbin's (1998) *Basics of Qualitative Research*. The method has also taken a more social constructionist and less rule-bound emphasis with the work of Kathy Charmaz (2014).

Grounded theory is based on the idea that one moves from a general description of a social phenomena to generating middle-range theory or explanation that is grounded from the data. Such approaches, particularly as it appears in its classic (1967) form, highlight the need to delay the literature review phases of the research until the findings and analysis are complete (Thornberg, 2012). It appears as though both writers, but particularly Strauss (from the famous Chicago School of Sociology), were strongly influenced by American social theory during the 1960s that sought to reject, and move beyond, hypothetico-deductive grand theoretical traditions as they were not seen as empirical enough and the theories were not grounded enough in what people were discovering in the data. As such, the general philosophy of grounded theory has more in common with the American pragmatism of writers such as John Dewey and Charles Pierce (Bryant, 2009).

Grounded theory approaches to methods suggest that any theoretical rationale/explanation is 'grounded' in the data, so the crude explanation for this is that theory emerges inductively – the common complaint of most grand theoretical schemes is that the theories are accepted almost a priori. However, this is not necessarily the way that grounded theory was originally formulated, but in some iterations this is certainly seen as received wisdom. A basic principle of data collection and analysis for the grounded theorist is that it can be seen as an iterative process: one collects qualitative research data to shed light on a particular issue. As a theoretical position is constructed from the data, the researcher may return to collect more data to refute or develop the theory. As such, a form of generalisable theory from the data hopes to account for the phenomenon.

One of the key aspects of Glaser and Strauss' reasoning was the notion of abductive reasoning, that the strength of grounded theory approaches comes from the cyclical and iterative process of sampling, collecting data, analysis, further sampling, data collection, analysis, and so on, refining the development of theory from the empirical data. This idea is also based on the premise that in research we should think about linking examples, events and observations in our research data to cases of larger social phenomena. This means essentially that we need a repertoire of pre-existing ideas, theories of the world, and understandings from literature, to link those examples or cases to (Atkinson, 2017). The ideas or 'themes', as they are sometimes known, do not emerge out of thin air (they are not empty and devoid of wider theoretical connections); they link explicitly to them. The point with grounded theory is to remain fairly open and not to narrow the focus of the research too much at the earliest stages.

Why grounded theory for public health research?

Grounded theory satisfies a need for a more systematic approach to collecting and analysing qualitative data; it can help build up a more unified theory of social action and behaviour so that complex public health issues can be understood. Given more public health calls for evidence-based practice, there is a need for high-quality qualitative research that takes a more systematic approach and grounded theory as a general approach can fulfil that need.

BOX 6.7 HIV DISCLOSURE IN VULNERABLE POPULATIONS (THAPA ET AL., 2018)

This study explored HIV disclosure processes, the ways in which a person's HIV status is declared to others, and wanted to find out how this could be done in order to reduce the stigma of HIV status. The authors used a grounded theory study to help develop a theoretical model to explain those processes. The study took place in a district of Nepal with one of the highest prevalence rates of HIV infection.

A key method in this approach was 'theoretical sampling' (see Chapter 7 for further explanation), an exemplary grounded theory approach. From the grounded theory, the authors developed a theory to improve understanding on the contextual factors and mechanisms that influence HIV disclosure, so as to influence future interventions to reduce stigma.

Phenomenology

In the twentieth century, phenomenology has emerged as a philosophical perspective to understand human consciousness, particularly in the writings of such philosophers as Husserl (1859–1938), Heidegger (1889–1976) and Merleau-Ponty (1908–1961), but it is also a qualitative methodology which we consider here, and it is often best not to mix the two up (see Paley, 2017, on this issue). Different terms are sometimes used to describe the use of phenomenology in qualitative research, such as descriptive phenomenology, interpretive, hermeneutic, and so on, but the research process is often very similar. It is popular as a methodology for nursing and health services research in particular, which can be attributed to its focus on the meaning for patients with particular illness experience (Stott et al., 2018). Phenomenological research studies are usually either descriptive or interpretive. Descriptive phenomenology aims at providing collective descriptions of experienced phenomena, in ways that offer an objective account of reality – to achieve that, the researchers' influence must be 'bracketed' out (removed) from the account (Reiners, 2012). In interpretive phenomenology, based on what is called the 'hermeneutic' tradition, objectivity is seen as impossible and, therefore, the aim is to achieve some critical though subjective interpretation and description of human experience.

The aim of phenomenological research is to explore the common meaning for a group of individuals of their 'lived experience'. Paley (2017) has called this 'meaning attribution' and is considered to be a distinctive element of much phenomenological research, as opposed to other qualitative studies, though what it means in practice is much harder to decode. Much has been made of the term 'lived experience' as a phenomenological trope, and in some ways it is problematic as it is hard to think of a non-lived experience, but the term is about trying to make sense of the embodied and existential experience of a phenomenon as it is impacting on the individual (as opposed to talking about past experience or events leading on to something as in the case of narrative/biographical research). The phenomenon could be an object of human experience (e.g. obesity, or giving up smoking, or living through substance misuse, or a disrupted life event such as illness). The question for the research then becomes, 'what does it mean to experience… obesity, etc?' Phenomenological research then provides a very deep understanding of the nature of one's experiences and that can be built up over a number of cases to understand the 'common' experience of the phenomenon, and, as such, can be a very structured methodology.

Why phenomenology for public health research?

> ### BOX 6.8   HEALTH PROMOTION INTERVENTIONS RELATED TO MOBILE HEALTH TECHNOLOGIES FOR UK TRUCK DRIVERS (GREENFIELD ET AL., 2016)
>
> Greenfield et al's study focused on professional truck drivers in the UK and the known risk for various health conditions such as cardiovascular disease, obesity, diabetes and stress. The aim was to explore truck drivers' perception of using 'wearable' mobile technology devices (such as smart watches), and their potential as an intervention for a high-risk group.
>
> A key method in this study was the use of phenomenology to understand the 'lived experiences' of using mobile health from the perspective of truck drivers. They describe the purpose of the method to reduce individual experience to a description of the universal essence of the phenomenon. They took what they called a psychological phenomenological

approach, which focused more on the participants' descriptions and less on the researcher's interpretation (known as a hermeneutic approach).

Four focus groups were conducted with truck drivers (each containing between 5 and 12 participants). The findings suggested that wearable devices made the truck drivers more aware of their lifestyles, more vigilant towards cardiovascular health, and could be a possible motivator to change lifestyle, though concerns were raised about privacy and whose interest would be served by truck companies providing such mobile health devices.

Within public health, issues like obesity or physical activity, come to take on common-sense meaning and researchers may assume that everyone knows what it is. Yet, we need to understand that lay people may attach a very complex set of meanings to those public health concerns. It is important for reseachers to explore these meanings; as such, phenomenology can help to make researchers more attuned to lay understandings, and thereby hopefully be able to design more appropriate and acceptable interventions on the basis of these meanings.

Conclusion

Qualitative methods approaches research issues with different questions, sometimes helping us to answer the 'why' or the 'how', helping us to explore understandings, experiences, behaviour and beliefs. Some methodologies are better at providing contextual and holistic understanding of public health issues. Qualitative research can be used creatively in combination with quantitative methods, as well as being used as a stand-alone approach.

Further reading

Atkinson, P. (2017) *Thinking Ethnographically*. London: Sage

Charmaz, K. (2014) *Constructivist Grounded Theory* (Second edition). London: Sage.

Moses, J. and Knutsen, T.L. (2012) *Ways of Knowing: Competing methodologies in social and political research*. Second edition. Buckingham: Palgrave.

7 ACCESSING AND SELECTING CASES IN QUALITATIVE RESEARCH

—————— CHAPTER SUMMARY ——————

This chapter explores **access** and **sampling** in **qualitative research**. We start by exploring access as the first stage of a research process. The chapter discusses the journey towards building research participant 'engagement'; we consider the **ethical** and **practical** measures involved in approaching the setting, negotiating access, then selecting cases. Key approaches to case selection and sampling in qualitative research are outlined (e.g. **convenience sampling, purposive sampling, theoretical sampling, snowballing**), and the pros and cons of each discussed. A key question for many students undertaking qualitative research is to know whether sample numbers are important in qualitative studies and what implications this will have for their research. Pragmatic guidance is given for dissertation students or those undertaking research in practice.

Introduction

'Access' is a very important first stage upon which the success of a research project hangs. It is about gaining entry to the research field and achieving traction once in, with the intention of selecting cases, then collecting and analysing data, with a view to reliably addressing a research question. Access refers to the process of transition into the field. The research will be concerned to seek out potential cases that will become the objective for sampling and a source of data. A case can be an individual or collective unit; it can denote people, events or occurrences (Charmaz, 2014). This implies that qualitative data – usually verbatim, textual or pictorial – can arise from different sources, commonly directly from people (individually or collectively), but also from a wide range of audio-visual sources.

Gaining access to cases is a pragmatic and ethical process. Established sampling proto-cols reflect the range of philosophical and methodological traditions in qualitative research (see Chapter 6). However, as well as the pragmatics, research access in qualitative research involves building relationships with stakeholders, gatekeepers and potential par-ticipants (or cases) to achieve the research goals. The research process is fundamentally a social one, where rapport, tact, diplomacy and honesty are crucial tenets. Unlike quantita-tive research, sampling is much less concerned with generating numbers of cases and much more with accessing rich data through a 'social contract' between the researcher and the research context. In the ensuing sections, we explore how this process manifests for different research designs.

Accessing the field

Research access may be defined in terms of the accessibility of the setting and the degree of self-disclosure of the researcher. With regard to the latter, researchers may operate overtly or covertly (Gilbert, 2015) – intentionally or unintentionally masking their research intentions and/or their personality and character. Covertness has also been described as 'deception' (Calvey, 2017) and 'systematic concealment' (Bell and Newby, 1977: 118). Here, we don't advocate or recommend intentional deception in qualitative research, but it is important to recognise that researchers are likely to 'front manage' how they present themselves to research gatekeepers and stakeholders and how they express and articulate their research problem, possibly oversimplifying the research purpose and goals to ease transition into the field. For example, qualitative research that aims to inves-tigate 'health' and 'wellbeing' could seem ambiguous when it lacks clear explanation and definition. Notably, Giddens (2009: 37) suggested that 'some of the most valuable data that have been collected by sociologists could never have been gathered if the researcher had first explained the project to each person encountered in the research process'.

Research access is an ethical and relational process, where a researcher's accountability extends to explicitly respecting the values of participants and understanding the potential consequences of the research (Cunliffe and Alcadipani, 2016). Access involves more than a series of procedural protocols, and is principally about the nature of the relationships involved:

> '... the form of the research relationship can have a major impact on the nature of access, the degree of transparency and trust between participants, the perceived outcomes of the research, and the agency attributed to researcher and/or research participants.' (Cunliffe and Alcadipani, 2016: 541)

Agency here refers to how much the researcher is faithful to research participants' inten-tions, feelings, knowledge and abilities to make informed choices and to become actively involved in the research process. It is a 'transactional' process of, 'reciprocal agency in which the relationship is a contractual one of give-and-take, trade-offs, and compromise, involving a "bargain" over outcomes that benefit both the researcher and the organization.' (Cunliffe and Alcadipani, 2016: 541–2)

Access thus involves a process of social transition as the researcher seeks social access to the research setting. Cassell (1998: 93) suggested that this requires 'a thick skin and a certain imperviousness to rejection', given that entering a new or unfamiliar setting or group can be daunting and make one feel exposed and vulnerable. The individual may then find it necessary to '… adopt a role or identity that meshes with the values and behaviour of the group being studied, without seriously compromising the researcher's own values and behaviour' (Cassell 1998: 96–7). Brannen (1987: 167), likewise, equated entry into a new research setting as a 'period of initiation', as one enters the world of others and has to learn to interpret and fit into that world. For qualitative research that seeks to recruit human participants or cases, this involves acquiring privileged access and insight into people's lives and experiences across varied settings and situations. It affords the opportunity to explore and seek to understand health and social issues within people's lifeworlds, at the level of their everyday experiences. The complex character of public health means that opportunities to undertake qualitative research are limitless, especially given the personal, social and cultural situatedness of public health issues.

When planning to undertake primary qualitative research – whatever the setting or context – it is therefore important to reflect carefully on the whole process, considering this as 'transition' into the field. Qualitative research with human participants involves stepping into other people's lives, whose experiences may be similar, tangential or very different to ours. One participant in Dickson-Swift et al.'s (2008: 330) study commented,

'[research participants] … are actually allowing you into their lives, they are telling you personal information that might be quite hard […] the reality is that it is more than just words … it's their life, their experience.'

Just as it would be inappropriate and impolite to walk uninvited into a stranger's house unannounced and uninvited, this is equally the case with qualitative research. The researcher hopes to become a 'welcome guest' rather than an inquisitor or voyeur, while acknowledging any potential disruption or demands their presence could bring to bear on those who could become involved in the research. Researchers should therefore employ etiquette while engaging with gatekeepers and recruiting participants so as to yield a productive research partnership.

Recruiting research participants is therefore more than a technical, pragmatic exercise of appealing to volunteers. It is about acquiring access through building relationships with the goal of eliciting meaningful, reliable findings that genuinely represent the views and experiences of research participants. Access is an ethical process that requires the researcher to invest at a personal and social level in the research relationship from the outset, in a reflexive and sensitive way.

BOX 7.1   ACCESS: ISSUES TO CONSIDER (FONTANA AND FREY, 2005)

Access requires operationalising emotional and social assets, and employing emotional intelligence to manage interpersonal relationships as they manifest, judiciously and empathetically. Fontana and Frey (2005) suggest that this means considering the following:

- How to access the research setting
- How to understand the language and culture of participants
- How to present oneself
- How to locate key informants or gatekeepers
- How to gain trust
- How to establish rapport.

Emic perspective

A key guiding principle in qualitative research is to achieve an 'emic perspective' or insider's normative view of reality; this is fundamental to understanding how people perceive the world around them. For this reason, access is an inductive process that requires the researcher to strive to forge constructive relations with gatekeepers, stakeholders and potential research participants, so as to be able to acquire deep 'indigenous' insight into people's lives from an emic perspective, which is only possible if trust, respect and rapport underpin relationships with key actors in the research setting.

This means getting to know people to the extent that it is possible to elicit reliable and trustworthy data that can be verified by participants and that arise from undertaking the research ethically. The researcher builds the research relationship through active dialogue, listening, establishing rapport and positive regard, exercising empathy and striving for mutual respect. Moreover, as Morse and Field (1998: 78) emphasised, this is important because:

'Data collection can be an intense experience, especially if the topic that one has chosen has to do with the illness experience or other stressful human experiences. The stories that the qualitative researcher obtains in interviews will be stories of intense suffering, social injustices, or other things that will shock the researcher.'

With investment of time and perseverance, it becomes feasible to seek and elicit rich data concerning the social phenomena one is interested in exploring. Relationship building is thus the key to access, ahead of formal measures to operationalise the research. There are obvious links with methodologies commonly used within health promotion and within the caring professions, including employing active listening, striving for unconditional positive regard, working with groups and teams, and community participation and engagement.

In such instances, researchers must strive to work cooperatively and collaboratively with people to enable them to have agency and voice. In this respect, qualitative research can play an empowering role, as the research subject becomes an active participant.

Participation

It is also important to consider the notion of 'participation', a concept central to the ethos of public health and health promotion. Referring to community participation, Agarwal (2010: 100) argued that full participation is 'a dynamic interactive process in which all stakeholders, even the most disadvantaged, have a voice and influence in decision-making'. This definition is just as valid when recruiting human participants, where an essential ethical tenet is that they must be able to make an informed, free decision whether or not to volunteer or opt into a research project, to participate and to withdraw should they choose to (see Chapter 14 for a further discussion of ethics).

Fundamentally, procedures for selecting research participants must be equitable. Furthermore, prior to giving consent to participate, human participants must be provided with all relevant information about the research in formats they can interpret and comprehend, and not be coerced into participating nor be exposed to any kind of inhumane treatment. A further principle, implied by Agarwal's definition, is that of active participation, where all 'stakeholders' – including research participants who have a stake in the research – have the power to influence decisions governing the research. This is consistent with recent developments in public involvement in research. In this respect, Rose (2014) argues that researchers should avoid equating 'research participant' with 'research subject', the latter being a term that implies status difference.

Researcher status

A key investment within qualitative research is the researcher's own personal commitment and involvement. Instead of perceiving a dualistic relationship between researcher and research participant and, moreover, as a one-way 'fishing exercise' where the researcher is merely intending to ask questions and listen, the aim is to develop a reciprocal relationship (Nielsen, 1990). In this regard, Gadamer (1976) argued that researchers should not endeavour to 'mask' their own personal values but, rather, use the potentially new relationship opportunity to 'fuse horizons' or create new, less predictable outcomes.

This more-equal relationship predictably brings greater trust and respect, and ultimately greater integrity for the research outcomes. Oakley (1981) supported empathy and personal involvement as core ingredients for an equitable research relationship – also described as taking a 'reflexive' stance – where the researcher is conscious of their own social status as researcher and the corresponding influence this may bring to bear on the research (O'Connell Davidson and Layder, 1994). By being reflexive, researchers acknowledge that we are part of the social world we study (Hammersley and Atkinson, 2007), necessitating non-hierarchical, positive identification between researcher and research participant (Nielsen, 1990; Mies, 1993). The researcher then becomes as much a subject of the research as the researched.

Self-perception, self-awareness and presentation of self are therefore significant in this process. Goffman (1956) argued that in attempting to explain social relations in any given context, researchers should examine how individuals present themselves to others; as an 'actor' one may feel compelled to present to others an idealised impression of oneself to suit the circumstances and to fit in. So, within any given research situation, researcher and researched act and associate with others consistent with the social consensus. This is likely to happen where a researcher is operating within an unfamiliar social context.

BOX 7.2 ACCESS AND ENGAGEMENT

When planning to undertake qualitative research involving human participants within an institutional setting (e.g. school, hospital, clinic, custody setting, workplace), having first reviewed the qualitative research evidence and developed the research rationale, research question and methodological approach, it is prudent to develop an engagement strategy by considering realistic responses to the following questions concerning 'access':

How will you identify and select an appropriate institution?

- *What is it about this institution that is special and relevant?*
- *Will this choice of setting be consistent with your research question?*

Who do you envisage to be the research participants?

- *Why these participants specifically?*
- *Do you consider them to be stakeholders?*
- *Will their involvement be consistent with your research question?*

Who can/should you approach to discuss the proposed research with?

- *Are these external and/or internal informants?*
- *What makes them legitimate informants?*

(Continued)

(Continued)

- *Do they have authoritative/governance status?*
- *What would be their 'stake' in your research?*
- *How should you engage and communicate with them?*
- *Will you need to educate potential stakeholders or gatekeepers?*
- *What information should you share with initial contacts and in what format?*

Are there any ethical or governance barriers to overcome?

- *Are there safeguarding or other issues to consider?*
- *Is there a physical cost (e.g. travel)?*
- *Will I require specific training or supervision?*
- *How much engagement with stakeholders and gatekeepers should you have before applying for formal ethical or governance approvals?*

What concerns might stakeholders and gatekeepers have about your research, and how would you respond to these?

- *Time/duration*
- *Location*
- *Numbers of participants*
- *Degree/level of active involvement in research*
- *Safeguarding, mental capacity, informed consent, etc.*
- *Staff resource implications*

What other potential challenges or barriers should you address before embarking on the research?

Gaining entry

A useful starting point when planning qualitative research is to try to visualise the process, mapping out the key challenges, 'gateways' and milestones. These are likely to be physical, institutional, bureaucratic, legal, social and personal. Successfully acquiring gatekeeper consent – which will include research ethics approval – will necessitate working out the complexities of access. From whom should permission be sought? Whose consent is required? Are there research governance or legal requirements to overcome? Are there safeguarding protocols? Does one have appropriate personal and social skills? This process is illustrated below (see Box 7.3).

BOX 7.3   THE RESEARCH JOURNEY

Phase 1

Develop the rationale

- *Review existing evidence*
- *Identify setting and population*
- *Devise research question*
- *Determine methodological approach*
- *Decide inclusion and exclusion criteria*

Phase 2

Check the feasibility

- *Review researcher skills mix*
- *Governance and ethical approvals*
- *Consult with stakeholders*
- *Identify and approach gatekeepers*

Phase 3

Commence engagement

- *Educate gatekeepers*
- *Negotiate access requirements*
- *Recruit champions*
- *Develop and distribute promotional materials and participant information*
- *Appeal for volunteers*
- *Drop-in Q&A sessions*
- *Acquire informed consent*
- *Recruitment of participants*

Developing relations with stakeholders, gatekeepers, ethics and governance panels and, eventually, research participants should human participants be involved, is a process of socialisation and education, where the researcher or research team must make sense of the research to all those whom they encounter before and during the research project. It will be necessary to explain the research to different contacts with differing levels of knowledge and understanding, who may feel bewildered about the notion of 'research', and who will make differing interpretations of the research topic and question. Moreover, it is unlikely they will have the same knowledge and understanding of the research evidence that has framed the research question. A key challenge is therefore to convey what one wants to do in such a way that it is accurate yet not overly complex. Informed consent then becomes somewhat contested when it is necessary to convey 'in lay language' the rationale and philosophical basis for the research.

BOX 7.4 EXPRESSING AND ARTICULATING THE RESEARCH

Educating gatekeepers and stakeholders

> *How do you explain your research question, methods, outcomes and risks?*

Informing ethics committees

> *How do you articulate potential risks and justify potential 'costs'?*

Recruiting participants

> *How do you convince potential volunteers that it is within their interest to volunteer?*
> *What will participants gain from becoming involved?*

Informing participants

> *How do you articulate what you will require from participants, the nature of their involvement and the potential costs and benefits?*

Consenting participants

> *How do you undertake the consent process?*
> *Do you consent for separate phases of the fieldwork?*

Selecting cases

The term 'sample' derives from the Latin and Old French for 'example' or 'specimen', but such a definition implies an intention to collect cases that typify or represent a larger population. This perspective is consistent with the quantitative rather than the qualitative research paradigm. The term 'case selection' is commonly preferred in qualitative research, since the concern is not with numerical units or cases; rather, the objective is to elicit deep understanding, rich insight (Guba and Lincoln, 2005) or thick description (Geertz, 1973) of phenomena, individuals or events. This is achieved through purposively seeking cases that will yield data that reliably answer the research question.

Qualitative research tends to involve small numbers of cases selected purposively and then studied intensively, usually following a sequential rather than pre-determined process. The intention is to seek cases that adequately explain, describe, and interpret the phenomenon of interest in depth (Maxwell, 2013). The sampling strategy is shaped by the theoretical framework and research rationale. In developing a sampling strategy and expressing this adequately in the overall research design, one must give detailed consideration to the following:

- Sampling definition – that it is congruent with the methodology
- Sampling approach – how case selection will be undertaken
- Sample size – how many cases will be required
- Time frame – staging of case selection.

In this discussion, we continue to use the term 'sampling' to denote case selection to remain consistent with the majority of the qualitative research literature.

Sampling definition

Qualitative sampling necessitates selecting cases in such a manner as to elicit and acquire rich understanding of the phenomenon that forms the focus for the research question. The methodology usually determines the case, the sampling approach and the sample (Creswell, 2009). A phenomenological study will research human experiences and meanings people attach to these, and involve sampling individuals as cases who share the common experience. A grounded theory study will take an inductive, incremental approach to sampling, gathering cases (usually individuals) who contribute to the emerging theory. Ethnography seeks to understand socio-cultural factors within specific settings, the objective of sampling being to gather cases that illuminate and describe the culture of the setting; cases are likely to include people (individuals and groups), observed events or occurrences, field notes and other forms of observed data. Essentially, qualitative research methodologies fall within the interpretivist paradigm, and therefore case selection is concerned with seeking out the best way to interpret the phenomenon that forms the focus for the research question.

Sampling approach

Qualitative sampling is commonly described as 'purposeful', the objective being to intentionally seek cases perceived to have the potential to maximise the possibility of obtaining appropriate data and new leads (Glaser, 1978; Cresswell and Plano Clark, 2011). Patton (2015: 264) describes this in terms of seeking out 'information rich cases' to achieve deep understanding of phenomena, '... those from which one can learn a great deal about issues of central importance to the purpose of the inquiry'.

Another way to think about this is to compare sampling with the behaviour of a dog intent on following a scent, or alternatively, as anthropologist Gluckman (1964 in Evens and Handelman, 2006: 94) put it, to 'follow your nose wherever it leads you'. Gluckman advocated such an approach in ethnography, introducing the 'Extended Case-Method' approach, also termed 'situational analysis'. This is an inductive rather than predictive process of case selection. Three broad categories of sampling are commonly described across the literature – 'convenience' (sometimes termed 'selective'), 'purposive' (sometimes termed 'judgement'), and theoretical, which is associated largely with grounded theory approaches (Marshall, 1996; Coyne, 1997). Patton (1990) argued that all qualitative sampling is essentially purposeful since it involves actively selecting the most appropriate cases to answer the research question, while remaining consistent with the methodology. In his view, purposive sampling (synonymous with 'purposeful' sampling) involves selecting 'information-rich cases … from which one can learn a great deal about issues of central importance to the purpose of the research' (Patton 1990: 169). This is bearing in mind the fact that the process can be, and often is, unpredictable.

BOX 7.5 PURPOSIVE SAMPLING TYPES (PATTON, 2015)

Patton (2015) devised forty purposive sampling types within the following eight broad categories:

1. *Single significant case sampling*

Selecting single, in-depth cases to provide rich insight of a phenomenon. This is commonly used with biographical research where the focus is on single cases.

2. *Comparison-focused sampling*

Selecting cases to compare and contrast concerning a phenomenon of interest.

3. *Group characteristics sampling*

Selecting cases that provide specific insight into a group's experiences or features in relation to a phenomenon of interest, typical of phenomenological research.

4. *Concept or theoretical sampling*

Selecting cases as exemplars of emerging constructs or theories, as with grounded theory approaches.

5. *Instrumental-use multiple-case sampling*

Selecting multiple cases relating to a phenomenon of interest across several contexts to attempt to generalise findings and inform developments in practices, programmes or policies.

6. *Sequential and emergence-driven sampling strategies during fieldwork*

Selecting cases inductively to build the sample during fieldwork, one case leading to others sequentially, following leads and new directions. This is usually termed 'snowball sampling'.

7. *Analytically focused sampling*

Selecting cases later on in the research to support and deepen the qualitative analysis and the interpretation of patterns and themes. This is usually undertaken at the analysis stage.

8. *Mixed, stratified, and combination sampling strategies*

Selecting cases to meet multiple inquiry interests and needs, to deepen focus, and for triangulation purposes, common with ethnography.

Such broad typologies can be confusing, especially when distinctions become blurred or are misinterpreted (Coyne, 2008). Choice of sample strategy should be underpinned by careful methodological considerations. It is also important to stress that qualitative research often uses a combination of sampling approaches as part of the overall sampling strategy; for instance, combining convenience sampling, snowball sampling, intensity sampling and theoretical sampling. This is sometimes termed 'combination' or 'mixed' sampling.

Convenience sampling

Patton (2002: 228) described this as a 'fast and convenient' sampling approach, commonly used but the least rigorous. Sometimes viewed as a quick and indiscriminate approach to undertaking qualitative research, it involves selecting the most accessible cases and tends to be economical on time and resources. It can therefore elicit poor quality data.

Purposive sampling

Purposive sampling involves a range of techniques used in qualitative research to select cases based on judgement of what would constitute an appropriate sample. The techniques described below are derived from Patton (2002: 235–41).

- Typical Case Sampling

This describes the practice of selecting typical or 'average' cases, where it is judicious to consult with key informants on what is likely to constitute a typical case (Patton, 2002: 236).

- Criterion Sampling

Similar to 'typical case sampling', this approach involves selecting, as comprehensively as possible, 'all cases that meet some predetermined criterion of importance' (Patton, 2002: 238).

- Critical Case Sampling

This approach seeks to facilitate 'logical generalisations' with the reasoning that 'if it happens there, it will happen anywhere,' or, vice versa, 'if it doesn't happen there, it won't happen anywhere' (Patton, 2002: 236).

- Homogenous Sampling

This sampling approach involves selecting cases that are alike and share common characteristics or group affiliation, where common themes are likely to emerge from the data (Patton, 2002: 235).

- Intensity Sampling

This approach involves selecting 'information rich cases' considered exemplars that can provide deep insight into the phenomenon of interest (Patton, 2002: 234).

- Sampling Politically Important Cases

This is where special cases are intentionally selected or avoided that have political importance or sensitivity, which may occur when stakeholders signal an important line of enquiry (Patton, 2002: 241). Selection of a politically significant case may also have greater research impact (Elmore, 1991).

- Heterogeneous (or 'Maximum Variation') Sampling

This approach is used to identify cases that are likely to vary markedly from one another, in terms of uniqueness or individuality. This enables the research to identify how salient shared characteristics across cases emerged from their heterogeneity (Patton, 2002: 235).

- Extreme or Deviant Case Sampling

This approach involves selecting highly unusual 'illuminative' cases (Patton, 2002: 232) considered as outliers or that appear to be the 'exception to the rule'. This can lead to a richer, more in-depth understanding of a phenomenon and to lend credibility to the research findings.

- Confirmatory and Disconfirmatory Sampling

A confirmatory case is an additional case that fits with the already emergent themes, confirming and building the findings, adding richness, depth and credibility. A disconfirmatory case is essentially a deviant case that does not fit with others and may offer a rival interpretation or place limits on the findings (Patton, 2002: 239).

- Snowball or Chain Sampling

This approach involves seeking additional, new information-rich cases through key existing informants or participants. This 'chain' of participants can become typically heterogeneous and variable in quality/richness as different contacts are solicited (Patton, 2002: 237). Snowball sampling is a procedure whereby the researcher recruits a research subject through a contact who can vouch for the researcher's legitimacy (Gilbert, 2015). This is particularly useful in situations where potential subjects are likely to be sceptical of the researcher's intentions (Hedges, 1979). However, this technique requires the researcher to be able to draw on a network of reliable contacts, and certain subjects will likely be missed.

- Stratified Purposeful Sampling

This approach is used to select a relatively homogenous sub-sample (or 'stratum') of cases within the wider sampling frame, to capture and add integrity and credibility to thematic variations (Patton, 2002: 240).

- Combination or Mixed Sampling

This sampling approach is commonly used in larger, more complex studies, especially ethnography, where it is prudent to combine two or more sampling strategies to facilitate triangulation, bring flexibility to the research process and increase validity (Patton, 2002: 240). It is also useful when sampling different participant types, such as service users, service providers and stakeholders.

- Opportunistic or Emergent Sampling

Similar to the snowballing approach, this is an inductive, organic approach to sampling that enables the researcher to take advantage of unforeseen opportunities as fieldwork progresses, and therefore to select cases as they 'appear' and as themes begin to emerge (Patton, 2002: 240).

- Purposeful Random Sampling

This is a less common approach that involves taking a random sample of a small number of cases from a larger population. It is used to add credibility to the results of a larger quantitative study (Patton, 2002: 240–1).

Theoretical sampling

Glaser and Strauss (1967) developed the notion of theoretical sampling for their grounded theory methodology (see Chapter 6). It involves selecting cases that maximise theoretical development. Strauss and Corbin (1998: 73) later defined theoretical sampling as distinctive from other forms of purposive sampling, whereby case selection occurs as 'theory' is constructed from the data in the form of themes and sub-themes that begin to form theoretical constructs concerning the phenomenon of interest. It is an iterative, *theory driven* process, cases being selected 'as they are needed rather before the research begins' (Glaser, 1992: 102). Cases are selected that generate as many themes and sub-themes as possible and, as the sample builds, so the relations between these become clearer and the integrity (or validity) of the data is strengthened. Theoretical sampling, data collection, coding and analysis occur simultaneously and when to stop sampling is contingent upon reaching theoretical saturation – when no new themes can be constructed (Coyne, 2008).

Sample size

What is an appropriate sample size? This is a very common question students ask when first embarking on qualitative research. However, it is actually not that important a question for a qualitative study. Qualitative sampling is not so much about getting the right number of participants, as this would infer that the purpose is to represent a population. More important is to achieve high-quality, rich data that lead to a robust research output, rigour of method being of most importance. The character of the sample therefore depends upon methodology, scope and focus of the study, and the type, quality and richness of data required. An adequate sample size for a qualitative research study is therefore one that effectively answers the research question. Hardon et al. (2004: 64), in a report for the World Health Organization, provided an explanation that reflects much of the qualitative research literature: the aim of sampling being to achieve valid, meaningful data and subsequent data analysis by accessing the most appropriate rich cases; it is not to gather cases that are representative of a host population. Sample size therefore depends upon the research question, the purpose of the study and the methodology.

The most commonly cited criterion for adequate sample size is 'data saturation' or 'data redundancy'; this means that data collection should end when there is no new information forthcoming from data collection (Charmaz, 2003; Glaser, 1992; Glaser and Strauss, 1967; Lincoln and Guba, 1985; Merriam, 2009). Data saturation is more feasible with a tightly focused, precise research aim and question. A more complex, inductive study that perhaps takes a grounded theory approach or uses ethnography can take longer to achieve saturation given the potential uncertainty or unpredictability with the direction and focus of the research (Suri, 2011). A further point to note is that data saturation can also be considered in relation to a single case, where the focus of data collection is with an individual – such as with a biographical study – with data collection ending when no new data emerges from the case, possibly across a series of interviews with the one participant.

Another pragmatic, but less satisfactory criterion in terms of achieving depth and validity, is to consider how much resource is available to undertake fieldwork when time and access are limited (Hardon et al., 2004). Thus, a time limit may be imposed on the research, which means that only so much data can be collected, whether or not data saturation is achieved. This is common practice given that most research has to be curtailed by resource and timing constraints. In such instances, it is important to find other ways to enhance richness and depth, and thereby increase the integrity and credibility of findings.

Given the range of methodological options available to qualitative researchers, the research sample can be very small – in single figures – or larger depending on the complexity of the research design. For instance, some more complex sampling strategies would imply a larger sample, especially where there is some level of stratification, heterogeneity, triangulation or comparative component, bearing in mind that number of cases does not necessarily equate with quality. A sample size of ten may be adequate for a homogenous sample (Sandelowski, 1995), while 20–30 cases may be required to achieve data saturation when using a grounded theory approach (Creswell, 2013; Marshall, 1996). Biographical or narrative research requires very few cases given the specific focus on individuals' narratives. Ethnography will often triangulate different data sources and types (e.g. observation, interviews, focus groups) and may therefore sample more heterogeneously across a relatively large number of cases. A case study approach may typically recruit 15–30 cases (Creswell, 2013). Nonetheless, it is worth noting that inconsistency does arise across the literature regarding appropriate sample size and character.

It is also worth noting that excessive sampling is not necessarily productive if depth and richness are compromised. Sampling for the sake of increasing numbers may lead to excessive and unnecessary repetition of data, be a waste of resources, while not achieving sufficient deep insight into a phenomenon for effective data saturation, and it may be unethical to recruit more research participants than are required (Sandelowski, 1995). Moreover, a sample should not be so large that it becomes difficult to extract rich data nor so small such that it is difficult to achieve data saturation where this is the objective (Sandelowski, 1997; Flick, 1998). There is consensus that it is inappropriate to predict sample size in advance although there is often a pragmatic need to provide sample size estimates for funding proposals and applications for ethical approval (Cohen et al., 2000; Glaser, 1998).

Conclusion

Essentially, it is important that a sample strategy is *relevant* to the research purpose and question. When making decisions about research design, especially the sampling approach, it is worthwhile reviewing previous study designs investigating similar phenomena or cases. The sampling strategy should have a clear rationale that includes procedural detail regarding adequacy, with clear explanation of why the cases are relevant to the research question. To summarise, the following key objectives should underpin the sampling strategy:

- Provide clear, detailed description of the sampling strategy.
- Provide a clear methodological rationale for the sample strategy.
- Consider the range of sampling approaches available.
- Ensure the sampling strategy is adequate to address the research question.
- Provide full explanation of sample character (types of cases), sample size (numbers of cases), and sampling technique(s).
- Evaluate sample adequacy in terms of providing depth and validity.

Further reading

Cunliffe, A.L. and Alcadipani, R. (2016) The politics of access in fieldwork: Immersion, backstage dramas, and deception. *Organizational Research Methods,* 19(4): 535–61.

Gilbert, N. (2015) *Researching Social Life* (Fourth edition). London: Sage.

Patton, M.Q. (2015) *Qualitative Research & Evaluation Methods: Integrating theory and practice* (Fourth edition). London: Sage.

8 COLLECTING QUALITATIVE DATA

═══════════ CHAPTER SUMMARY ═══════════

This chapter explores the different ways qualitative researchers think about data and what counts as data. Methods of **primary data collection** are considered, including **observation, interviews** and **group interviews** (focus groups), as well as **visual data** and **online methods**. The suitability of these methods for different situations, and pros and cons of each, are illustrated using real examples, drawing on our own research experience.

What are qualitative data?

In qualitative research, the term 'data' can be problematic since it infers that research is concerned with collecting immutable 'facts' or 'statistics', usually in numerical form. In this regard, 'data collection' is a positivist notion, which makes the task of collecting qualitative data somewhat contested. The positivist paradigm assumes that facts are immutable, fixed, clearly identifiable and objectively measurable. By contrast, the social constructionist stance may question the authenticity of the very facts used to define and problematise health and wellbeing, suggesting they may be contestable or open to interpretation (see Chapter 6 for an example of this). Indeed, Guba and Lincoln (2005), among others, argued that 'facts' are values based, every fact implying a value. A randomised controlled trial, for instance, might be used by a researcher who values the methodology and makes a judgement to research a particular phenomenon using RCT. Likewise, an epidemiologist will measure 'relative risk' to determine the risk of a health event occurring among one group relative to another. Beck (1992: 172) argued that such attempts to deduce 'risk' in a population constituted a 'moral scientific judgement'. So, for instance, the assertion that one community is likely to have a greater prevalence of type-2 diabetes may be accurate from an epidemiological point of view, but the very assertion that this might be a possibility and something worth investigating will be a value-based judgement.

BOX 8.1   WHAT ARE 'DATA'?

With the advent of computing in the 1950s, data became commonly understood as units of numerical information that could be processed, transmitted and stored. However, the etymology of 'data' is actually very different; in seventeenth-century Latin, the term 'datum' – literally translating as 'a thing *given*' – implies a transactional relationship, though not necessarily a numerical one. Indeed, 'datum' is the neuter past participle of the verb 'dare', 'to give'. Philosophically speaking, therefore, data are 'things known' or 'assumed-to-be facts', which enable us to reason or make deductions.

Qualitative public health researchers tend to ask different questions, considering that health phenomena do not exist in isolation from the contexts and social determinants in which they prevail. Thus, in investigating type-2 diabetes, rather than assume this to be an uncontroversial objective and a *fait accompli* epidemiological exercise, a qualitative researcher might question the motive and desire to investigate type-2 diabetes from a biomedical, preventive stance and the epidemiological approach taken – e.g. measurement of relative risk. An altogether alternative approach would be to investigate values, attitudes and/or beliefs associated with health, illness, diet and nutrition within the particular social setting, especially given that type-2 diabetes is just one health concern among many that prevail within a complex cultural and social milieu of health and wellbeing. Moreover, an inductive approach to data collection – that seeks to elicit 'indigenous' knowledge and facts through exploring values, beliefs and experiences – will arguably yield deeper insight into health, wellbeing, diet and nutrition, which a biomedical 'frame' such as 'type-2 diabetes' will inhibit.

In qualitative research, therefore, 'data' are not sought through deterministic, reductionist (deductive) techniques but emerge in a less certain inductive way, given that the nature of the 'findings' may not be known at the outset. Data are representations of context that manifest through consensus between researcher and researched. They 'are subject to continuous revision, with changes most likely to occur when relatively different constructions are brought into juxtaposition in a dialectical context' (Guba and Lincoln, 2005: 113).

Deductive reasoning begins with a rule and proceeds through a case to arrive at an observed result, which either demonstrates the rule or falsifies it. Induction, by contrast, starts with a collection of given cases and proceeds by examining their implied results to develop an inference that some universal rule is operative. The inductive rule gains certainty with the multiplication of cases. Abduction starts with consequences and constructs reasons.

Qualitative data therefore tend to be much less tangible, fixed and measurable, in the conventional sense, than quantitative data. As with all phenomena within the social world, data are constructed through social relations and cultural practices, including at the site of data collection. Essentially, they comprise symbolic linguistic or visual material that carries subjective or intersubjective (social) meanings. The focus of enquiry is likely to be a social phenomenon or an experience that the researcher may choose to describe, interpret or

BOX 8.2 INTERSUBJECTIVITY

Intersubjectivity has been extensively debated within psychology, sociology and anthropology, and is a central theme of phenomenology. It describes interaction, or *discourse*, between two or more individuals, or what Habermas (1987) referred to as 'communicative action'. Intersubjectivity is that dialogic space where two or more individuals share knowledge reflexively. Schutz (1962 in Reich, 2010: 40) referred to it as the 'enigma of how man can understand his fellow man', which Reich argued depends upon the capabilities and co-operation of the parties involved. Communicative action includes language, discourse, conversation and any symbolic action through which people share meaning and purpose. The challenge for the qualitative researcher is to not only tap into research participants' intersubjective worlds but to become part of it in a reciprocal relationship.

interact with. Research data are therefore manifestations of the social context, expressed verbally, textually or visually.

However, it is important not to overstate or valorise the validity of qualitative data, but to recognise their subjectivity and the limits to what may be interpreted from expressed, recounted or observed experiences and narratives, especially given that qualitative research does not necessarily seek the 'truth'. Indeed, 'acceptance of limits requires an acknowledgment that speech is no more pure or authentic than other forms of data … [which] make it impossible to capture a truth or essence in the data' (Jackson and Mazzei, 2012: 16).

What we have established here is that the realm of qualitative data does not involve fixed truths in a reductionist, 'scientific' sense, where facts may be isolated and individually classified. Rather, as Foucault (in Foucault and Gordon 1980) argued, all knowledge is socially constructed and therefore the role of the researcher is to make knowable objects intelligible (*connaissance*). This involves collecting 'knowledge' that is authentic to participants and to the social context, by capturing accurately those subjective and intersubjective meanings attributed to experiences, existences and behaviours that are consistent with participants' beliefs and identities. The challenge is to do this in a robust, accountable way, such that one is as confident as possible in the findings.

Qualitative data are collected in many different ways, depending upon the research question and objectives, the purpose of the research, the research methodology and what is feasible within the research setting. As discussed in Chapter 7, defining the 'case' is important in determining the kind of data that will be gathered and the location and duration of data collection. Data can occur in the form of words or pictures and, as with any art form, are open to interpretation. Take, for instance, this excerpt from Mary Shelley's *Frankenstein*; not knowing the source could very easily lead to a different interpretation than that implied by the author:

'Once my fancy was soothed with dreams of virtue, of fame, and of enjcyment. Once I falsely hoped to meet with beings, who, pardoning my outward form, would love me for the excellent qualities which I was capable of bringing forth. I was nourished with high thoughts of honour and devotion. But now [...] I am quite alone. [...] I desired love and fellowship, and I was still spurned. Was there no injustice in this? Am I to be thought the only criminal, when all human kind sinned against me? [...] I, the miserable and the abandoned, am an abortion, to be spurned at, and kicked, and trampled on. Even now my blood boils at the recollection of this injustice.'

Not only are Shelley's words open to interpretation – depending upon the reader's perspective and standpoint – but the social, cultural and historical context must be considered since these frame the narrative in the place and time that it was written. One common assumption about the leading character of the story is that he is a 'monster'. It is poignant that Percy Shelley, the author's husband, in a later review of the novel, suggested that there is no monster in the story; rather, he asserted, 'treat a person wicked and he will become wicked' (Tropp in Bloom, 2007: 14). If we think about the central role of social determinants in understanding and interpreting public health concerns – for example, childhood obesity – there is an interesting parallel here.

Consider an image of someone sleeping rough; we subjectively draw upon our reserves of knowledge and understanding, our values and beliefs, social norms and cultural traditions to interpret it. How we perceive and interpret the image depends on these frames of reference; is this a homeless person or is it perhaps a person experiencing homelessness? 'Homelessness', while describing the phenomenon of being without a home, may not accurately reflect the perspective of the individual depicted here.

The underlying argument here is that facts, truths and data are essentially subjective and value-based, giving them fluidity and 'slippage' of meaning. Was Shelley's main character actually a 'monster' or was he an ostracised individual who had become socially excluded? Tilford et al. (2003) have debated how seemingly common-sense concepts – like 'health' and 'wellbeing' – are indeed socially constructed and culturally derived. 'Health', they argue, is a value rather than a fact; its meaning is contested and varied and its linguistic usage reflects personal, social and political values. Strategies to promote or improve the public's health therefore have to reconcile that the meaning of health is constantly shifting, based on beliefs about what we think to be true and values that pertain to what we want or desire to be true.

Qualitative data, likewise, are socially located and culturally derived in the sense that what we may experience in an interview scenario or when interpreting an image or an observed event are expressions of people's values – what they consider to be salient to the given time and place. Researchers furthermore bring their own social and cultural character (or 'baggage') to the research setting and interpret experiences against what they think to be true and – depending upon their reflexive stance – desire to be true. Phenomena of central interest to researchers are therefore always essentially contested. This *existentialist* perspective thus emphasises focus on *being* and *existence* within the given time and place (e.g. what it means to experience homelessness) rather than on the *essence* of the phenomenon (e.g. the character of the homeless person). This has an important bearing on the types of data we seek to collect and how we then proceed to collect them.

Hence, what we intend to collect as data is as important a concern as how we go about collecting it. Cogitation over what we want to collect provides us with our 'bearings' on how we should set about accessing it. Thus, thinking about *what* we want to research and arriving at an appropriate research question can enable us to deduce that we may be less concerned with a health behaviour or health indicator *per se* and more concerned with the experience, meaning, social context or values associated with the phenomenon. These become our primary concern from which we can endeavour to derive meaningful interpretations.

Collecting qualitative data

Decisions over data collection methods are contingent upon the research question, the methodological approach, the 'case', the character of the data, and issues of access and feasibility. For secondary-based qualitative research that utilises evidence synthesis methodologies, the data source will likely be published or grey literature (this is discussed further in Chapter 13). This section examines those data collection methods most commonly used in primary qualitative public health research, where human participants are involved. Table 8.1 provides a summary of how the 'case', the 'data' and data collection methods vary by methodology, adapted from Creswell and Poth (2018).

Table 8.1 Data collection methods by selected methodological approaches

Methodology	Phenomenology	Grounded Theory	Ethnography	Action Research
Case	individuals who share a common experience	individuals who share something in common	individuals who share a cultural space	individuals who share a cultural space
Data	• spoken word • non-verbal communication	• spoken word	• spoken word • written word • non-verbal communication • behaviour	• spoken word • written word • non-verbal communication
Roles	• researcher-led	• researcher-led	• researcher-led or participant-led (e.g. auto-ethnography)	• participant-led (peer researchers)

(Continued)

Table 8.1   (Continued)

Methodology	Phenomenology	Grounded Theory	Ethnography	Action Research
Data Collection Methods	• one-to-one and/or small group semi-structured interviews • participant and/or researcher reflective diary/journal	• one-to-one and/or small group semi-structured interviews • researcher reflective diary/journal	• participation and observation • one-to-one and/or small group semi-structured interviews • participant and/or researcher reflective diary/journal	• participation and observation • one-to-one and/or small group semi-structured interviews • participant and/or researcher reflective diary/journal
Recording Technique	audio, video, written	audio, video, written	audio, video, written	audio, video, written

Source: Adapted from Creswell and Poth, 2018: 149

Key to Creswell's analysis is the notion that a single method – e.g. an interview – can vary in character and purpose, depending on the respective methodology, the research question and the type of data. As discussed previously, the nature of the 'case' – which could be an individual, a group or a social setting – is significant, since this determines the focus of data collection. For instance, when considering the phenomenon of homelessness, the 'case' can take various forms; for example, 'a homeless individual', 'a group of homeless people', 'people directly or indirectly affected by homelessness' or 'a social setting in which homelessness manifests'. Moreover, the 'data' themselves will constitute spoken and/or written words captured through audio or digital recordings or handwritten notes, journals or documentation, representing participants, stakeholders, gatekeepers, the researcher and even people absent from the research setting (e.g. within documentation).

A flexible approach towards selecting and operationalising data collection methods may be necessary, provided the research design is developed to meet the research objectives. Arguably, as inferred by Table 8.1, one's choice of data collection methods is steered less by methodological convention and more by the research objectives and may depend upon by what is feasible and expedient. Furthermore, the research may be undertaken by research participants themselves, using peer research techniques, which is common with action research and auto-ethnography.

Data collection approaches for qualitative research usually involve direct one-to-one interaction with individuals or, at a collective level, with groups. Of central concern is the active relationship the researcher must foster with stakeholders, gatekeepers and research participants, since data collection is essentially an exercise in communication, with active participation and listening being central to the process. This 'participatory approach' (Cotterill, 1992: 594) 'aims to produce non-hierarchical, non-manipulative research relationships which have the potential to overcome the separation between the researcher and researched'; the key is to endeavour to reduce power differentials through building rapport with research participants. Added to this, an important method that runs through most qualitative research designs – and brings greater trustworthiness and rigour to data collection and analysis – is 'reflexivity'. Qualitative researchers should engage in reflection on the research process – before, during and after fieldwork – giving active thought and critique to all stages of the research process, especially during data collection. Reflexivity is discussed further in Chapter 10.

Primary data are accessed through the various mediums of communication available to the researcher, usually active engagement in *participation, observation* and *conversation*. Consequently, researchers must harness a range of social skills to access participants' social spaces and realise, from an emic point of view, how participants explain and interpret their circumstances or those phenomena that concern them.

BOX 8.3 EMOTIONALLY INTELLIGENT RESEARCH

Qualitative data collection is an active rather than passive exercise. Its success depends on effective communication between researcher and researched and building productive relationships. This requires the qualitative researcher to be perceptive, empathic and reflexive. Data collection is not a 'smash and grab' exercise but should aim for social, emotional and interpersonal connection with participants within the research social setting. Higgs and Dulewicz's (2016) seven elements of Emotional Intelligence, adapted here, provide a useful way to conceptualise the range of interpersonal skills applicable to qualitative researchers:

Self-awareness – awareness of own feelings and self-belief in managing and controlling emotions within a research situation.

Emotional Resilience – ability to perform consistently under pressure, even when faced with personal criticism or rejection, and to adapt to the imperatives of the research setting and to the needs and demands of research stakeholders.

Motivation – energy and drive to remain focused on the research objectives and towards attaining rich, meaningful outcomes, despite unanticipated challenges.

Interpersonal Sensitivity – awareness and capability to cope with personal, consensus, institutional and political values expressed by research stakeholders, and to maintain open-mindedness and suspend one's personal values and pre-judgements.

(Continued)

(Continued)

Influence – ability to influence others to participate voluntarily and engage effectively in the research process, and to perceive the benefits of participating.

Intuitiveness – versatility and intuitiveness in live data collection scenarios, and ability to actively listen, participate and exploit complex or confusing situations.

Conscientiousness – being consistent in words and actions, professional and organised, and showing commitment to ethical standards and modes of engagement.

Methods of qualitative data collection

Qualitative data collection generally falls within two categories – primary and secondary. Primary data collection seeks to gather audio or visual material from a 'live' research setting, usually involving human participants. Secondary data collection most commonly encompasses any stored data, usually transcripts or field notes taken from a previous study and used to undertake re-analysis, or it may comprise secondary documentation that is relevant to the research context (e.g. minutes, case notes, records, etc.). Secondary data can also include published qualitative research that is analysed using evidence synthesis methodologies (see Chapter 13). Here we discuss the collection of primary qualitative data as was summarised in Table 8.1.

Commonly, a qualitative study will seek to acquire verbatim data (or speech), visual data (or observations) and reflexive data (usually field notes/journals). Whichever is utilised, the method involves active engagement in the research setting (Holstein and Gubrium, 1995) and the product or output is generally textual in the form of a transcript or written narrative description that is then analysed.

Interviewing

Qualitative interviewing has evolved as a means of getting close to individuals or groups to understand, interpret and represent their perspectives and experiences. Unlike questionnaires, which are essentially quantitative instruments used to ask prepared open and closed questions, a qualitative interview is a dialogic, interactional and collaborative 'conversation with a purpose' (Burgess, 1984: 102; Fontana and Frey, 2005: 696). With a questionnaire, the researcher has absolute control, whereas qualitative interviewing involves a more egalitarian relationship, with control bestowed to the participant. The goal of qualitative interviewing is to engage in dialogic exchange or conversation with individuals or groups to achieve understanding of the phenomenon of interest from their emic perspective.

BOX 8.4 MEANING OF THE WORD 'INTERVIEW'

'*Interview*' originates from the sixteenth-century French verb '*s'entrevoir*' meaning '*to see each other*', from '*entre*' – '*between*' – and '*voir*' – 'to see'. In qualitative interviewing, '*voir*' (to see) is interpreted in its deepest sense, being concerned with intersubjective perception rather than objective observation; it reflects the emic viewpoint (and 'point of view') of the interviewee. '*Entre*', moreover, implies connection or partnership between agents engaged in interview, as opposed to a more detached 'shaking of hands'.

Theoretically, qualitative interviewing can involve any number of people; usually, it is a one-to-one or group technique, depending on the purpose of data collection. Interviewing is commonly described along a continuum between 'structured' and 'unstructured', the most common approach being 'semi-structured'. *Structured interviewing* tends to ask a series of relatively focused, predetermined questions, and allows little scope for diversion or variation. The interviewer controls the interview and plays a neutral, facilitative role, using open and closed questions. This approach is suited to telephone and online interviewing, and interviews conducted 'on the hoof' where there is limited opportunity for full conversation or digression. *Unstructured interviewing*, by contrast, provides much greater latitude, being open-ended and entirely inductive. It is most commonly used in ethnography where the researcher is seeking to build relationships with people to understand rather than to explain (Spradley, 1979). Douglas (1985) described this approach as 'creative interviewing' because it is likely to be somewhat unpredictable and the researcher must be creative and adaptive. An unstructured approach will not tend to rely upon predetermined questions or even topics to guide the process; instead, the researcher will ask questions and probe for clarification and illumination in a spontaneous way, seeking understanding from participants while in the field.

An inductive research design – a grounded theory study, for instance – might take a less structured approach, while a more focused, 'deductive' research design – for example, a study that takes a realist or pragmatic epistemological stance – might take a more structured approach to interviewing. The research context might require a more structured approach especially where time or access are limited.

Here, we choose to prioritise the semi-structured approach, which is generally accepted as highly applicable to most social research contexts. *Semi-structured interviewing* allows greater latitude than structured interviewing while maintaining focus around the research problem. There is scope to digress, investigate further, probe and illuminate. The interview is dynamic in the sense that it can respond and adapt to the narrative emerging from the individual or the group. It is cumulative and iterative in that what the participant says and how the conversation unfolds informs the direction of the interview (Galletta, 2013). While the researcher sets the 'agenda', the key objective is therefore to facilitate communication and to seek to yield rich, meaningful accounts that help to inform one's understanding and lead to accurate interpretation of the phenomenon under investigation.

One-to-one Interviewing

One-to-one interviewing involves striving to generate a conversation based on trust, empathy and, in the Rogerian tradition, to facilitate a process whereby the researcher strives to give unconditional positive regard to the interviewee. The purpose is to achieve a productive relationship that generates rich insight or 'thick description' (Geertz, 1973). Gadamer (2006: 305) described this as a meeting of minds or 'fusion of horizons', the 'horizon' being 'superior breadth of vision' that necessitates looking beyond the superficial.

Oakley's (1981) seminal work on feminist interviewing advocated an egalitarian process of establishing rapport and trust between interviewer and interviewee. The interviewer, she argued, should be empathic and prepared to self-disclose, communicating commitment and positive regard to the interviewee. Qualitative interviewing can therefore become an intimate experience, as it requires 'give and take', where both participants reveal things about themselves openly and reciprocally. A successful and fulfilling interview is one where the interviewee feels at ease and where an evident 'connection' has been forged between interviewer and interviewee (Lyons and Chipperfield, 2000).

Group interviewing

Group interviews are commonly referred to as 'focus groups', although this term can be misleading, as it is also associated with marketing and polling techniques used to elicit public opinion. Unlike these, group interviewing shares similar goals with one-to-one interviewing in terms of building relationships to elicit deeper insight into perspectives or experiences that are salient to participants. It provides the conditions for participants to engage in critical reflection and to explore common experiences, viewpoints and beliefs that may not surface in a one-to-one situation. Group interviews are essentially collective conversations that enable researchers to explore group dynamics and group characteristics in relation to the construction of meaning and the practices of social life (Kamberelis and Dimitriadis, 2005). They provide access to intersubjective, interactional dynamics that constitute social practices and discourses and are a useful tool for exploring social values and consensus within a group. For these reasons, as with one-to-one semi-structured interviewing, a group interview is not generally used to question individuals *per se*, but to encourage participants to talk to each other, 'exchanging anecdotes, and commenting on each other's experiences and points of view' (Barbour and Kitzinger, 1999). Thus, a group interview can, on the one hand, provide verbatim data concerning the phenomenon of interest, while, on the other hand, provide a window into the character of the group captured through observation.

Group interviewing can also perform a political function in terms of giving voice to a group, through facilitating dialogue. Kamberelis and Dimitriadis (2005) remind us of the emancipatory collective pedagogic work of Freire (1970), whose 'culture circles' were essentially focus groups intended to cultivate 'conscientization', commonly associated with community empowerment as a health promotion methodology. Dialogic focus groups generate ideas through 'praxis' – or critical reflection – as a means towards a sense of collective purpose. In this regard, group interviews can be useful for generating social interaction, observing peer relations and studying social norms.

Group interviewing can be more structured or less structured. As with one-to-one interviewing, empathy, flexibility and active listening are important, while it can also be necessary to take an objective, facilitative stance to steer the group process. This means directing the questioning and course of the conversation while simultaneously responding to and balancing needs of participants, particularly when faced with dominant or recalcitrant individuals. Group size should be sufficient to enable all participants to engage in discussion.

A key advantage of group interviewing is that it can be an efficient way to capture the perspectives of multiple participants on a single occasion, although this approach may not always achieve the richness and depth of one-to-one interviewing. The synergy and dynamism of a group can also elicit valuable data on social norms and values, especially since these are expressed not only through participants' words but also through body language, non-verbal gestures and group banter. Group interviews are useful for testing out ideas and for recruiting participants for follow-up one-to-one interviews. They can also offer an additional method for triangulation.

Interview design

The interview strategy – whether for one-to-one interviewing or group interviewing – should be focused and flexible, guiding participants towards the phenomenon of interest. Rather than having a list of questions to ask, a non-prescriptive topic guide provides direction and focus for interviewing, to facilitate the conversation and to tap into participants' thoughts and opinions (Smith and Osborn, 2007). This approach enables the interviewer to 'break the ice', to build trust and to develop rapport, nurturing the conversation as the interviewee gradually assumes the lead. General conversation at the start of an interview is considered a useful way to generate rapport.

'Funnelling' is one technique often used to direct a semi-structured one-to-one or group interview, whereby the interviewer gradually brings the focus of the conversation to the salient issues pertinent to the research question (Smith and Osborn, 2007; Creswell and Poth, 2018). This approach involves posing general, non-threatening, exploratory questions early on and, as rapport builds and participants grow in confidence, the questioning becomes focused on more sensitive, searching or opinion-based issues (Aroni et al., 1990). An interview or focus group might therefore begin with an open question to establish the conversation and that participants are liable to feel confident and comfortable speaking about. For instance, an opening question might inquire about immediate situational or contextual issues, e.g. 'what is this place?' Later questioning might then explore participants' feelings and opinions – e.g. 'what do you think of this place?' Funnelling means gradually shifting the direction of the interview from the general to the specific, the goal being to access participants' values, attitudes, opinions and beliefs. However, this deeper level of 'access' is only likely to be possible having first built trust and rapport.

Attempting to make sense of an individual or group's account, especially if it reflects an unfamiliar cultural, social or institutional context, can be bewildering, and therefore requires persistence and perseverance to ask searching questions, digress, seek clarification and reflect. An interview guide should facilitate conversation but be sufficiently flexible to enable divergence from planned questions whenever encountering new ideas or emergent themes. The scheme in Table 8.2, adapted and developed from Galletta (2013) and Silverman and Patterson (2015), distinguishes three phases of interviewing:

Table 8.2 Phases of qualitative interview design

Opening Phase	Main Phase	Concluding Phase
Establish a comfortable environment; welcome and thank participant(s); briefly summarise the purpose of the interview; clarify salient ethical issues.	Ask *descriptive questions* concerning meaningful events or situations.	Return to any issues where you felt that further clarification or illustration might be possible.
Invite participant(s) to introduce themselves outlining why they chose to participate.	Ask *example questions* to illustrate an event or situation.	Return to any issues (junctures) where you saw potential to probe further.
Begin with two or three uncontroversial *experience questions* relevant to the research that make it relatively easy for the participant[s] to begin talking.	Ask *experiential questions*, encouraging the participant[s] to recall and reflect upon (or evaluate) an experience.	Pose additional questions to test the veracity of any tentative emergent themes that have come to mind during the interview.
Where prudent, probe and seek clarification or elaboration to maintain momentum, flow and confidence of the participant[s].	Ask *clarification questions* to improve the accuracy of the account, enhance the richness of the narrative and seek further clarity.	Ask participant[s] if there is anything else they would like to add that was not asked about during the interview.
Be alert for any meaningful junctures in participants' accounts that might be worth returning to later.	Ask *opinion questions* to uncover participants' values, attitudes, emotions and beliefs.	Signal that the interview is now ended and invite any general questions about the research.
Continue to prompt wherever there is opportunity for the participant[s] to continue building their narrative.	Ask *comparative questions* to juxtapose and challenge participants' accounts against alternative scenarios or perspectives.	Thank participant[s] for their involvement and emphasise their valuable contribution to the research.

While listening, keep a mental or written note of tentative themes/ideas as they emerge to follow up.

Participatory observation

'Observation' in qualitative research is an active participatory experience rather than a passive process, 'participant observation' being commonly associated with ethnography. All qualitative research involves some observation, whether or not we choose to call it 'data collection', which occurs through watching, listening and experiencing to glean understanding of how research participants 'naturally' behave, act and interpret a given situation. In this sense, observation is an active endeavour on the part of the researcher; it is 'autobiographical' in the sense that the researcher becomes the instrument of data collection and operates reflexively. This can mean participating in the experiences of the researched and reflecting on the experience via field notes and journal or diary keeping. Reflexivity is an important method that transcends the qualitative research process and is discussed in Chapter 10.

Participatory Observation is used here as distinct from *Participant* Observation since the purpose is not so much to observe participants in a detached, objective way, but to become involved with participants. Essentially, the goal is [1] to attempt to understand and interpret the world as research participants do, and [2] to reveal and explain taken-for-granted, routine, common-sense features of participants' everyday existences (Brewer, 2000: 60). As discussed previously in Chapter 7, privileged access, along with sensitivity and diplomacy, are essential to be able to strike a balance between getting close to and identifying as far as is feasible with research participants while maintaining some degree of distance. A partly detached or 'bracketed' stance may be necessary to enable critical reflection upon what is experienced as a participant researcher, which May (1997: 138) described as 'reflexive rationalisation' where the researcher continuously interprets and applies new knowledge gleaned as a gradual process of theorisation.

BOX 8.5 PARTICIPANT OBSERVATION WITH YOUNG OFFENDERS (DE VIGGIANI ET AL., 2013: 38–9)

Participant observation was used while carrying out ethnographic research with young offenders involved in a creative music programme. Hand-written field notes recorded observations and perceptions of the experience, of the group dynamics, of the organisation of the sessions, of participants' behaviour and their reactions to tasks. They observed and recorded social interaction between participants and musicians. Observations were structured in three ways:

- **Capturing what was visible:** e.g. room layout and size, availability of natural light, furniture layout and seating, availability of refreshments, participants' locations, group dynamics, physical barriers, locations/proximity of staff, etc.

(Continued)

(Continued)

- **Capturing how sessions were organised:** e.g. warm-ups, introductions, use of names, facilitation skills, instructions, inclusion strategies, engagement techniques, engagement barriers, staff involvement, timing/scheduling, use of breaks, allocation of roles, tasks and instruments/equipment, management of disruption/unexpected events, etc.
- **Capturing what was audible:** e.g. conversations, interruptions, banter, emotional expression, outbursts, humour, anger, attitudes, engagement between musicians and participants, active/passive communication/dialogue, etc.
- **Capturing what could be sensed:** e.g. atmosphere, emotions, attitudes, tension, enjoyment, sense of achievement, dissatisfaction, frustration, etc.

Willig and Stainton Rogers (2012) suggest that detailed field notes should include near-verbatim quotations from participants and concrete descriptions of the setting, people and events involved, focusing on key episodes and experiences specific to affected individuals or groups. Banister (2011: 67) suggests that field notes should comprise 'reflections, personal feelings, hunches, guesses and speculations as well as the observations themselves and anything else observed (and these different aspects should be clearly differentiated). Descriptions should be reasonably full, allowing the writer to remember the observation from the accounts later, and the reader should be able to visualise it reasonably accurately.' The following scheme, adapted from Banister (2011), is a guide for recording observations, bearing in mind that this should not be a 'tick box' exercise nor a definitive judgement about person characteristics:

- **Describe the context** including impressions of the physical setting, space, date, and time, weather, lighting, temperature, constraints and barriers, etc.
- **Describe the participants** including impressions of status, roles, identities, dominance and subordination, age, gender, ethnicity, social class, clothing, physical characteristics, etc.
- **Describe the observer** in terms of status, role, degree of participation/involvement identity, gender, social class, ethnicity, etc.
- **Describe the actions of participants** and impressions of them, including attitudes, responses to the situation, verbal and non-verbal behaviours, utterances, roles, peer relationships, etc.
- **Interpret the situation**, attempting to explain how it is perceived by participants, other actors or gatekeepers and researchers.
- **Consider how different interpretations** might be given of the situation.
- **Describe emotions** as a participant observer and impressions of the situation.
- **Write up the scenario**, drawing on verbatim quotations and vignettes.

Conclusion

Choice of data collection methods in qualitative research depends upon a number of factors including methodological requirements, the research question and objectives, and situational factors relating to local protocols, ethical and governance requirements, the nature of the population and issues of access. However, as has been discussed in this and the previous chapter, qualitative research involves building relationships with key stakeholders, and the methods described above require open, reciprocal, dialogical relations to be established to achieve depth and richness in data collection. This chapter has focused on interviewing and participatory observation, these being the most commonly employed data collection approaches in qualitative public health research. In Chapter 10, we discuss the issues of rigour and quality in terms of how to operationalise qualitative research methods to produce robust and convincing findings.

Further reading

Creswell, J.W. and Poth, C.N. (2018) *Qualitative Inquiry and Research Design: Choosing among five approaches* (Fourth edition). London: Sage.

Jackson, A.Y. and Mazzei, L.A. (2012) *Thinking with Theory in Qualitative Research: Viewing data across multiple perspectives*. London: Routledge.

Silverman, R.M. and Patterson, K.L. (2015) *Qualitative Research Methods for Community Development*. London: Routledge.

9 QUALITATIVE DATA ANALYSIS

═══════════════ CHAPTER SUMMARY ═══════════════

In this chapter we introduce the basic principles of **qualitative research analysis**, and the relationship between **methodology**, **data** and **analysis**, as well as the ways in which **data analysis techniques** can address some of the key criticisms of qualitative research. Differences in fundamental approach to quantitative research are discussed and some of the key principles of ensuring robustness in qualitative research, such as avoiding **anecdotalism** and constant comparison. Some of the specialist qualitative data analysis strategies are alluded to, paying particular attention to **thematic analysis**.

Thinking about analysis

Making sense of prodigious amounts of data, especially qualitative, is probably the most difficult job that a researcher has to do. Thinking about 'data' and 'analysis' as two separate processes or stages is perhaps a contributing factor to that. Data analysis is often seen as a separate and distinct stage of the research project, and indeed we can see this in the way that descriptions of projects or project proposals and protocols typically divide up the stages of research (e.g. sampling, recruitment, data collection, data analysis). It is also a neat feature of this text (and many others), a concession perhaps to ease navigating the methods.

Yet, thinking about your data – yet to be 'collected' – and thinking about how to interpret it and explain it (using theory) is something that will take place at the earliest stage of the project, even if one decides to conduct a grounded theory project. When discussing ethnographic research, Atkinson (2017) has a good point when he says that accumulating data should not be considered a category separate from analytic reflection: 'We do not spend time "in the field" just accumulating "data", only to embark on thinking at some subsequent stage in the research process' (Atkinson 2017: 167). Qualitative data analysis, in essence, is using what we know, which is always informed by theoretical traditions and prior acquaintance with the field, to inform what we find out in our data.

Completing a research project, whether a large-scale one or a student dissertation proj-ect, will usually involve producing large amounts of data. The nature of that data will vary from project to project, and in quantitative research it is inevitable that a significant pro-portion of the data will be numerical or can be reduced to numerical data. The task of the researcher then is to reduce that large numerical data set to meaningful statements about the research, often in straightforward statistical (e.g. percentage) terms that allow the reader to judge the meaningfulness of the outcomes of the study (see Chapter 4). Reducing a large volume of data to more manageable summaries of what that data means is important as it gives us an understanding of the relationship between the key variables in a study. Data analysis can be a creative process, and often the challenge for quantitative researchers is how best to present this statistical data in a way that best shows the contrasts between data.

Qualitative research studies frequently produce a large volume of descriptive data, such as conversational accounts from individuals, verbatim transcribes of interviews, field notes and descriptions of events, places, and time. For example, conducting an interview that takes an hour could translate into 20–40 pages of written transcript (Pope et al., 2000). Again, similar to quantitative research, the analysis of that data will involve *reducing* and making *meaningful* those individual accounts. However, what can make it more difficult and challenging for qualitative research is that there is more of an interpretive process than with quantitative studies, as what is meaningful and important is a process that must be agreed upon by the researcher, there is less of a common set of guidelines and rules about how that is to be agreed.

Therefore, the task of data analysis in qualitative research is often to provide an inter-pretive account of what someone (e.g. a research participant) has said, sometimes in isolation, but more often than not, in comparison with what others have said on the topic of interest. It can be a difficult process to document, given that it involves a rather subjec-tive interpretation of data. There are both simple and complex strategies for analysing qualitative data, and the emphasis in this chapter will be on outlining the more straight-forward and pragmatic approaches to analysis, providing some examples within the public health research field, and with some reading suggestions for taking it further.

Key features of qualitative data analysis

There are some fundamental differences between qualitative and quantitative data analy-sis, and it is worth highlighting those here so as to see the different mind-set in approaching data.

Although this is in some ways a generalisation, quantitative research analysis will typically involve a hypothetico-deductive model of analysis – data is collected and then analysed in two distinct stages. You can then repeat the process if necessary or use falsifica-tion to try and disprove your emerging hypothesis.

In contrast, in qualitative research the process of data analysis is frequently (though not always – see 'framework analysis' later in the chapter) inductive – data is collected and analysed in combination, so that critical decisions can be made about what data to collect as the research progresses (this is especially the case in grounded theory methodological approaches). The inductive approach also implies that researchers do not work with pre-existing theories of social action (a priori); theoretical accounts may develop during the analysis. There are some approaches to qualitative data analysis that replicate broad quantitative approaches. For example, some forms of content analysis will allow the researcher to describe the coded data using descriptive statistics by counting the words or instances of codes in the data (Hsieh and Shannon, 2005); this is frequently referred to as a quantitative analysis of qualitative data.

In qualitative research we see that there is a critical interplay of data and analysis, to generate theory or a meaningful account of the data. In terms of developing accounts of the data, in quantitative research theory is focused on proving/disproving/falsifying at the start of the research design, for qualitative research this process is more emergent – that is, the aim is for the best, most credible account: 'there should always be a dialogue between ideas and data, between the concrete and the abstract, the local and the generic' (Atkinson, 2017: 166).

Moreover, regardless of methodology there are some key principles to qualitative data analysis that can act as a guideline for your analysis:

1. Data does not 'speak for itself', despite what some research papers may try to imply; all research data needs some analytical story that connects it up and provides theory, context and comparison for the reader. It is important in data analysis to try to be transparent about how conclusions are drawn.

2. Qualitative research is not an exact science. There is rarely an exact replication in most qualitative data analysis process (that is, each study is unique). Qualitative data analysis should avoid being too procedural or mechanistic, a flaw that is understandable given the need for some objectivity, but rigour can be obtained by other means. Some exceptions to this might include conversation analysis, which methodologically does use some very precise techniques that require less emphasis on *context* (see point 3 below).

3. There are no absolute rules for qualitative data analysis, which for the inexperienced researcher can be intimidating. There are 'guidelines' for analysis, and researchers may vary on how forensic they are in their interpretive analysis and approaches. Barbour (2013) argues that in the process of analysis the qualitative researcher can either take a broad-brush approach (thinking about the bigger picture) or a more forensic approach that may involve, for example, line-by-line coding and detailed analysis. Neither of these approaches is necessarily the correct one, but they suit different purposes for qualitative research and the appropriateness of one may depend on the underlying methodology as well as the story one wishes to tell.

4. For the majority of qualitative research, the wider context is a key part of the interpretive framework for analysis, and that context might involve reflecting on social, cultural, political and economic lifeworlds that exist outside of the data itself. Qualitative data analysis thus requires both *contextualisation* and *familiarisation* and both can be achieved with time. So, if your interpretation will differ according to familiarity and other contexts, how

will your description change and how will that affect your analysis? These are some of the key questions that researchers may address. Qualitative data analysis is therefore rarely just about the words on the page, though this may be a feature of poorly conducted, largely descriptive, qualitative research.

5. The research paradigm leading the study (e.g. positivist, realist or social constructionist) will lead the researcher to different conclusions about the validity of the interpretations and will impact on what the researcher counts as true (or more valid/credible) interpretations.

6. Lastly, the researcher's own identity and positioning plays a role in the interpretation process, and qualitative research should at least acknowledge the role of identity, representation and reflexivity in the analytical process.

So, we can firmly agree that qualitative researchers differ in their approach to data analysis, and some ethnographic researchers take a slightly different approach that focuses more on the wider context of social life. Others may argue that it is important to focus on the development of theory in leading the analysis. In more ethnographic (i.e. anthropological) accounts it is more common to seek fewer examples of individual lives (than more), as wide-scale social, political, economic transformations may be found in individual lives. The practice of generalising from averaging large samples of individuals' experiences (to demonstrate representativeness) is seen as problematic. For example, the psychoanalyst Devereux argues that to generalise by averaging large numbers of individuals' traits, or seeking common denominators or representativeness, is a 'corruption of identity' (see Dawson, 2017). This approach also takes as its inspiration a psychoanalytic view of individuals and the relationship between inner psychic life and external societal events.

Being pragmatic: avoiding anecdotalism and improving validity

As we noted in Chapter 6 it is a feature of some qualitative research that it seeks to enhance quantitative studies, perhaps in the use of mixed methods, or that the researchers do not see a fundamental difference in the research endeavour, so qualitative researchers should critically examine their practices and methods in a similar way to any quantitative study. In line with this thinking, a common concern among qualitative researchers is avoiding what David Silverman and others has called 'anecdotalism' (Silverman, 2015). The goal of good qualitative data analysis, for writers like Silverman, is to improve validity, which is fundamentally the relation between one's account of a particular phenomenon and the thing itself that is being represented in that account. Validity, therefore, is a problem of representation, and anecdotalism is seen as a particular threat to validity (see also Chapter 10).

The problem of anecdotalism refers to the way that qualitative researchers may provide segments of data or examples (e.g. sometimes an entertaining story or particularly stand-out narrative) to tell the story of the research data in written-up publications. This has also been referred to as 'cherry picking', and it is viewed by some qualitative researchers as a particularly heinous crime! If the data segment used does not reflect the complexity of the data, or is used when more contradictory data is ignored, it could be argued that the researcher is not doing justice to the whole data set. The example used may not be 'representative' of the whole data set, and it may therefore threaten its validity or truth-telling quality.

Clearly, the practice of cherry picking falls somewhere on a continuum between only selecting and presenting on very small aspects of the total data and ignoring the rest, and the practice of identifying some data trends and findings that may not be numerically significant, (i.e. that a finding may not occur that regularly in the data), but are selected as the researcher, the one who is embedded in that social reality and context, comes to view it as particularly significant given the totality of their experiences. The latter is a practice that is unlikely to be unusual in qualitative research, and particularly in ethnographic research, as the researcher is keen to provide thick description accounts (see Chapter 10), ones they have consciously selected for the research.

Qualitative methodologists like Silverman (2015) take a largely pragmatic and empirical approach to qualitative research, and are keen to ensure that qualitative researchers treat their research and their data with the same rigour and critical mind-set as a quantitative researcher, but that is not necessarily straightforward. In order to achieve this, a qualitative researcher must be alive to the possibility that their research is too subjective, guided by specific agendas, and not imbued with the spirit of objectivity that accompanies other scientific endeavours. One of the problems of this approach is that it is hard to avoid in some ways, as what separates qualitative research from investigative journalism or travel writing (as in comparison to ethnography) is quite debatable. We hope for greater objectivity in our accounts of the social world from a researcher, but it is not always easy to achieve. Even in the more 'scientific' world of laboratory science it has been argued that not being selective in the process of interpreting results is hard to achieve all the time (for example, see Bruno Latour and Steve Woolgar's (1986; 1988) ethnographic work on laboratory science).

In order to try and achieve this, Silverman and others (e.g. Glaser and Strauss, 1967) suggest we must adopt specific analytical techniques – what is referred to as analytic induction – that may be common to all qualitative analysis. Analytic induction is a way of systematising the analytic process; Silverman describes the general process of forming hypotheses and theories about the data as the analysis proceeds (i.e. grounded in the data) – to do this properly we must also use a range of techniques such as constant comparison, comprehensive data treatment and deviant case analysis.

Analytic induction (Silverman, 2015)

Constant comparison

Put forward originally in grounded theory as a comparative method (Glaser and Strauss, 1967), a common technique of almost all qualitative research (though the term is not always used explicitly) is constant comparison (see also Chapter 10). This principle suggests comparing all parts of the qualitative data set, and comparing on different levels – e.g. comparison of individuals, settings, contexts and instances. Constant comparison involves looking for the patterns in the data, thinking about where else one might find a comparable case when we find something of interest (e.g. in the comparative literature, and not just across the data set). As one generates analytical categories to explain segments of data the researcher seeks other examples in the larger data set, and adds new categories as nuances in the data are discovered.

What is interesting about this idea is that some qualitative researchers argue that while comparing, when you find higher numbers of instances of something, that it is more important and demonstrates the significance of a category in the data. Yet, we know that trying to infer statistical/numerical value to qualitative data is often a mistake. With more experienced qualitative researchers it may be less the numbers of times an issue arises in the data that is important, but the significance that instance holds when compared with other similar examples in the data. The technique often involves finding another case that exemplifies an emerging theory and seeking out cases across the data.

Comprehensive data treatment

Put simply, this refers to the way that qualitative researchers code data from transcripts and the way in which they code data. For those who insist on this it means that all parts of the data must be inspected and coded to avoid accusations of 'cherry picking'. If a particularly revealing part of the data is reflected on in the development of a theory or interpretation, then to ensure that data is explored comprehensively all relevant data to this interpretation must be inspected and analysed to ensure a level of generalisability across the data set (this is not to be confused with generalisability outside of the setting). Comprehensive data treatment then is ensuring all parts of the data are coded to ensure that the researcher has not been selective.

'Deviant' (negative) case analysis

Comprehensive data treatment also involves some element of seeking negative cases or data that does not fit an emerging theory or interpretation (see also Chapter 10). The aim of this stage is to explore why this deviant case exists, not to see this unusual case as an 'outlier', but to explore whether the emerging theory would need modification or serious amendment to reflect the deviant case.

Qualitative analysis can aim at building up a theory to account for the data, and in grounded theory that aim is made quite explicit. However, we can argue that theory development is an important part of all qualitative analysis, as it is important in our analysis not to jump to conclusions too quickly, to build up theory on the basis of careful and intensive analysis and interpretation of data. In a world that increasingly relies upon, and values, somewhat superficial take-home messages and sensational reporting of research findings, it is important to emphasise how careful and considered analysis is what may distinguish good from merely ordinary qualitative analysis.

Grounded theory and data analysis

In Chapter 6, we provided some discussion of grounded theory methodology and its importance to the way that many qualitative researchers think about how they analyse data. Many of the key principles about data analysis that are increasingly being taken for granted, particularly in applied fields, have their origins in grounded theory and the work of Glaser and Strauss (1967). A key principle of grounded theory approaches, in their purest sense, has been that any theoretical propositions must arise from the data and that they must not act a priori as a way of influencing how we think about the data.

This is a good idea in principle, and one that encourages some degree of objectivity and 'value-free' thinking about your data, but very often it is impossible to do, given that researchers tend to enter into any researcher endeavour with pre-dispositions, ideas, theories and hunches about their field, and the nature of the research subject. To set aside those pre-dispositions in the process of analysis is not only unachievable but also probably undesirable. Some theoretical framework, operating at a surface level perhaps, will be influential in how researchers interpret their data and conduct their analysis. As such, increasingly, researchers that use grounded theory talk about using the methodology in a modified way, taking what is valuable in the approach, and discarding less popular or less usable guiding principles. However, grounded theory language of analysis is prevalent throughout much qualitative analysis description.

The use of cases

As we discussed in the qualitative sampling chapter (Chapter 7), the use of cases is more common with qualitative research, as some of the formal 'statistical' rules around sampling do not apply in the same way. In grounded theory methodological approaches, there is a clear relationship between sampling (case selection) and analysis. As the research progresses and more data is collected the grounded theory researcher will engage in open coding, but as the researcher begins to develop and focus on theoretical sensitivity, then the coding and the analysis will align with this sensitivity. This will also aid the process of further sampling and case selection (as in theoretical sampling). The sample used, and the data collected and analysed, is then all completed in the aim of achieving greater theoretical sensitivity and to test the emerging theory.

Thematic analysis

Thematic analysis has become the most commonly used qualitative data analysis method, but there are varying approaches available. Thematic analysis has proven to be a very popular approach to qualitative data analysis, and seems to transcend scientific disciplines. It is most commonly viewed as an approach to coding data (see Ryan and Bernard, 2000), and one that has been a cornerstone of grounded theory approaches, as opposed to being a method of analysis in its own right (though this is put forward as a possibility by writers such as Braun and Clarke, 2006), but such is its ubiquity that we outline simply aspects of the approach here. There is a range of good how-to guides to doing thematic analysis or coding, which we will not replicate here, but summarise some of the use when thinking about public health research.

One of the criticisms of those doing thematic analysis is that researchers rarely report in depth the process of doing the analysis, or the mechanics behind how they came to their 'themes' in the process, and much of this critique currently focuses on the extent to which themes are found (emerge in the analysis) or are constructed (made) by the researcher. Of course, the simple answer to this question is that themes are constructed by the researcher as it is not an objective or value-free process, but the more difficult answer reveals more complexity here. In trying to avoid merely a subjective and self-referential account of social reality, some researchers have argued for a case that a theme reflects an underlying reality as it is not just a category to summarise a semantic field (taking a more realist or positivist approach). In aiming to establish some wider significance to their analysis and findings, such researchers may argue that they are uncovering social reality (and therefore highlighting 'emerging' themes) as opposed to the relativist position that they are only constructed. Such debates about the relevance and importance attached to how best to not only 'do' thematic analysis but also how best to construct a language about it, are unlikely to be resolved soon as we recognise that qualitative researchers come from different disciplinary traditions and ways of thinking about social reality, objectivity, researcher values, and so on.

BOX 9.1 THEMATIC ANALYSIS IN A PUBLIC HEALTH STUDY (FIELDEN ET AL., 2011)

The authors conducted a qualitative focus group study of children's understandings of the causes and consequences of obesity. A thematic analysis approach proposed by Braun and Clarke (2006) was adopted to identify 'themes' from focus group data. The thematic analysis approach in this case was used thus:

- A 'contextualist' approach to analysis was used – that is, meanings and interpretations are not exclusively individual and that the wider social (and cultural) context is important in 'framing' those experiences.
- The focus was on 'identifying' themes in the analysis of data.
- Obesity is framed as a 'real' problem for the participants (not socially constructed), but that society also plays a role in shaping that meaning-making for the children.
- Initial thoughts and ideas were considered during the transcription process.

(Continued)

(Continued)

- Transcripts were re-read and tapes listened to again to immerse themselves in the data – to gain familiarity (or closeness with the data).
- A coding phase was used to 'identify features of the data' and used the whole data set.
- Another stage involved 'searching for themes'.
- Thematic maps were developed.
- Themes were refined – 'any themes that did not have enough data to support them or were too diverse were discarded'.
- Themes were defined and named, accompanied by detailed analysis.
- Writing involved choosing transcript examples (data) that best illustrated the theme.

The process outlined in many examples of thematic analysis are very similar, though may acknowledge some slight differences between them. This will ordinarily take a number of key steps (see Braun and Clarke, 2006 and Box 9.2 below), which can be seen as rather mechanistic, but at the very least has the benefit of outlining a process of thinking for the researcher.

BOX 9.2   STEPS IN THEMATIC ANALYSIS (BRAUN AND CLARKE, 2006)

1. Immersion and familiarisation: this stage is about getting to know your data. Some level of immersion is expected (reading and re-reading). At this stage you would be encouraged to read in-depth both the individual level data transcripts (if interviews were conducted) and compare them across the data set.
2. Coding: this process is discussed in more detail below, but in general refers to fixing the meaning for a segment of data (a word, sentence or passage) using a specific word or phrase. This word or phrase ('code') might be influenced by your theoretical leanings and interest (theory-driven) or not as in a more inductive strategy (data-driven).
3. Developing and refining 'themes': at a broader level of analysis is the development of themes in your data. This will inevitably involve some constant comparison as you compare aspects of the whole data set in order to think 'what is this about?' A theme will be the development of that idea into something more tangible. A theme will also at some level be offering an explanatory context for the data.
4. Organising themes and writing-up: once you feel that you have exhausted all possibilities in the development of codes and themes, then moving on to writing up and considering how these themes are ordered in the presentation of data is an important stage.

The process outlined above is quite familiar to those doing qualitative research, but there are some issues with it that are worth pointing out. The first of which is that it can seem overly mechanistic and underplays the value of creative interpretation in analysis. Also, when researchers use language to say that they are identifying themes in the data then we can usually surmise that both the data and the theme are 'out there' in the world ready to be discovered, and that the purpose of the research is to uncover that social reality. Often in this situation the researchers who conducted the interviews may not do the analysis, as it is a view that this will improve inter-rater reliability or other such measure that suggests we are encountering a serious and scientific process. Other social scientists critique this as 'scientism', suggesting that such practices of routinisation of qualitative data analysis or the use of formulaic strictures barely hides its positivist leanings (St. Pierre and Jackson, 2014; Okely 2010).

The process of refining themes is interesting and worth noting, as it is common for researchers to discard a 'theme' that is not properly supported by the data, but it is not always clear why researchers do this. One suspects it is to avoid Silverman's accusation of anecdotalism, lack of comprehensive data treatment and constant comparison, but it is sometimes ideas or thoughts on the fringe of the data set (at the margins) that are the most valuable – just because one particular idea that the researcher sees as important does not have enough data to support it does not mean it is not important. It just means that there is not enough data to support it. If the researcher kept collecting data, would they have found more to this idea or theme to help it develop? We should also take into account that not all data is worthy of analysis, just because there may be a lot of one particular type of data does not make it important. In some ways, this plays to the view that good qualitative research is both contextually rooted, conducted over a longer time than most qualitative studies, involves a researcher who is fully immersed in the field, and draws not only on interview/focus group data.

BOX 9.3 'IN VIVO' AND 'IN VITRO' CODING: THEORY DRIVEN VS DATA DRIVEN (SALDANA, 2016)

In more scientific terms, 'in vivo' (Latin for within the living) and 'in vitro' (Latin for within the glass) are familiar in biochemical experimental studies. In grounded theory qualitative research, the terms 'in vivo' and 'in vitro' are used to highlight different, though complementary, approaches to coding.

In 'in vivo' coding the words or phrases that participants use are adopted as the specific 'code' for the research; the researcher views the phenomena through the eyes of

(Continued)

(Continued)

the participant. This may happen at an early stage of the research process, or to ensure greater sensitivity to the analysis. This is also often referred to as an 'emic' form of analysis, as the codes used stay closer to the words of the participants.

In 'in vitro' coding, more abstract, sometimes technical and/or conceptual terms more familiar to the professional researcher may be used. This is also referred to as an 'etic' level of analysis, as codes become more abstract they lose their sensitivity to the participants' lifeworld. Qualitative data analysis will try to strike a balance between the two.

Coding

One of the key tasks of most, if not all, qualitative research is to ascribe meaning to the segments of descriptive data that you find in your transcripts, fieldnotes, observations, and other qualitative data sources. There is no commonly accepted method of coding data, no best way to analyse the data (Saldana, 2016). The qualitative researcher can make decisions about a) how much of the data to code, b) how far the coding strategy and terms used stray from the 'original' words and phrases used by the participants of the research, and c) when to start the coding process in the research journey. Each of those decisions may be influenced by methodological principles. A 'code' for the data is a means of 'fixing' the meaning of a segment of data – it is driven by the researcher or person doing the analysis, and once fixed has implications for how each segment of data is interpreted.

It is frequently argued that coding is not analysis (St. Pierre and Jackson, 2014), but it does constitute an early (and significant) part of the analytical process, as assigning words and phrases to segments of data reveals a lot about how the researcher thinks about that data. One of the reasons textbooks on qualitative data analysis tell us a lot about coding is that it is genuinely one of the areas of qualitative data analysis where we can give some guidelines, more in line with a positivist approach to thinking about data. Indeed, coding has been described as a 'positivist, quasi-statistical analytic practice... that has, unfortunately, been proliferated and formalized in too many introductory textbooks and university research courses' (St. Pierre and Jackson, 2014: 715). This is a good point, and not reflected on too much in more applied fields, but it is a debate that has clearly incensed those qualitative researchers that are more social scientifically inclined.

Coding is the organisation of raw data into conceptual categories. Each code is effectively a category or 'bin' into which a piece of data is placed. As Miles and Huberman (1994: 56) note:

Codes are tags or labels for assigning units of meaning to the descriptive or inferential information compiled during a study. Codes are usually attached to 'chunks' of varying size – words, phrases, sentences or whole paragraphs.

For example, in grounded theory there is the view that researchers initially code using participants' own words in the coding scheme, which, it is argued, will improve the way the researcher 'sensitises' to the local understanding and meaning. For instance, if a participant in a study mentions the words 'sad', 'unhappy', or 'upset', then these terms are used for the coding scheme. It is important that their words are not initially re-framed using second or third-order concepts deriving from the researchers' own conceptual framework.

In many ways this is an important strategy, and it builds upon grounded theory principles about starting with the raw data and trying not to be influenced by existing literature, concepts and theoretical frameworks, all of which may influence the coding process.

In a study that uses pre-existing categories and conceptual precepts, the data is analysed and coded more or less according to those categories. Coding itself can be broad-brush (coding larger segments of data) or more forensic, coding down to individual words or phrases. The decisions about which approach to take will depend on the nature of the research as well as the researcher's predisposition to analyse the data in a particular way, but more important will be the view that the researcher should try not to code mechanistically, but to be creative in their approaches and to be alive to different possibilities (leaving room for varying interpretations in the early stages of analysis).

From codes to categories and themes

'A grounded theory is generated by themes, and themes emerge from the data during analysis, capturing the essence of meaning or experience drawn from varied situations and context' (Bowen, 2006: 2). We need to be wary of this kind of statement, as it promotes a view about the analytical endeavour that is misleading. It is a statement that many methods textbooks contain, and, we suspect, even more research papers that use qualitative methods. What the authors usually mean is that in the process of reading and absorbing the data, the authors/researchers made some conceptual linkage between the data and other sensitising concepts. By saying they emerge, I do not think that any qualitative researchers actually think that such 'themes' arise like a phoenix from the data ashes, but the phrase does give that impression. Rather, the ideas about how to organise the data (e.g. themes or 'categories') are constructed from the data and are formulated by the researcher, emerging is just shorthand for 'as researchers we discovered there was a link between x data and x ideas/concepts'.

BOX 9.4 BLUMER AND 'SENSITISING CONCEPTS' (1954)

In a well-known paper, the sociologist Herbert Blumer argued the case of 'sensitising concepts'. These are ideas that can help us to provide a perspective on our research, which may help the way we interpret our data. We do not work in a conceptual vacuum when

(Continued)

(Continued)

we research a particular issue, and so these 'sensitising concepts' act as a starting point for more in-depth analysis; they provide guidance and direction as to where to look particularly in the analysis of data. For example, the concept of 'social capital' was drawn up based on previous research and helped in the analysis. They are often used in grounded theory, as 'Sensitizing concepts provide starting points for building analysis to produce a grounded theory' (Bowen, 2006: 7).

Other notable approaches to qualitative analysis

There are many other approaches to qualitative data analysis; for example, in phenomenological studies interpretive phenomenological analysis (IPA) is frequently used as it pays more attention to the overarching methodological concerns of phenomenology (Smith et al., 2009). Narrative methods of analysis emphasise the meaning that individuals ascribe to life events and take the importance of individual stories at their core. Narrative research is an increasingly popular method in research on health in the social sciences, one that provides an implicit critique of medical science and notions of objectivity (Riessman, 1993; Czarniawska, 2004; Elliot, 2005).

In more policy-oriented, evaluation and applied qualitative research a 'framework analysis' approach may be more suitable (Ritchie and Spencer, 1994; Ritchie and Lewis, 2003) as it helps to ensure rigour and transparency. Framework analysis has similarities with thematic analysis – it is a step-by-step procedural approach – but the fundamental difference is that it is largely deductive in that the thematic framework is identified early on in the research study. At the start of the study, a priori themes are identified by the researchers, drawing on their knowledge and understanding of the research area, and this influences the development of the interview questions. In the analysis, the researchers seek out the a priori themes in the interview data, but where data cannot be found to 'fit' the themes they are usually discarded or the themes are modified (see Daivadanam et al., 2014 for a good public health example that uses both deductive and inductive methods). It has also been acknowledged as a good approach to use if involving non-experts (other key stakeholders) in the data analysis process (Gale et al., 2013).

The use of computer software to aid analysis

Increasingly, qualitative researchers make use of computer software, programs such as NVivo, to help them with the analysis. But, we need to be clear that the software programs do not help the researcher with the analysis itself; it cannot make analytical decisions, but merely act as an aid to help the researcher both *organise* the data and help to establish some *patterns* in the process of analysis. Writers, such as Okely (2010), suggest that information technology has been used to elaborate purely quantitative routes to knowledge while neglecting more creative and free association-based approaches, and there is a danger that computer programs will encourage a more procedural approach to qualitative analysis.

Prior to the use of computer software for this purpose, qualitative researchers would do this by hand, making use of highlighting pens, a pair of scissors and a decent floor or desk space to spread out the data and seek patterns. Indeed, this is the way that many researchers still work, as having some 'hands-on' familiarity with the data is a very useful exercise. Just as many writers/authors have not made the transition to writing directly on to the computer keyboard, preferring instead to write long-hand into their notebook, many qualitative researchers also prefer to take this low-tech 'feel' approach to their analysis. In this respect, we suggest Barbour is correct in saying that we must learn the principles of qualitative data analysis before finding our way around any computer software package. If this is not done, 'there is the very real danger that your analyses are driven by the properties of the package rather than the other way around' (Barbour, 2008: 195).

Conclusion

Data analysis for a qualitative study can be a daunting task, but there are carefully laid-out approaches and procedures that you can follow, regardless of the overarching methodology, and these can provide some rigour and transparency to the process. However, one must try to be creative, and not to take too straight-jacketed an approach, regardless of whether one is being led by more inductive or deductive methods.

Further reading

Braun, V. and Clarke, V. (2006) Using thematic analysis in psychology. *Qualitative Research in Psychology*, 3(2): 77–101.

Daivadanam, M., Wahlström, R., Sundari Ravindran, T.K. Thankappan, K.R. and Ramanathan, M. (2014) Conceptual model for dietary behaviour change at household level: A 'best fit' qualitative study using primary data. *BMC Public Health*, 14: 574.

Pope, C., Ziebland, S. and Mays, N. (2000) Qualitative research in health care: Analysing qualitative data. *BMJ*, 320.

10 QUALITY AND RIGOUR IN QUALITATIVE RESEARCH

================= CHAPTER SUMMARY =================

In this chapter we explore how to think about **quality** and **rigour** in **qualitative research**. As qualitative research becomes more commonplace, particularly in public health research, there is also an increase in the reporting and publication of **qualitative research studies**. Medical public health has traditionally relied on more epidemiological studies and researchers in public health have less confidence in knowing how to assess the strengths and weaknesses of qualitative research and to examine their particular claims. This chapter, therefore, explores how we might assess quality such as in the form of specific guidelines, and we will summarise developments in this area. More specifically, we highlight the contested nature of 'quality' and the complexity of issues of **knowledge judgement** within different methodological traditions.

Introduction

Referring to qualitative research, Buchanan (1992) argued that its quality lies in the power of language to discover things about ourselves and our common humanity. In previous chapters, we have examined how qualitative research methodologies provide access to people's social worlds and experiences, through observation, conversation and interpretation, within subjective and intersubjective contexts. Qualitative methodologies also involve the researcher as an integral part of the social world – a co-participant, a co-creator, a co-researcher – which necessitates consideration of how to conduct research appropriately and ethically, and how to communicate and represent research outputs with integrity, while retaining an inherently social relationship.

A common criticism levelled at qualitative research is that it lacks 'scientific rigour', that it can be anecdotal, impressionistic and that it is strongly subject to researcher bias

(Mays and Pope, 1995; Koch and Harrington, 1998). However, while qualitative research is indeed subjective and interpretivist, various techniques are employed to ensure rigour, legitimacy and quality. These involve being extremely thorough, attentive to detail and transparent in all elements of research design and at all stages of the research process, particularly in ensuring veracity and confirmability of research outputs. Hammersley (1992) suggested that research quality may be evaluated on the basis of the adequacy of the evidence, on the efficacy of the main claims, and on whether they are true beyond reasonable doubt. Douglas (1976) argued that this is best achieved by being 'tough-mindedly suspicious', 'checking out' and 'testing out' what has been found. Fielding (1993) proposed that a 'test of congruence' could be performed to demonstrate the researcher's competence in interpreting the rules, mores or language of research participants. Researchers should acquire, '... systematic understanding which is clearly recognizable and understandable to the members ... and which is done as much as possible in their own terms' (Fielding, 1993: 164).

As discussed previously, 'trust' is a core principle of qualitative research – especially in terms of developing positive, reciprocal relations with research participants and stakeholders. Equally important is the need to produce *trustworthy*, verifiable 'data'. Guba and Lincoln (2005) challenged the use of conventional quantitative rules and techniques of rigour to evaluate qualitative research, arguing for an alternative approach consistent with constructivist and interpretivist methodologies. They identified *trustworthiness* rather than rigour as a benchmark for qualitative research, comprising *credibility* as opposed to internal validity, *transferability* as opposed to external validity, *dependability* as opposed to reliability, and *confirmability* as opposed to objectivity. In this chapter, we refer to Guba and Lincoln's categories, given the greater flexibility and applicability they afford qualitative research.

Reflexivity

Before discussing *trustworthiness*, it is necessary to explore briefly the notion of *reflexivity*, a core principle that threads through all qualitative research designs. Qualitative research requires careful interpretation and representation, and therefore depends upon an active reflective process, bearing in mind that it does not take place in a neutral, apolitical, asocial and ideology-free space (Alvesson and Sköldberg, 2009). Rather than conforming to a technical or formulaic process, a reflexive approach means keeping a close eye on the veracity of the research while engaging in active critical reflection upon one's role, identity and social status as a researcher, specifically attending to intentional and unintentional effects on the research (O'Connell Davidson and Layder, 1994). Guba and Lincoln (2005) argued that reflexive practice should transcend all aspects and phases of research, from choice of research problem through to final reporting on the findings. To be reflexive means to be strongly self-aware so as to minimise bias or prejudice and to forge non-hierarchical, reciprocal relations with research participants. As we discussed in Chapter 8, qualitative research, therefore, requires harnessing one's skills of emotional intelligence,

'On the basis of a limited identification … [reflexivity] creates a critical and dialectical distance between the researcher and his (sic) "objects". It enables the correction of distortion of perceptions on both sides and widens the consciousness of both, the researcher and the "researched".' (Mies, 1993: 69)

Harding (1991: 163) advocated 'strong reflexivity', where research participants are:

'… conceptualised as gazing back in all their cultural particularity … [and where] … the researcher, through theory and methods, stand[s] behind them, gazing back at his own socially situated research project in all its cultural particularity and its relationships to other projects of his (sic) culture …'

High-quality qualitative research seeks to capture 'emic' representations of the social world or of social phenomena as participants would perceive them to be (Hammersley, 1992). This should involve a combination of genuineness, directness (having physical and social presence), informality and honesty (McCall and Simmons, 1969).

Trustworthiness

Qualitative research does not seek to reveal absolute truths or realities. Rather, social reality is socially constructed and expressed through people's everyday experiences (Guba and Lincoln, 2005). Qualitative researchers are therefore concerned with uncovering these various constructions that represent the meanings people attach to situations. They are therefore necessarily and unavoidably personal, subjective and idiosyncratic. This means that verification of the research process and outcomes requires both *methodological rigour* and what we term *democratic rigour*. The former implies the need to select and use research methods in a robust way, while the latter implies the need to attain a sense of defensible community or stakeholder consent. Trustworthiness implies, therefore, the need to attend to the quality of the research process – that the research technique is sound – and to ensure that what is elicited is legitimate and 'true' to those stakeholders involved and affected.

Credibility

To be credible literally means to be believable; it infers that the research must be designed and carried out with honour, transparency and legitimacy, and be feasible and ethical. Credibility raises questions about the overall veracity of the research and provides a hallmark against which four key dimensions are evaluated: [1] credibility of research design, [2] researcher credibility, [3] credibility of method, and [4] credibility of findings and conclusions. All should be evidenced throughout reporting on the research process and outcomes. Credibility of research design arises from the strength of the rationale for the research, established when identifying the research problem and question, and subsequently from the theoretical and conceptual frameworks that drive the research methodology. In other words, it concerns whether the research design is best suited to the research question, which includes consideration of whether the research is appropriate and ethical. The second dimension – the credibility of the researcher – concerns the skills, capabilities and character of the researcher; not only should the researcher be capable and equipped to undertake the research but be positively disposed towards the research and research participants in terms of value position and attitude. For instance, if researching young people's sexual behaviour, it may be inappropriate to employ a researcher who holds strongly skewed views. The third dimension concerns the credibility of the methods, whether these are consistent with the methodology and research design, and in terms of their execution. The fourth dimension concerns the credibility of the emerging data; that they reflect what participants expressed and are accurately interpreted and represented.

The following checklist, adapted and developed from Charmaz (2005: 528) and Miles and Huberman (1994: 279), captures these dimensions of credibility across the various stages of the research:

	CREDIBILITY
Research Design	• Is the research question credible and appropriate? • Does the research rationale justify the research methodology? • Has the feasibility of the research been established? • Is the research ethical from the perspectives of stakeholders? • Does the researcher have credible understanding of the research problem?
Access	• Has the researcher established genuine relations with key stakeholders? • Has trust and rapport been genuinely established? • Has adequate time been given to learn sufficient about the setting / context? • Has there been time to establish adequate relations within the setting?
Recruitment & Sampling	• Is there a credible recruitment and sampling strategy? • Are recruitment and sampling ethical from the perspectives of stakeholders? • Are recruitment and sampling consistent with the research methodology?
Data Collection	• Is there a credible data collection strategy consistent with research methodology? • Is data collection undertaken robustly, transparently and faithful to the method? • Is the process of data collection adequate in depth and breadth?
Data Analysis	• Is the data analysis method described explicitly and accurately? • Is the data analysis method congruent with the research methodology? • Are contradictory, deviant or divergent data included or dealt with? • Is the analysis process transparent in terms of evolving themes or categories? • Are the emerging data credible in terms of breadth and depth? • Are techniques used to confirm associations applied, e.g. triangulation?
Interpretation of Findings	• Are strengths and limitations of association across the data discussed explicitly? • Is the account of the findings credible and convincing to stakeholders?

Figure 10.1 Credibility

Source: Adapted and developed from Miles and Huberman 1994:278, Charmaz 2005:528 and Creswell 2013:179–217

Transferability

Generalisability is used in quantitative research to measure external validity or the degree to which research findings are repeatable, generalisable and representative of a similar or larger population. In qualitative research, to avoid confusion with this definition, the term *transferability* is used to refer to the extent that an account, observation or theme is comparable to others, usually within the same research study, a linked study or a study that is very close in character and design. Thus, generalisability in qualitative research tends to remain within or local to the primary data and the sample population, and it is considered inappropriate to apply the findings of a qualitative study to a wider population. This is an area of controversy within qualitative evidence synthesis, where published qualitative studies are compared, as we discuss in Chapter 13.

The following checklist, also adapted from Miles and Huberman (1994: 278–9), captures key indicators of transferability within the context of a qualitative research design.

	TRANSFERABILITY
Research Design	• Does the research question infer that the research outcomes may be comparable, illustrative or confirmatory of wider evidence of trends? • Does the research orientation and methodology lend itself to comparable or transferable outcomes (e.g. realist or pragmatic epistemology, or a mixed methods design)?
Recruitment & Sampling	• Is sufficient detail given about the sample (e.g. inclusion criteria, participant characteristics, demographic details, social context, etc.) to permit adequate comparison with other groups of cases (samples)? • Have limiting features of sample selection (e.g. inclusion and exclusion criteria) been applied and explained? • Are details of limiting characteristics of the final sample identified and discussed? • Is there sufficient diversity (heterogeneity) within the final sample to allow broader applicability?
Data Collection	• Are data collection methods adequate to achieve breadth and depth and enable transferability of themes beyond the study (e.g. methods triangulation)?
Data Analysis	• Are the data sufficiently rich / in-depth to enable comparison with others' data where strong similarity can be evidenced?
Interpretation of Findings	• Do stakeholders and other researchers perceive the findings to be consistent with their own experience? • Do the findings confirm or show congruence with prior theory or research? • Is adequate detail described about research processes to enable detailed comparisons with others' research? • Are the limits to transferability discussed and acknowledged explicitly?

Figure 10.2 Transferability

Source: Adapted and developed from Miles and Huberman 1994:278, Charmaz 2005:528 and Creswell 2013:179–217

Dependability

Dependability is referred to in quantitative research as *reliability*. In simple terms, it refers to the accuracy and stability of both the research methods and the findings. It concerns whether the research methods are dependable and consistent in what they purport to do, pragmatically and ethically, over time and between situations. For example, it would be used to evaluate consistency of interview technique across a sample of participants or to evaluate the degree to which themes and categories are stable in terms of accurately reflecting the data, the setting, the phenomenon and the sample (Morse, 2015). Dependability is also important in terms of the execution of methods, especially with regard to the reliability of the researcher in undertaking the research (Miles and Huberman, 1994; Kirk and Miller, 1986). Unlike with quantitative research, the researcher is intimately involved in executing the research methods and must, therefore, be able to demonstrate and evidence their dependability and consistency in the research process.

In terms of dependency of method, stability is not always desirable, since qualitative research designs can be more structured and pre-planned or less structured and organic in terms of process, depending upon design and methodology. As we have discussed previously, varied degrees of control, direction and structure may be applied to methods due to methodological imperatives. This is typical when comparing designs that use unstructured, semi-structured or structured interviewing, or more direction or less direction during sampling. For instance, a highly inductive, constructivist grounded theory study that uses theoretical sampling and semi-structured interviewing may have weaker dependability of method than a realist descriptive phenomenological study that employs more deterministic sampling, data collection and data analysis strategies. Nonetheless, the dependability of the researcher to conduct the research consistently remains important regardless of the research methodology or design. The checklist below summarises key dependability criteria:

Confirmability

Confirmability is similar to dependability in that it is also concerned with consistency and reliability. As with dependability, the role of the researcher is important in terms of executing the research, analysing data appropriately and drawing conclusions from the findings. Research quality is evaluated in terms of being able to show and evidence that fieldwork is undertaken impartially and that the findings are reliable and not anecdotal.

In terms of the execution of field work, impartiality may be recognised as prejudice, bias or coercion that can be intentional or unintentional and occur when negotiating access, during recruitment or sampling, during data collection or data analysis, and during interpretation and discussion of the findings. Essentially, a poorly planned and executed project, where lack of strategic clarity and detail can lead to a loose operational process

	DEPENDABILITY
Research Design	• Is the study design congruent with the research question and objectives? • Are the methods (the research process) congruent with the research methodology? • Is there congruence between the epistemological position and the research design? • Is there logic and congruence between methods – sampling, data collection, data analysis? • Is the researcher's role and status explicitly described and consistent in terms of epistemology, methodology, executing the methods and relations within the research setting? • Are potential conflicts of interest or ambiguities addressed or reconciled?
Recruitment Sampling & Data Collection	• Are recruitment, sampling and data collection methods congruent with the overall research design and methodology? • Are the methods undertaken consistently according to methodological conventions? • Is sufficient detail provided about the processes of recruitment, sampling and data collection to evidence dependability? • Is sufficient attention given to researcher reflexivity during all stages of recruitment, sampling and data collection in attending to potential for bias or compromise in consistently executing the methods? • Are limits to achieving dependability in recruitment, sampling and data collection acknowledged, justified and explained? • If multiple field workers are involved, do they share comparable recruitment, sampling and data collection protocols?
Data Analysis	• Are data analysis methods congruent with the overall research design and methodology? • Are data analysis methods undertaken consistently according to methodological conventions? • Is sufficient detail provided about the data analysis process to evidence dependability? • Is sufficient attention given to researcher reflexivity during data analysis in terms of attending to potential for bias or compromise in consistently executing the methods? • Are limits to achieving dependability in data analysis acknowledged, justified and explained? • Are coding checks made and do they show adequate agreement? • Are data quality checks made (e.g. for bias or deceit)? • Do multiple fieldworkers' accounts converge? • Do the findings reveal meaningful themes or parallels across data sources (informants, contexts, times)? • Is peer review used during fieldwork and data analysis?
Interpretation of Findings	• Are the findings consistent with the research question and objectives? • Does the research answer the research question?

Figure 10.3 Dependability

Source: Adapted and developed from Miles and Huberman 1994:278, Charmaz 2005:528 and Creswell 2013:179–217

through which the methods are executed, will very likely suffer from superficiality and reliance on anecdotal data. This can happen when the researcher has underestimated what may be involved in designing a robust qualitative study, where rationale, methodology and method have not been properly thought through, and the methods not clearly aligned with the methodology.

Anecdotalism and prejudice can manifest at any stage of the research process (see Chapter 9 for a further discussion of anecdotalism). During sampling, these may involve 'cherry picking' of cases; for instance, due to convenience or opportunism that may be legitimate but arise because a gatekeeper has directed the researcher to a specific case or because recruitment has been unsuccessful in producing typical volunteers. During data collection, prejudice can occur when the data collection technique is misused, particularly where the values of the researcher influence the course of data collection; this may manifest as the posing of leading or loaded questions or asking a limited range of questions with anticipated answers. During or before data analysis, anecdotalism can occur if researchers attempt to predict themes and categories rather than allow these to develop, or to select specific data that stand out but are not representative of the breadth of the data (see Chapter 9). At the discussion stage, likewise, there may be a tendency to exaggerate or over-emphasise research outcomes (Bryman, 1988; Silverman, 2015; Morse, 2015).

Confirmability criteria are summarised in the checklist below.

Techniques for enhancing quality and rigour

In the sections above, we presented a typology of criteria designed to increase trustworthiness, focusing specifically on *credibility, transferability, dependability* and *confirmability*. This is useful in terms of working out the key questions used to appraise qualitative research. In terms of application, various techniques are commonly employed to address these criteria that can be integrated into a qualitative research design. Creswell (2013) offered a useful summary of these, terming them 'verification' and 'validation' procedures. Importantly, their use will vary according to methodological approach. For instance, ethnography might use more verification techniques, given the potential for using several sampling and/or data collection methods. A smaller, more discrete study in a single context or setting might use fewer techniques.

Prolonged engagement

The more time a researcher can spend in the research setting in ongoing engagement with potential recruits, and then with actual participants, the greater likelihood of building relationships that lead to rich data. Trust, rapport and reciprocity will strengthen credibility, dependability and confirmability at each stage of the research since this enables the

	CONFIRMABILITY
Research Design	• Is there consistency and coherence between the research design, methodology and methods that correspond with the research question? • Does the preliminary literature review provide an adequate rationale for the research question and design? • Has the researcher been explicit and reflected upon how their personal values, attitudes, beliefs, assumptions and prejudices may impact on the research process?
Access	• Is access achieved without prejudice or coercion? • Have potential vested interests been anticipated and managed (e.g. on the part of the researcher or of stakeholders)? • Has the site and population been selected without prejudice? • Have measures been implemented to mitigate the influence or potential coercion of gatekeepers or stakeholders? • Are unavoidable restrictions / off-limits data sources acknowledged and explained?
Recruitment & Sampling	• Are recruitment and sampling methods adequate for producing rich, confirmable data? • Are recruitment and sampling undertaken strictly to protocol and consistent with methodological requirements, mitigating against prejudice and anecdotalism? • Have appropriate ethical issues been addressed during recruitment and sampling (e.g. consent, confidentiality, privacy, non-coercive approach, etc.)? • Has the influence of gatekeepers and stakeholders been mitigated with regard to access to and selection of cases? • Have measures been instituted to ensure potential cases are recruited voluntarily and without coercion? • Are the recruitment and sampling methods described in sufficient detail to follow as an "audit trail"?
Data Collection	• Are data collection methods adequate for producing confirmable data? • Is data collection adequately executed to produce confirmable data? • Have ethical issues been addressed in terms of executing data collection (e.g. consent, confidentiality, privacy, non-coercive approach, etc.)? • Have sufficient trust and rapport been established to achieve rich, confirmable data? • Are data collection methods described in sufficient detail to follow as an "audit trail"?
Data Analysis	• Is the data analysis method adequate for producing confirmable data? • Is data analysis adequately executed to produce confirmable data? • Have measures been used to check the veracity and confirmability of the analysis (e.g. member checking, re-analysis)? • Has the full range of data been exhausted in the analysis and is the range of exhibited raw data adequate in representing the full range of cases? • Are the emerging data adequate to produce confirmable results (themes, categories, theories, etc.)? • Are all raw data retained, archived and available for re-analysis?
Interpretation of Findings	• Are the conclusions explicitly linked with the findings from data analysis? • Are competing hypotheses or rival conclusions considered?

Figure 10.4 Confirmability

Source: Adapted and developed from Miles and Huberman 1994:278, Charmaz 2005:528 and Creswell 2013:179–217

researcher to learn about and understand the culture, the language and social norms, and to interpret what is going on with greater accuracy. Sampling and data collection are then informed by increased understanding of the social context, and it is more likely that the researcher will be able to operationalise and execute the research methods appropriately, ethically and consistent with research objectives. Prolonged engagement in research settings is a luxury for most qualitative researchers, being particularly important in ethnography. Many factors can impede this, including governance and ethical barriers, professional or organisational protocols, and research funding or educational deadlines.

Persistence

While the purpose of prolonged engagement is to maximise opportunities within the research setting, persistence is less about duration and more about intensity. Prolonged engagement enables the researcher to identify phenomena, events and issues that are central to the research problem; it provides scope. Persistence, on the other hand, means focusing on the salient issues in detail.

Thick description

Thick description characterises the process of giving close attention to detail in both the execution of the research and in how it is described. Thick description enhances transferability in the sense that a theory that has a strong connection with all or most cases (breadth) and that is supported by rich data (depth) has much greater applicability and relatability. Thick description may be contrasted with 'thin description' that would essentially be tantamount to providing an insufficient, superficial or misleading account of a phenomenon. Thick description, therefore, comprises detailed commentary, interpretation and reflexivity.

Triangulation

Triangulation means combining two or more theoretical perspectives, settings or sites, investigators and/or methods in a research design to achieve deeper, more complex understanding of the phenomenon in question (Denzin, 2006; Flick, 2002). Denzin and Lincoln (2013) also described this in terms of constructing a 'montage' around a central issue or phenomenon. Again, this approach is commonly used with ethnography where time and opportunity enable triangulation of multiple methods within a complex setting where the researcher is learning about the culture. Theoretical triangulation may be used to frame and rationalise the research using two or more theoretical perspectives. For instance, gender and inequality theories might provide epistemological and ontological lenses for the research. Equally, more than one theoretical perspective may be used to interpret the findings. Triangulation of setting or site might occur where the research involves more than one group or scenario within a setting or within two or more settings that have close connection, similarities or characteristics. The purpose is not so much to increase generalisability but more so to enrich the investigation and achieve deeper understanding of the phenomenon. Investigator triangulation involves more than one investigator in one or more stages of the research. Again, the purpose is to achieve greater accuracy through more credible, dependable and confirmable processes and outcomes. For instance, two researchers might undertake data collection, either working together as a pair or independently, which can provide opportunity for debriefing and maximising researchers' skills. Method triangulation involves using two or more methods, which can be sampling methods, data collection methods or data analysis techniques. However, it is important to note that each method has its own purpose in the scheme of the research. This means that using multiple methods of data collection, for instance, is not to produce increased aggregative output but to yield different forms of data, alternative dimensions across the findings and a deeper, richer and dependable understanding.

Constant comparison

Constant comparative method is a data analysis technique commonly used in grounded theory research (see Chapter 9 for further discussion). It involves checking consistency and accuracy of interpretations while coding by constantly comparing one interpretation or theme with others to ensure consistency and completeness in the analysis. This is an ongoing iterative and inductive process involving simultaneous theoretical sampling, data collection and coding, with themes evolving that are closely integrated with and representative of the emerging data. It is common practice to develop a list of codes and to attempt to define and produce brief summaries for each, enabling comparison and further refinement of clear delineated themes and categories.

'Deviant' (negative) case analysis

A deviant 'negative' case describes data (i.e. a primary observation, occurrence, articulation, perspective, etc.) that seems to contradict or differ markedly from others, therefore prompting questions about its veracity and meaning within the context of one's emerging theories (see also Chapter 9). It is an active process that involves intentionally seeking out such instances. If a negative instance is identified, it is then necessary to re-examine all the data in the light of this occurrence and attempt to explain why the case occurred in this untypical way. The emerging theory is then reconsidered and modified until it 'works' for all cases. This approach can lead to richer, more complex theory development and involves refining the analysis until it explains and accounts for most cases.

Peer review

Peer review – also termed 'peer debriefing' and 'inter-rater reliability' – is the inclusion of some objective evaluation of the research process by a peer who is external to the research. This involves asking tough questions about the research design and process and is an opportunity for the researcher to talk about the research, to reflect on the process and to debrief. This is a useful process at any stage, including at the design stage when decisions are being made about the research question, ontological and epistemological stances, methodological preference and choice of methods. It has an important role in verifying that methods are executed ethically and accurately, and ultimately during data analysis when developing themes, categories and theories, interpreting the findings and expressing the overall implications of the research. Sometimes a peer reviewer can be used to repeat the coding as a further check on the confirmability and dependability of the findings; this relies upon a clear coding system so that an independent coder approaches the analysis in the same way.

Member checking

Member checking is another way to seek external validation of the findings. It is often interpreted as the returning of interview transcripts to research participants to check for accuracy of their accounts. However, it is much more than this; it is a valuable technique for soliciting research participants' views on the credibility of the data and of the researcher's interpretations. Moreover, it is one way to ensure that research participants are more fully involved and able to be more legitimately represented within the research. It is a further tactic for building trust and ensuring trustworthiness. Member checking can, therefore, be used during data collection as well as during the analysis and write-up phases. During data collection, it involves checking out credibility, dependability and confirmability of observations, issues and utterances across participants. This is an inductive process as, for instance, an issue could be raised with one interviewee, which prompts the interviewer to raise the issue with subsequent interviewees.

Audit trail

All qualitative research should be developed with complete transparency across the whole research process. Somebody reading the research should be able to see what was done, how it was done and how decisions were made along the way. There should be sufficient clarity about the research process to allow others to learn from it and to see how the research question and objectives were operationalised through the methodology and methods. This also means that discussion of the research findings and their implications can be traced back through the research process, such that the reader has complete faith in the decisions that were made. In other words, it should be possible to see dependable connections between the selection of cases, data collection, data analysis and findings, interpretations and conclusions.

Conclusion

Ensuring quality and rigour in qualitative research means thinking about both processes and outcomes. This means attending to the early stages of decision-making – one's values going into the research and one's decisions about the research question, ontology and epistemology, methodology and methods – to the execution of the methods and to the interpretation and presentation of results. A key principle that applies to all qualitative research study is transparency, especially as qualitative research is undertaken in a spirit of trust. The qualitative researcher is often a privileged guest who is seeking to enter others' worlds and is obliged to represent their views and experiences with accuracy and integrity.

Further reading

Alvesson, M. and Sköldberg, K. (2009) *Reflexive Methodology* (Second edition). London: Sage.

Miles, M.B. and Huberman, A.M. (1994) *Qualitative Data Analysis: An expanded sourcebook* (Second edition). London: Sage.

Morse, J.M. (2015) Critical analysis of strategies for determining rigor in qualitative inquiry. *Qualitative Health Research*, 25(9): 1212–22.

PART 3

MIXING IT UP: COMBINING METHODS AND EVIDENCE SYNTHESIS IN PUBLIC HEALTH

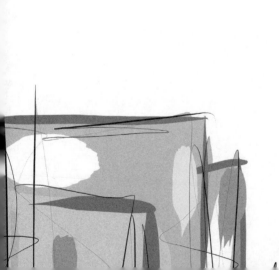
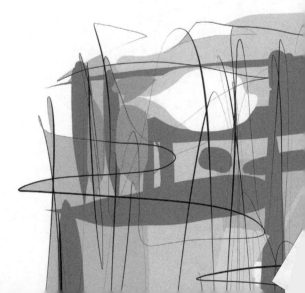

11 MIXED METHODS RESEARCH AND EVALUATION DESIGN

═══════════════ CHAPTER SUMMARY ═══════════════

Mixed methods research and **evaluation design** implies both a method and a methodology for research studies that purposefully bring together both quantitative and qualitative research in a single study. This chapter explores **mixed methods research** from the perspective of whether this provides a more coherent understanding of a research issue than either qualitative or quantitative research can in isolation. We discuss the different ways that research may be mixed methods, through **exploration** (combining or integrating methods in a single study), **triangulation** (to help corroborate findings), and **explanation** (one set of findings help to explore arguments for and against mixed methods). In this chapter we also consider different mixed methods designs for public health, focusing on **sequential** and **concurrent mixed methods design**, providing key examples where appropriate.

Mixed methods research – what is it?

As you will have seen, earlier chapters in this book describe quantitative and qualitative research paradigms and explore a range of quantitative and qualitative research methods (Chapters 1 to 10). Chapter 1 examines quantitative experimental and observational studies and describes how these study designs generate numerical data. Quantitative research traditionally follows positivist philosophy, which has an underlying belief that reality can be measured and observed objectively. For example, we might conduct a randomised controlled trial (RCT) to assess the effectiveness of a community-based physical activity intervention designed to reduce childhood obesity. Chapter 6 is concerned with qualitative research methods, which involve the collection of non-numerical data, such as interview, focus group, or observational data. In contrast to quantitative research, qualitative research usually takes an interpretive stance, which aims to explore complex human and social phenomena through consideration of multiple viewpoints, contexts and meanings. For example, a qualitative researcher might undertake a study to understand children's perceptions of obesity so that it may be better prevented, or they might explore social constructions of childhood obesity and how it has been perceived in society over time. As a brief refresher, Table 11.1 summarises some of the key strengths and limitations associated with quantitative and qualitative approaches to research. On first look, quantitative and qualitative research may seem entirely distinct in philosophy, design and outlook, and you might be sceptical about *how* and *why* some researchers seek to combine quantitative and qualitative approaches to undertake mixed methods research. Through this chapter we will explore the principles and methods of mixed methods research, with a specific focus on how mixed methods research is relevant for those interested in public health.

Table 11.1 Summary of the strengths and limitations of quantitative and qualitative research

	Strengths	Limitations
Quantitative research	Large sample sizes increase opportunities for producing generalisable findings.	May not explain the full complexity of human experience or perceptions.
	Statistical methods, if used appropriately, are considered reliable.	Seeks to identify 'what', but does not always uncover 'why', 'how', 'for whom'.
	Can be used to generate systematic and standardised comparisons.	May give a false impression of homogeneity in a sample.
Qualitative research	Can generate in-depth and rich data.	Qualitative researchers set out to produce generalisable findings, but as a result of this the findings may have a limited impact at public health policy, practice and implementation levels.
	Appropriate for situations where a detailed understanding about a phenomenon is sought.	Conclusions need to be carefully positioned and grounded in the data.
	Events are explored within a specific socio-cultural context.	Qualitative research can face criticism for producing 'unreliable' findings (e.g. different findings might be observed on a different day or if research conducted with different people).

The recent publication of Creswell and Plano Clark's *Designing and Conducting Mixed Methods Research* states that a researcher 'collects and analyses both qualitative and quantitative data rigourously in response to research questions and hypotheses, integrates (or mixes or combines) the two forms of data and their results, organises these procedures into specific research designs that provide logic and procedures for conducting the study, and frames these procedures within theory of philosophy' (Creswell and Plano Clark, 2018: 5). Simply put, mixed methods research seeks to better understand a research problem than could be expected from the utilisation of a quantitative or qualitative approach alone. While Creswell and Plano Clark are arguably the most well-known writers on mixed methods research, it should be acknowledged that the field is broad and there exists debate about how mixed methods research is defined and conducted (Greene, 2007; Guest and Fleming, 2015; Hesse-Biber, 2010; Morse and Niehaus, 2009; Tashakkori and Teddlie, 2010; Teddlie and Tashakkori, 2009). The *Journal of Mixed Methods Research* is another excellent source for further reading material.

Why is mixed methods research relevant for public health?

In recent years, mixed methods research is increasingly recognised for its potential to overcome some of the limitations associated with quantitative and qualitative research (Table 11.1), and this is particularly true in the case of public health research (Kaur, 2016; Padgett, 2012). Public health research is faced with tackling complex issues and health inequalities that are often influenced by a multitude of individual-, social-, and environmental-level factors, and it is possible that these may not be comprehensively understood through the application of quantitative or qualitative approaches alone.

For example, let's imagine you are interested in undertaking a quasi-experimental (or non-randomised) study to examine the effects of a school-based body image intervention. This utilisation of a quantitative study design has its benefits: 1) the design might help to reduce the potential impact of confounding on results; and 2) if the study is representative and adequately powered it might be possible to draw conclusions about the generalisability of the findings at a population level. Despite these qualities, as a researcher involved in this study you would be unable to say anything about: a) how the intervention was received by pupils and their teachers (i.e. did they like it, was it 'acceptable'?); and b) whether it was feasible to implement the intervention in the school setting. This is where a qualitative study component could be useful. For example, qualitative data generated from focus groups or interviews with relevant stakeholders could explore these issues in detail.

Now let's imagine you are interested in learning more about men's experiences of living with the hepatitis C virus. You might conduct qualitative interviews with a sample of affected men and generate a rich and in-depth overview of men's beliefs, perceptions and views. However, it is possible that due to a small sample size and an inability to generalise to a wider audience, the findings may have limited impact at public health policy and practice levels. As such, it might be desirable to conduct subsequent quantitative research, drawing upon key findings from the initial qualitative enquiry, to assess the magnitude of experiences faced by men affected by hepatitis C virus.

It is useful at this point to note that the analysis of data from separate quantitative and qualitative studies that address the same research question does not constitute mixed methods research, as there is no attempt to integrate approaches at any stage of the research process.

Sevens steps to consider when designing a mixed methods research study

Guest and Fleming (2015) describe sevens steps to consider when designing a mixed methods study, each of which is described in more detail below and is summarised in Table 11.2. The steps provide a useful and pragmatic framework, especially for those that may be new to mixed methods research and unsure where to begin.

Table 11.2 Seven steps to designing a mixed methods research study

Step	
1	Develop the research question
2	Justify need for utilising a mixed methods approach
3	Identify the types of data to be collected
4	Define the research design
5	Draw a schematic of your study, depicting how each component relates to another
6	Review diagram
7	Review the overall mixed methods design

Source: Guest and Fleming, 2015

Step 1: Develop the research question

Based on what you have read so far you might be wondering how to go about conducting mixed methods research, particularly given the need to integrate seemingly distinct quantitative and qualitative methods and data. Broadly speaking, qualitative researchers ask 'how' and 'why' and use verbs such as 'describe' or 'explore' to allow researchers to focus on a phenomenon of interest (Chapter 6), while in contrast, quantitative researchers tend to write clearly defined research questions, often with specific populations, interventions/exposures and outcomes (Chapter 1).

As we have seen in earlier chapters, regardless of the quantitative or qualitative approach taken, the careful development of a research question is a crucial aspect of the conceptualisation of a research study. This is also the case for mixed methods research, in which the development of the research question is important for shaping the overall study design. While it is generally accepted that good quality research stems from a clearly defined research question, writings on what constitutes a 'good' research question when it comes to undertaking mixed methods research are relatively limited.

As you will doubtless have noticed, the process for developing a research question for quantitative research differs from the development of a qualitative research question (Chapters 1 and 6). When it comes to mixed methods research, you would do well to first consider the following questions:

- What is already known about my chosen topic? (You should consider existing quantitative, qualitative and mixed methods literature.)
- Where are the evidence 'gaps'? What do we *not* know yet?
- Is the use of one research question and approach enough to address the knowledge gaps, or would the integration of quantitative and qualitative questions and methods better inform the evidence base?

Once you have considered these questions, and decided that a mixed methods research study is right for you, you might find that you are asking yourself:

- How can I develop a mixed methods research question that combines quantitative and qualitative questions?
- How can I ensure that I 'do justice' to both approaches?
- Should I write multiple separate questions, to highlight both quantitative and qualitative aims?

Unfortunately, the simple answer to these questions is that there is no 'right' answer; it is an area that is open to debate. For further information on this debate, try Collins et al. (2007), Plano Clark and Badiee (2010) and Tashikkori and Creswell (2007).

For instance, Tashikkori and Creswell (2007) recommend that before determining your research question you must consider the following three options. Table 11.3 presents these options, with hypothetical examples:

1. The first option is to construct separate quantitative and qualitative questions, followed by a question that relates specifically to the use of mixed methods. The later 'methods' sub-question is recommended in order to explicitly present the researcher's intention to undertake mixed methods and to clarify from the outset how the methods will be mixed in the proposed study.
2. A second option is to write a research question that is overarching, covering all aspects of a programme of work. This is sometimes known as a 'hybrid' or 'integrated' question.

The overarching question may include sub-questions that are specific to quantitative and qualitative approaches. This approach is most often seen in studies that utilise a convergent design (see Creswell and Plano Clark's three-item typology).

3. The third possibility is to write a series of research questions as your research develops. If you intend to conduct qualitative enquiry at the start of your mixed methods study, then you will need to develop a qualitative research question. Findings from the initial qualitative aspect of the study may identify an issue that could be examined using quantitative methods and, as such, a quantitative research question is required. Guidance indicates that this approach is most commonly observed for studies that utilise a sequential design (see Creswell and Plano Clark's three-item typology).

We feel it is important to recognise at this point that it is not always desirable or appropriate to integrate quantitative and qualitative approaches. As discussed throughout this book, when developing a research project, the focal point for all decisions should revolve around the research question. If your research question can be adequately addressed through the utilisation of quantitative or qualitative methods alone, then it is arguably unnecessary to include an additional quantitative or qualitative angle to your research.

Table 11.3 Options for writing mixed research questions (with hypothetical examples)

	Brief description	**Example**
Separate questions only	The researcher constructs separate quantitative and qualitative questions.	**Example 1** • Is there an association between social isolation and time spent playing online games? [Quan] • What is the lived social experience of individuals who play online video games? [Qual] **Example 2** • How do parents of obese or overweight children understand childhood obesity? [Qual] • What factors influence parents of obese or overweight children to engage in a family-centred weight-management programme? [Quan] These examples may be followed by a 'methods' question such as: • Do the quantitative and qualitative findings converge? • How do the follow-up qualitative findings help explain the initial quantitative results?

	Brief description	Example
'Hybrid' or 'integrated' questions	The researcher writes an overarching research question, covering all aspects of a programme of work. This may include sub-questions that are specific to quantitative and qualitative approaches.	What is the impact of a community-based exclusive breastfeeding intervention delivered in disadvantaged communities in the UK? • Sub-question 1: Is the community-based exclusive breastfeeding intervention effective in increasing the uptake of exclusive breastfeeding for new mothers from a disadvantaged community? [Quan] • Sub-question 2: What are stakeholders' experiences of the intervention (perspectives of mothers, fathers, and intervention deliverers)? [Qual]
Series of questions as research develops	The researcher writes a question that has developed as a result of the research process.	• How do internal labour migrants in Nigeria experience 'health'? [Qual] • What are the determinants of internal labour migrants' health in Nigeria? [Quant] • How do these determinants influence internal labour migrants' health in Nigeria? [Quant]

Step 2: Justify need for utilising a mixed methods approach

Step 2 is chiefly concerned with ensuring that the utilisation of mixed methods is appropriate in the context of the public health 'problem' or 'issue' under investigation. There are many reasons why mixed methods research might be appealing to the public health researcher, possibly more reasons than you might have already considered. Tariq and Woodman identify five reasons why those involved in health research might be motivated to undertake mixed methods research (Tariq and Woodman, 2013). These are summarised below, with specific reference to a hypothetical public health research question:

'What are the outcomes and experiences of inactive older adults participating in a 12-week physical activity programme?'

1. **Complementarity**

    Description: Use of data obtained from quantitative or qualitative methods to illustrate the results from the other.

    Example: A quantitative survey might identify positive changes in older adults' physical activity over time. Qualitative interviews might reveal the facilitators associated with these changes in behaviour.

2. **Development**

    Description: Use of results from one method to inform and aid development of the application of the other method.

Example: Focus group data might identify barriers to physical activity participation including features of the environment (e.g. safety concerns associated with night-time programme delivery). This might inform development of a comprehensive quantitative survey identifying barriers and facilitators to participation that include individual-, social- and environmental-level factors.

3. **Initiation**

Description: Use of results from different methods to identify incongruence to generate new insight into an issue.

Example: Results from a quantitative survey might suggest high self-reported physical activity but objectively measured physical activity levels might be much lower. Qualitative interviews with programme participants might be used to identify reasons for discrepancies between self-reported physical activity outcomes and objectively measured physical activity.

4. **Expansion**

Description: Examining different aspects of a research question that requires use of different methods.

Example: One aspect of the study might involve a quantitative assessment of physical activity and mental wellbeing outcomes using validated measures, while participant experiences of the programme might be best explored using qualitative methods (e.g. interviews or focus groups).

5. **Triangulation**

Description: Use of data obtained by both methods to corroborate findings.

Example: Quantitative survey data might indicate a significant positive change in participants' mental wellbeing outcomes following completion of the 12-week programme. These findings might be corroborated by interviews with participants who describe perceived improvements in self-confidence and self-worth following receipt of the programme.

Step 3: Identify the types of data to be collected

Methods for collecting quantitative and qualitative data are described earlier in this book (Chapter 3: Quantitative data collection and Chapter 8: Qualitative data collection) and we recommend that you refresh your memory with these chapters before reading on. You may be pleased to hear that the types of data described in those chapters are likely to be relevant to a mixed methods study. However, the procedure for collecting data for a mixed methods study does require some careful thought. The key issues to consider are as follows:

- Determining sampling procedure and sample size
- Types of data to be collected

Determining sampling procedure and sample size

As described in earlier chapters of this book (Chapter 2: Quantitative Sampling and Chapter 7: Qualitative Sampling) there is a range of sampling approaches at your disposal, and your choice of sampling methods will most likely depend on your research question. One of the key questions or concerns raised by students undertaking a piece of quantitative or qualitative research is 'How large should my sample be?' The same question is often raised by those undertaking mixed methods research.

As you will know from earlier chapters in this book, the size of a study sample varies according to the research question and research design. For example, quantitative research studies often apply statistical methods to calculate a sample size that is large enough to detect a statistically significant difference in a target outcome, should a difference truly exist in the wider population (Chapter 2). Conversely, in qualitative research a sample is generally considered large enough if the researcher reaches a point where no new information is emerging. This is known as data saturation (Chapter 7).

In an ideal world, when undertaking mixed methods research the target sample size should reflect the minimum sample size required to satisfy the needs of both the quantitative *and* the qualitative aspects of the research. Having said that, we must be mindful that student research projects are often limited in terms of time and available resources, and, as such, it is important to consider a sample size that is feasible to achieve. The way you identify and recruit your sample is probably more important than the total number of people that you ultimately include in your sample.

Types of data to be collected

Before conducting your mixed methods study, you will need to spend some time considering the types of quantitative and qualitative data you intend to collect to address your research question(s). A brief comparison of data types associated with quantitative and qualitative research studies demonstrates that this list is extensive (Creswell, 2005). For qualitative research, you might collect data from the following:

Interviews; focus groups; observations; videotapes; diaries; documents; photographs; emails; blogs.

For quantitative research, data types might include:

Survey; structural interviews; observational data (with pre-defined measurement categories); objectively measured behaviours (e.g. accelerometers that measure actual physical activity): attendance data.

In mixed methods research, data collection occurs concurrently (i.e. quantitative and qualitative data are collected at approximately the same time) or sequentially (i.e. quantitative or qualitative data are collected first, and the results inform the second phase of the quantitative or qualitative data collection). Concurrent data collection treats quantitative and qualitative data independently, while sequential data collection considers quantitative and qualitative data as connected or related to each other.

Neither concurrent nor sequential data collection methods are free from the possibility of encountering issues in a real-world scenario. We recommend Chapter 6 of Creswell and Plano Clark's text: *Collecting Data in Mixed Methods Research* (2018) for a detailed and useful overview of potential issues.

Step 4: Define the research design

A number of typologies (or classifications) have been proposed that describe ways of integrating quantitative and qualitative methods into one research study (Creswell and Plano Clark, 2011, 2018; Greene, 2007; Guest and Fleming, 2015; Hesse-Biber, 2010; Morse and Niehaus, 2009; Tashakkori and Teddlie, 2010; Teddlie and Tashakkori, 2009). Creswell and Plano Clark's (2011) six-item typology has received the most attention and is most widely cited in the public health literature. However, in 2018 Creswell and Plano Clark published the third edition of their text *Designing and Conducting Mixed Methods Research* (2018), and put forward a consolidated typology of three core mixed methods research designs. It is this most recent typology that is described and explored later in this chapter. Before reading on to learn more about this typology, we recommended that you first consider the three following points:

1. Consideration of the methods that will be applied

   In earlier chapters we have emphasised the importance of developing a well-thought-out research question to determine appropriate research methods and to identify data sources and data collection strategies; the same is true in the case of mixed methods research. At this point, you might find it useful to refer back to *Step 1: Develop the research question* for a refresher.

   If you are conducting a piece of research for a student project you are probably facing time and resource restrictions. Designing, implementing and analysing data from a mixed methods research project is time consuming, and while it can add value to your research it is essential to consider the feasibility of completing a mixed methods project to a good standard in the time you have available. Furthermore, good quality mixed methods research, by its very nature, is ambitious in that it requires a combination of strong quantitative and qualitative research skills. As with all projects, support and guidance on undertaking mixed methods research should be sought from your supervisor or project team.

2. Consideration of the weighting of the methods to be applied

   The weighting of methods applied in mixed methods research essentially refers to the priority given to each method in a study. In the literature, this is generally referred to as 'weighting', but you may also read about 'priority' or 'dominance' of methods. These terms are interchangeable. It is important to acknowledge that the method (quantitative or qualitative) that is given less weighting in a study is not considered to be unimportant; it simply means that the way the reporting of study findings will focus on the more heavily weighted method. To illustrate an example of weighting specific to public health, let's draw upon one of the examples discussed earlier in *Step 2: Justify need for utilising a mixed methods approach.* A study might involve the administration of a large-scale quantitative survey to assess the impact of changes in older adults' physical activity following receipt of a 12-week community-based physical activity intervention. To better understand the impact of the intervention and identify factors influencing barriers and facilitators to participation, qualitative interviews might be conducted with a small sample of intervention participants. In this instance, the quantitative element of the study is more heavily weighted and would form the basis of the results.

Similar to the point above, decisions about how to weight methods should be grounded in the research question (i.e. which method is likely to provide the most insight to address the research question). In some cases, quantitative and qualitative methods will have the same weighting, while in other cases the weighting of the methods may change in response to emergent findings and data collected. As such, at the start of a study it is useful to discuss weighting with a supervisor or project team, but to also acknowledge the need for flexibility in methodological orientation if required.

3.   Consideration of the timing that methods will be used

The final question to ask yourself is 'In which sequence should I use quantitative and qualitative methods?' The most well-recognised approaches are sequential (i.e. quantitative methods are applied first, followed by qualitative, or vice versa) and concurrent (i.e. quantitative and qualitative methods are applied side-by-side at the same time). When using the sequential approach, the idea is that the data collected and analysed at the early stages of the project are used in some way to inform the subsequent data collection and analysis. For the concurrent approach, quantitative and qualitative data collection procedures are conducted separately and only integrated during analysis. As above, we recommend that you discuss your thoughts with your supervisor or project team and attempt to base your decision on the most appropriate approach for addressing your research question.

Creswell and Plano Clark's (2018) three-item typology of mixed methods study designs

Creswell and Plano Clark's (2018) three-item study design typology is summarised below, with examples of how each study design might be applied to address a public health research question. A more detailed overview of the typology, including sub-categories, is presented in Creswell and Plano Clark (2018) and it may be worth looking at this alongside the content presented here.

The examples presented below are neatly organised with clearly defined features. It is worth acknowledging at this point that when undertaking real-world research, things do not always go to plan and changes must be made in response to the situation at hand.

However, these three designs do provide a useful starting point and a common vocabulary to organise and describe your proposed plans for research.

1. **Convergent design**

    Key design features: Quantitative and qualitative methods are applied concurrently and independently analysed. The methods are only integrated during interpretation and reporting. The triangulation of quantitative and qualitative data enhances the validity of reported findings and promotes full and accurate interpretation of results.

    Hypothetical study and methods: A study aims to identify reasons for the delay in seeking healthcare among men experiencing illness. Researchers may employ concurrent collection of quantitative and qualitative data, with quantitative methods used to generate statistics on the delay in healthcare seeking, and qualitative methods used to reveal causes of the delay.

2. **Explanatory sequential design**

    Key design features: These studies begin with the collection and analysis of quantitative data, with qualitative methods used later to explore and better understand the results generated from the analysis of quantitative data. Application of an explanatory sequential mixed methods design is increasingly seen in the public health literature, and this study design is particularly useful for enhancing the strengths of quantitative and qualitative research.

    Hypothetical study and methods: A study aims to evaluate the effectiveness of a smoking cessation intervention for college students aged 16–24 years. Researchers may collect and analyse quantitative survey data from college students and use the results to explore factors influencing the quitting behaviour of those students identifying as smokers through qualitative focus groups.

3. **Exploratory sequential design**

    Key design features: These studies begin with the collection and analysis of qualitative data, with quantitative methods used later to answer epidemiological questions raised during qualitative analysis. The exploratory design is one of the most commonly used for mixed methods research. When contemplating conducting an exploratory sequential study, guidance suggests that a researcher should consider the extent to which the quantitative research will be informed by the initial qualitative work. Let's imagine you plan to pilot a validated survey tool with a new population study. It is possible that information on this already exists, potentially making the need for a qualitative study element redundant.

    Hypothetical study and methods: A study aims to better understand factors contributing to lower levels of breastfeeding initiation among mothers from lower socio-economic groups. Researchers may undertake focus groups with new parents to identify barriers to initiation. This might be followed by a quantitative study to determine how these barriers resonate with a wider sample, and whether or not these barriers differ from those parents from higher socio-economic groups.

Step 5: Draw a schematic of your study, depicting how each component relates to another

It is often the case that a visual representation of a concept or idea can be useful to aid understanding. This is particularly true in the case of mixed methods research, which, by its very nature, is more complex than a traditional quantitative or qualitative study design. Every project 'schematic' or visual representation will differ from the next.

Step 6: Review diagram

By this point, your research plans should be well formulated, and have included input from a project supervisor or team. Guidance suggests that the visual schematic of your proposed research should be simple, using concise language that can be interpreted by a layperson with little to no knowledge of mixed methods research. It is also recommended that the visual representation of the proposed plan fit on one-A4 page. You might benefit from sharing the proposed plans with a friend/family member/colleague at this stage.

Step 7: Review the overall mixed methods design

This final step provides an opportunity for individual researchers (and supervisors/members of the project team) to take one final look at the proposal before conducting the research. Phew – you're almost ready to conduct your research! At this point, the main consideration should relate to the feasibility of the proposed methods; after all, it is no good to develop a complex and methodologically sound mixed methods research plan, only to realise that the proposed tasks are unachievable in terms of available time and resources.

Data analysis and synthesis

Arguably, the most important and potentially trickiest phase to undertaking a mixed methods research study is the analysis and synthesis of quantitative and qualitative data. This chapter presents a brief introduction to recognised strategies for combining quantitative and qualitative data, but for a more detailed overview we recommend Sandelowski (2000).

Independent analysis of quantitative and qualitative data

In the public health literature, the most commonly used approach involves the analysis of quantitative and qualitative data, with each data set independently analysed, and followed by the integration of findings. As a researcher, you are essentially looking for aspects of data comparability and commonality, but only at the end of the study (Sandelowski, 2000). As the quantitative and qualitative data are considered distinct and confined to a specific research paradigm, analysis usually involves the application of techniques associated with either quantitative or qualitative methods. For example, qualitative focus group data may be best explored through thematic analysis, while application of a statistical technique might be appropriate for the analysis of quantitative survey data. An overview of these methods is presented in Chapters 4 and 9.

Integration of quantitative and qualitative data

A second approach to data analysis and synthesis is called 'integrative strategy' (Caracelli and Greene, 1993). Unlike the approach described above, where quantitative and qualitative data sets are kept apart during analysis, the integrative strategy involves the transformation of quantitative or qualitative data into the other. 'Quantitizing' is when researchers transform qualitative into quantitative data, through numerical coding of themes or constructs. Conversely, 'qualitizing' involves the transformation of quantitative data into qualitative themes or ideas. One of the benefits of transforming either data type is the ability to generate and extract more information about your topic of interest. If you would like to know more about some of the methodological challenges and opportunities associated with this approach, we recommend Nzabonimpa (2018).

For the purposes of this introductory chapter, let's return again to an earlier example that referred to a hypothetical research study aiming to answer the following research question: *'What are the outcomes and experiences of inactive older adults participating in a 12-week physical activity programme?'* We might 'quantitize' or transform data from qualitative focus groups with programme participants to generate a statement such as: 'Participants in eight out of 10 focus groups agreed that safety concerns associated with travelling at night were one of the main barriers to evening class attendance.'

The transformation of quantitative data into qualitative is less common, but it can be useful. With specific reference to the example above, we might use quantitative data on participant characteristics to create a portrait or typology of them. So, if most participants taking part in the physical activity programme are aged 55 to 65 years, we might describe them as 'young old'. Or, if most of the participants taking part in the programme scored highly to a scale of questions on mental wellbeing, the group could be described as having 'positive mental wellbeing'.

Mixed methods research: Challenges and opportunities

So far in this chapter we have focused mainly on the qualities associated with undertaking mixed methods public health research. We close this chapter with a summary of these benefits alongside some of the challenges that you may encounter on your mixed methods journey (see Table 11.4).

Table 11.4 Mixed methods challenges and opportunities

Challenges	Opportunities
There is continuing debate surrounding the compatibility of quantitative and qualitative paradigms.	Mixed methods have the potential to increase the validity of findings.
Combining quantitative and qualitative methods can be time consuming.	Mixed methods can be used to gain a deeper and broader understanding of the phenomenon under investigation.
Skills in quantitative and qualitative research methods are required.	Mixed methods can be utilised to gain a better understanding of a research problem than could be expected from the utilisation of a quantitative or qualitative approach alone (and can overcome the shortfalls of taking a single approach).
True integration of data is not easy, and there is no consensus on the 'right' way to achieve integration.	The integration of data can corroborate findings and allow researchers to draw stronger conclusions based on interpretation of mixed data.
The presentation of mixed methods results requires careful consideration (e.g. journals have relatively restrictive word limits, which may make it difficult to fully and accurately convey a study's contribution to the evidence base). Furthermore, mixed methods evaluation can be more difficult to publish, as quantitatively-orientated journals can comment 'there is no control group' and qualitatively-orientated journals may say the findings are not expansive enough or theoretically informed.	Mixed methods can help to identify, develop and cultivate new ideas for research.

Conclusion

This chapter introduced mixed methods research and evaluation design, and explored how it can be used to better understand a public health research problem than could be expected from the utilisation of a quantitative or qualitative approach alone. The chapter identified the different ways that research may be mixed methods, from 'exploration', to 'triangulation', to 'explanation'. A range of mixed methods designs has been examined, including relevant examples to guide the practical application of these methods in a public health context.

Further reading

Creswell, J.W. and Plano Clark, V.L. (2018). *Designing and Conducting Mixed Methods Research* (Third edition). London: Sage.

Sandelowsi, M. (2000) Combining qualitative and quantitative sampling, data collection, and analysis techniques in mixed methods studies. *Research in Nursing & Health*, 23(3): 246–55.

12 EVIDENCE SYNTHESIS APPROACHES: SYSTEMATIC REVIEWS

============== CHAPTER SUMMARY ==============

This chapter is divided into seven sections: introduction to **evidence synthesis**; approaches to **reviewing public health research; developing a research question; searching for relevant literature; assessing the quality of the literature; synthesising and interpreting findings** (including meta-analysis); and, a note on **writing for publication**.

An introduction to evidence synthesis

Parts I and II of this book are focused on primary research methods for public health. We have explored a range of quantitative and qualitative research designs, from the randomised controlled trial to ethnography. This chapter provides researchers with an alternative approach to research called evidence synthesis. Unlike primary research, which involves designing and conducting a research study from scratch, evidence synthesis is an example of secondary research, which involves the collection and analysis of data from research that has already been conducted. Evidence synthesis allows a researcher to gather and summarise evidence related to a specific topic to draw conclusions about the extent and quality of the existing evidence base. Evidence synthesis is associated with a number of advantages, for example:

- It is estimated that there are more than 2,000,000 health-related articles published each year. Summarising a large volume of evidence can be beneficial for health professionals, researchers and policy-makers who may be short of time.

- Evidence synthesis brings together the results of numerous studies, allowing researchers to draw more generalisable and transferable conclusions about a topic of interest, rather than relying on the results from a single primary study.
- Evidence synthesis can meet the pragmatic needs of funders and organisations who want to know the 'state of the evidence', but do not have resources at their disposal to explore the evidence base in detail.

Approaches to reviewing public health evidence

This chapter explores arguably the most well-recognised and most widely published form of evidence synthesis: the systematic review. In Chapter 13, we go on to explore two alternative approaches to evidence synthesis that have received increased attention in the field of public health in recent years; namely, meta-ethnography and realist synthesis.

An introduction to systematic reviews

Systematic reviews aim to identify, appraise and synthesise the best quality evidence in relation to a specific research question. There are three main types of review: those that combine evidence from quantitative studies, qualitative studies, and mixed methods studies. The most well known of these is the systematic review of quantitative evidence. In recent years, systematic review methodology has evolved beyond a traditional 'randomised controlled trial only' approach, with reviews now published synthesising results from observational studies, qualitative studies and a mixture of evidence from quantitative and qualitative studies.

Given the breadth and depth of the public health evidence base, the very idea of conducting a systematic review may seem overwhelming at the outset. It is certainly a big undertaking, but if each of the required steps is followed and enough time is set aside, then it can be a very rewarding piece of work.

What is meant by 'best quality evidence'?

Most textbooks and published systematic reviews refer to the importance of 'best quality evidence', but what exactly does this mean? As described in previous chapters there are numerous quantitative study designs and qualitative approaches for conducting public health research. At the start of a systematic review, it is helpful to consider these designs and approaches in relation to the traditional public health hierarchy of evidence (see Figure 12.1), which places systematic reviews at the top. We are introduced to the hierarchy of evidence in the main Introduction, and it is acknowledged that the rules and standards about the evidence hierarchy privilege a more positivist epistemological approach to research. As such, there is no universally accepted evidence hierarchy, and this is an ongoing debate to be mindful of as you undertake your research.

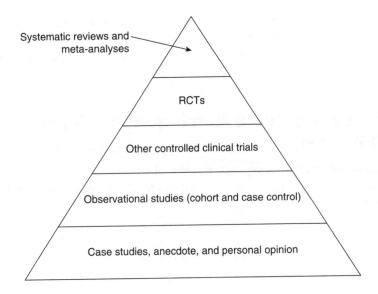

Figure 12.1   **Public health hierarchy of evidence**

Source: Figure adapted from Greenhalgh et al. (2014)

The hierarchy of evidence has been challenged for failing to appreciate that different study approaches and methodologies are required to explore different types of research question (Berlin and Golub, 2014). For example, it would be near impossible to examine fathers' experiences of attending a breastfeeding support group using an RCT design; an exploratory qualitative design would be much more suitable. Increased recognition for the role of alternative study designs and methodologies is now also apparent with regard to systematic reviews. Most published systematic reviews still collate findings from good quality randomised controlled trials, but there is now also a precedent for identifying and synthesising the best quality evidence from other types of studies.

Alternative approaches to evidence synthesis

Many alternative approaches to evidence synthesis have emerged that aim to overcome some of the limitations associated with systematic review. These have received a mixed response from the public health field, with significant debate regarding terminology, methods and reporting techniques utilised (Pawson and Tilley, 2004; Petticrew, 2009; Pope et al., 2007). Two relatively new approaches to evidence synthesis highlighted in this book are meta-ethnography (evidence synthesis of qualitative research) and realist synthesis (theory-driven evidence synthesis for policy development). Although newer and less well specified than the traditional systematic review, there is an increasing body of guidance on how to conduct these reviews and examples of published work applied to public health. Chapter 13 introduces these two alternative approaches to evidence synthesis.

Step 1: Develop the research question for a systematic review

A traditional systematic review typically follows four stages (see Table 12.1). Developing a clear and coherent research question is the first and most important stage of the systematic review journey.

Table 12.1   Steps to undertake a systematic review

Step	
1	Develop a research question
	• Inclusion and exclusion criteria
2	Search the literature
	• Construct the search strategy
	• Sift and sort the papers
3	Assess the quality of the literature
	• Defining 'quality'
	• Critical appraisal tools
	• Grading the quality of papers
	• Publication bias
4	Synthesise and interpret findings
	• Summarise search strategy outcomes
	• Data extraction
	• Data synthesis and interpretation
	• Strengths and weaknesses of the available evidence
	• Strengths and weaknesses of the findings of the review

It is easy to assume that once you have decided upon your topic area of interest, you can get straight on with searching the literature. This is not the case when conducting a systematic review; a poorly defined research question will almost certainly result in a more difficult to complete systematic review. When embarking on your systematic review it might be useful to consider the following two questions:

What is it that you are interested in finding out?

Try to answer this in your own words, without worrying too much about technical terms or correct language. A good strategy is to try to convey your ideas to a friend, colleague, or family member who knows nothing about your topic area of interest. This can help you to think through ideas simply by saying them out loud.

Has the answer to your topic area of interest already been published?

It is important to have a broad understanding about the published literature related to your topic of interest before making firm plans for your systematic review. One of the first tasks is to scope the literature to check that a review has not already been published in this area, as a systematic review should be an original piece of research. A search of the Cochrane Library (www.cochranelibrary.com) or PROSPERO, the International prospective register of systematic reviews (www.crd.york.ac.uk/prospero/), is a good place to start. It is worth noting that once you have fleshed out your plans for your systematic review you can register the review via the PROSPERO website.

In some cases, it might be appropriate to repeat a published review but this is only when the original review was published some time ago (let's say 10 years ago or more) and when there is clear justification for updating the evidence base. For example, in 2017 O'Connor and colleagues published the results of an updated systematic review of associations between proximity to animal feeding operations and health of individuals in nearby communities. This updated review was published seven years after the original review in response to the publication of a number of new studies during that time. The *British Medical Journal* has produced a useful set of guidelines on 'When and how to update systematic reviews' that may be of interest (Garner et al., 2016).

Once you have answered the two above questions you can then begin to frame a specific research question. Systematic reviews often use the 'PICOS' framework to generate a research question.

Population (P): What types of people are you interested in?

Try to narrow this down as much as possible. Men and women? Just men? Just women? What age group? A particular ethnic group?

Intervention (I) or Exposure (E): What is the indicator or phenomenon (intervention, exposure, risk factor) that you are interested in?

As above, try to be as specific as possible. The intervention could be a health promotion programme, a specific drug, a healthcare procedure or process. An exposure can be intentional or accidental. There may be no intervention or exposure component to your research question.

Comparator (C): What is the comparator group?

If you are looking at an intervention, what is the control or comparator group?

Outcome (O) What types of outcomes are you interested in?

This could be numerical (e.g. number of people who die or survive, or the incidence or prevalence of a condition or state of health), or this could be a categorical outcome (such as patient preference or levels of knowledge). Your outcome could be purely qualitative (e.g. participants' perceptions or attitudes). Some systematic reviews explore multiple outcomes. However, depending on available time and resources it might be most appropriate to focus on one outcome alone.

Study design (S) What types of studies are likely to have researched your area of interest?

If you are interested in a specific intervention, it is possible that there are published randomised controlled trials involving the intervention of interest. If you want to discover the prevalence of a condition or disease you will most likely seek to identify studies utilising an observational design. If you are interested in exploring people's perceptions, experiences or feelings, qualitative studies may be most appropriate to answer your research question. Generally, it is appropriate to focus on one study design to answer a research question; however, at times it can be useful to consider using more than one. Table 12.2 contains two example research questions that have applied the PICOS framework.

Table 12.2 Example research questions using the PICOS framework

Example 1. *What is the risk of malaria transmission in children under five years old who have been provided with, and use, permethrin impregnated bed nets, compared to those who have not been allocated to use permethrin impregnated bed nets?*	
Population	Children under five years old
Intervention	Provision and use of permethrin impregnated bed nets
Comparator	Those not allocated permethrin impregnated bed nets
Outcome	Risk of malaria transmission
Study design	Randomised controlled trials
Example 2. *What is the prevalence of depression among middle-aged men living in Australia that have received a diagnosis of type II diabetes since the year 2000?*	
Population	Middle-aged men living in Australia
Exposure	Type II diabetes diagnosis since 2000
Comparator	Not applicable
Outcome	Prevalence of depression
Study design	Any that include descriptive statistics

Inclusion and exclusion criteria

Once the PICOS framework has been generated it is time to define the criteria for including or excluding literature that is identified as you complete your systematic review of the literature. To start this thought process, it is useful to reflect upon each of the concepts from the PICOS framework in turn and to consider which study characteristics (participants, interventions/exposures, comparators, outcomes and study designs) will be eligible for inclusion. It is very important to keep a record of these criteria as they enable replication of your work and indicate the generalisability of your findings.

The eligibility criteria should also consider whether to exclude studies if they are not written in English or published within a certain time frame. For example, imagine you were interested in compiling articles that have reported results from the UK's National Child Measurement Programme (NCMP), a surveillance programme established in 2005 that measures the height and weight of children aged 4 to 5 years and aged 10 to 11 years to assess overweight and obesity levels. When searching the literature, only those papers published in or after 2005 would be eligible for inclusion as the NCMP did not exist prior to this date. It is important at this point to acknowledge any potential bias in implementing exclusion criteria. For example, limiting searches to studies written in English may miss important studies published in other languages.

Changing the research question or inclusion criteria

Guidance recommends that the research question for a systematic review be developed a priori (i.e. before the literature search begins). If not, it could be argued that interim findings and the personal interests of the researcher drive the review. This does not, however, preclude the researcher from conducting a scoping exercise to establish the extent of the literature in their area prior to the review (in fact, this is recommended).

Research questions for systematic reviews are generally conceived by a team of researchers, allowing for a discussion of the best approach for tackling a review. At the very least, it is important to discuss ideas with one other person to reduce the risk of generating a research question that is too broad or impossible to answer with the time and resources you have at your disposal. After embarking on a review, it may become apparent that there are too many articles that meet the eligibility criteria to analyse in the time available. At this point you may need to return to your research question and/or eligibility criteria to make modifications. This is something that should always be discussed with a colleague or supervisor.

Step 2: Search the literature

The ability of your systematic review to produce findings that are accurate and valid (please see Chapters 5 and 10 on quantitative and qualitative validity) will depend on whether or not you are able to identify the best available evidence that meets your eligibility criteria. A thorough and replicable search strategy is therefore essential.

Construct the search strategy

A search strategy is a set of terms that is used to search the evidence base for articles or documentation that meet eligibility criteria. It includes a set of subject heading terms and free text terms and is combined with Boolean operators (OR, AND and NOT) to generate a list of references. For example, consider the research question example presented earlier in Table 12.2:

> What is the prevalence of depression among middle-aged men living in Australia that have received a diagnosis of type II diabetes since the year 2000?

When breaking down this research question according to the PICOS framework we can begin to construct the search strategy. Each concept from the PICOS framework can usually be described using numerous terms (or synonyms). It can help to use a thesaurus or to look at the title and/or abstract of a relevant article to locate possible terms. The addition of 'Boolean operators' allows you to combine search terms in different combinations (see Table 12.3).

The search strategy needs to be sensitive enough to identify all the papers you are looking for but also specific enough to ensure that the list of references generated is manageable to complete the task at hand. This is clearly an important stage of the review process and it does require some degree of 'trial and error' testing across a range of electronic databases. Although this can feel time consuming, and at points frustrating, constructing a good quality search strategy is likely to save time in the long run. Most commonly, a search strategy is developed for testing in the electronic database MEDLINE and adapted to meet the entry requirements of other databases, where necessary. Ideally, the search strategy should be as similar as possible across databases and other sources.

There are two strands to searching the literature:

- A search of electronic databases.
- A search for published and unpublished articles that are located from sources other than electronic databases (e.g. websites, reports, newspapers). This is known as a search for 'grey literature'.

Table 12.3 Constructing the search strategy

	Concept	Synonym
Population	Middle-aged men	Middle-aged OR middle aged OR men OR man OR male OR father.
AND		

	Concept	Synonym
Exposure	Type II diabetes	Type II diabetes OR type 2 diabetes OR non-insulin-dependent diabetes mellitus OR NIDDM OR non-insulin-dependent diabetes OR ketosis-resistant diabetes mellitus OR ketosis-resistant diabetes OR ketoacidosis-resistant diabetes mellitus OR ketoacidosis-resistant diabetes OR adult-onset diabetes mellitus OR adult-onset diabetes OR maturity-onset diabetes mellitus OR maturity-onset diabetes OR mature-onset diabetes OR diabetes mellitus OR DM.
AND		
Comparator	Not applicable	Not applicable.
AND		
Outcome	Depression	Depression OR depressed OR depressive OR low mood OR anxiety OR sadness.
AND		
Study design	Any with descriptive data	Not applicable.

Searching electronic databases

Sadly, there is no one electronic database containing all publications ever produced. This means that a search of more than one database is required for all systematic reviews. A detailed record of all databases searched and when should be kept.

As a minimum, a search of MEDLINE and Cochrane Database of Systematic Reviews is recommended. Searches of other databases will depend upon the topic area of interest, as most databases tend to specialise in one or two specific areas of public health. Please see Box 12.1 for some of the most popular databases for sourcing public health research. When writing up the findings of a review, it is important to justify database inclusion decisions and to clarify why some databases were deemed to be unsuitable.

> ## BOX 12.1 FREQUENTLY USED DATABASES FOR PUBLIC HEALTH RESEARCH
>
> - Allied and Complementary Medicine (AMED)
> - BioMed Central
>
> *(Continued)*

(Continued)

- Campbell Collaboration
- Cumulative Index to Nursing and Allied Health Literature (CINAHL Plus)
- Cochrane Library
- EMBASE
- HMIC
- MEDLINE
- NICE Evidence
- PsycINFO
- PubMed
- SAGE Journals Online
- SportDiscus

Searching the grey literature

Not all literature is contained within electronic databases. There is a wide range of other potential sources for locating published and unpublished papers eligible for review that should be explored:

- Bibliography lists of key review articles and included studies.
- Contacting lead authors of key review articles and included studies.
- Looking in registers of unpublished research (e.g. UK National Research Register).
- Contacting experts working in the area of interest.
- Conference abstracts.
- Searching websites of key stakeholders known to conduct research in the area of interest (care is urged when taking this approach as some Internet sources are unreliable).
- Hand searching of specific relevant journal titles that are not included within the database search.
- Searching grey literature databases (e.g. ZETOC, System for Information on Grey Literature in Europe (SIGLE)).

Sift and sort the papers

Searching of electronic databases and the grey literature is likely to produce hundreds, if not thousands, of potentially eligible documents. At this point, a decision needs to be made on which ones meet the inclusion criteria that has already been defined. It is strongly recommended that all potentially eligible documents are exported to a reference management software package to maintain the paper trail required for each stage of a systematic review. There are numerous reference management software packages available (for example, RefWorks (www.refworks.com) or Mendeley (www.mendeley.com)) and the major databases allow for direct export from database to reference management software. Regardless of software package, it is recommended to label each export of references according to the database in which they were found (e.g. 'MEDLINE references'). Some of the smaller databases and grey literature sources do not have the capability to export references to a reference management programme. These references will need to be entered manually into the chosen reference management software package.

Once references are safely recorded in a software package it is possible to begin to whittle down the references according to review eligibility criteria. The decision to include a paper in a review is generally based on an initial assessment of the article title, followed by the abstract where necessary. It is recommended that all papers that appear to meet the inclusion criteria are added to a new folder (e.g. 'MEDLINE included references'). It is likely that in some cases it will not be possible to determine a paper's eligibility based on screening its title and abstract. In such instances, another folder is required allowing for further assessment of eligibility (e.g. 'MEDLINE full text assessment required').

In all likelihood, this part of the systematic review process will take the most time. It can feel tedious and at times confusing. At such times, it is useful to have a piece of paper to hand detailing the review research question and eligibility criteria as a quick reference tool for guiding your decisions.

Step 3: Assessing the quality of the literature

At this stage of the review, all eligible papers have been identified. Before the findings of each paper can be combined or synthesised they need to be critically appraised to determine their quality.

Defining 'quality'

'Quality' is a complex concept and is considered in numerous ways. Broadly speaking, it is an attempt to establish how near the truth the findings are likely to be, and how relevant the findings are to a particular setting or population group. It is very important that only those studies that are free from bias and error (or have attempted to reduce or minimise bias and error) are included in a systematic review.

Critical appraisal tools

To critically appraise papers included in a systematic review, a standardised critical appraisal tool is required to ensure that each paper is assessed in the same manner and with the same degree of attention to detail. Numerous validated critical appraisal tools have been published to support researchers with this task. The tool of choice will depend upon the study design(s) of the eligible papers included in the search history. The Critical Appraisal Skills Programme (or CASP) (https://casp-uk.net/casp-tools-checklists) has developed a free downloadable tool for most of the commonly utilised public health research study designs (randomised controlled trials, cohort studies, case-control studies, economic evaluation studies and qualitative research studies). These checklists can be found from the CASP website. An alternative framework that is widely used for assessing the quality of quantitative research is called GRADE (Grading of Recommendations, Assessment, Development and Evaluations) (Guyatt et al., 2011).

Evidence acquired from grey literature sources may differ in content from studies published in traditional academic journals. Where appropriate, it may be useful to locate a critical appraisal tool specifically designed to assess the quality of grey literature. There are many such tools available but the most well known is probably the AACODS checklist, which assesses papers according to six factors: authors' authority in the field; accuracy of reporting; coverage of study parameters and limitations; objectivity of study and consideration of bias; date of study; and study significance in the area of interest. This checklist was devised by researchers at Flinders University and can be found online.

At times, it may be appropriate to adapt a standardised critical appraisal tool to explore a specific aspect of the evidence base under review. This is something that should be discussed within the research team or with your supervisor. Any adaptation of a critical appraisal tool should be piloted with one or two papers included in the review, to ensure that any new questions are appropriate for application across all included papers.

Grading the quality of papers included within the review

To help to quantify the quality of included quantitative studies it is useful to grade or rank each paper. There is no single method for approaching the task of grading and it is a process that should be discussed and agreed upon by the research team.

A commonly used and simple grading system is 'ABC'. This can be applied to all papers, regardless of study design and is defined as such:

- *Studies rated 'A'*: A study that is well conducted and reported upon, with no major quality-based concerns.
- *Studies rated 'B'*: A study that raises quality-based concerns relating to the ways in which the study was conducted or reported, but not serious enough concerns to affect the validity of study findings.
- *Studies rated 'C'*: A study that raises serious concerns about the study design, conduct or reporting that may have negatively affected study validity.

If using this grading system, any study rated 'B' or 'C' should be discussed within the research team and a decision should be made on whether or not to exclude the study on quality-related grounds. If a paper demonstrates a lack of clarity regarding a specific aspect of study methods or results, it can be useful to contact the lead author for further details.

Many journals impose strict word limit restrictions or differ in their conventions for reporting, and this can result in some study details becoming lost at the point of publication.

Traditionally, systematic reviews of qualitative evidence do not include a grading system, as quantification of findings is not the aim of a qualitative systematic review. Despite this, it is useful to reflect upon the quality of eligible studies identified as part of a qualitative review of the evidence.

Ethical considerations for evidence synthesis

Evidence synthesis is a form of secondary research, drawing upon existing, publically available data. As such, formal ethical approval is not required. However, in undertaking an evidence synthesis it is useful to consult guidance on the ethical issues associated with evidence synthesis preparation and reporting (Wager & Wiffen, 2011).

A note on publication bias

Quantitative studies with null (no effect) or negative findings are less likely to be published than those that produce a statistically significant result (Thornton and Lee, 2000). This has serious implications for public health research, as it can distort the picture of the literature in relation to a given topic area, it can influence funding decisions, and it can lead to inappropriate research and teaching practices. When conducting a systematic review, this can be particularly problematic as there is a risk that relevant literature, not published in traditional peer-reviewed journals, is unaccounted for. One strategy to mitigate this is to search the grey literature in addition to electronic databases to try to locate evidence that has not been peer-reviewed. It is important to acknowledge that even by adopting this strategy it is possible that not all relevant literature is identified.

Step 4: Synthesising and interpreting findings

Following the identification and critical appraisal of eligible papers the next stage of the systematic review process is data synthesis. In short, data synthesis aims to bring together findings from different papers to produce an overall summary of the evidence base, whether this be an estimate of effectiveness or prevalence (if combining quantitative studies) or an understanding of a phenomenon (if combining qualitative studies).

Data synthesis consists of three processes:

- To summarise the outcome of the search strategy process.
- To extract data from each of the included studies.
- To combine extracted data in an appropriate manner to produce an overall summary of the evidence base.

Summarising search strategy outcomes

This is a purely descriptive process, providing an overview of the studies identified from searches of electronic databases and the grey literature. The first task is to construct a flowchart detailing how the final number of eligible papers for the systematic review was reached. As can be seen in Figure 12.2, a pathway from the total number of articles identified from the initial search of electronic databases and the grey literature, down to the final number of articles eligible for inclusion in the review, is clearly presented. As previously described, a detailed record of each stage of the search process is essential as it enables the replication of your work.

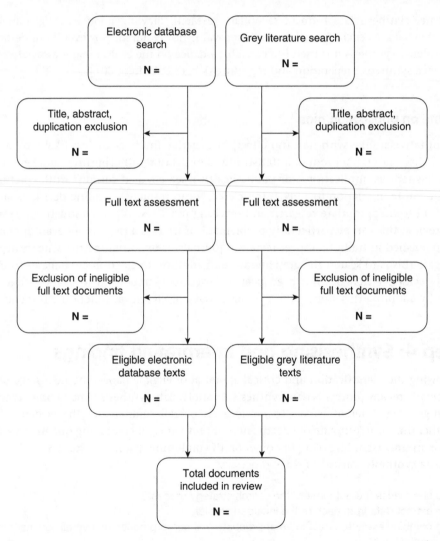

Figure 12.2 Flowchart summarising results from the search strategy

At this point it is also useful to provide a brief overview of the studies included in the review. The detailed specifics of each paper are provided at a later stage so this summary should be clearly and concisely conveyed. This may include the total number of studies eligible for the review, the range of sample size across studies, a description of study country of origin and a general comment on critical appraisal outcomes.

Data extraction

To ensure objectivity in the assessment of each paper, it is important that each paper is considered equally using a standardised approach. When reading included articles, there may be some that stand out more than others, or appear more engaging to personal interest, but it would not be appropriate to place too much emphasis on one paper over another.

Data extraction is the process by which the necessary information about study characteristics and findings from the included studies can be obtained. Extraction of data in a consistent and uniform manner is achieved using a data extraction form. The categories that contribute to a data extraction form are likely to vary from review to review and should be tailored to the review research question. As previously discussed with regards to critical appraisal, if a paper demonstrates a lack of clarity regarding a specific aspect of study methods or results, it can be useful to contact the lead author for further details.

At the very least a data extraction form should contain the following information:

- Study details (author(s), year of publication, country of origin).
- Study methods (study design, number of participants, gender split, recruitment strategy, follow-up procedure(s)).
- Interventions or exposures (what was done, how was it done, over what time period, using what staff or resources).
- Outcome(s) measured (list all outcomes relevant to the research question).
- Results (what was found – only include results relevant to research question, not all results).
- Authors' conclusions (how did the author interpret the results).
- Comments from the reviewer(s). It is common to record here the results from the critical appraisal. It is also useful to demonstrate personal views on the authors' interpretations.

Piloting the data extraction form

As with most aspects of the systematic review process, it is worth spending time piloting a data extraction form with one or two included papers. This is because you will likely find that some categories in the form work well but others do not work well at all. For example, you may find that the information you want to record does not have a designated space, or you may find that the question you are seeking to answer is too broad to allow for a concise response in the space available.

In theory, a good data extraction form should mean that you only have to read the paper once. You take details of all of the relevant information and from that point forward you need only refer to the data extraction sheet and not the full paper. In reality, this is not the case. You are extremely likely to need to return to the paper several times during the course of the review to clarify your understanding about certain aspects of the original research or to obtain information about things that were missed during the first data extraction attempt.

Single or dual data extraction

Reviews conducted by Cochrane require data extraction to be conducted independently by at least two members of a research team. These researchers are blinded to the original study authors and institutions from which the study was published. If conducting a systematic review alone, perhaps for a student dissertation, then this approach is unlikely to be feasible. Lone researchers are often faced with time and resource constraints, and there is a question about whether involving a second researcher in an assessed student project is appropriate. As such, single data extraction is recommended, with the caveat that the lone researcher/ student is explicit in describing the approach utilised and its associated limitations.

Data synthesis and interpretation

The third and final stage of data synthesis involves combining extracted data in an appropriate manner to produce an overall summary of the evidence base. The approach used to synthesise the evidence depends upon the types of studies included in the review and their key characteristics.

Synthesising findings from randomised controlled trials

Systematic reviews published by Cochrane tend to focus on the synthesis of data from randomised controlled trials (RCTs) and cluster-RCTs. However, unlike evidence-based medicine, where RCTs are commonplace, public health research draws upon a range of epidemiological study designs, often because public health research questions cannot always be easily answered using an RCT design (Petticrew, 2009). Conducting systematic reviews of studies applying other study designs is challenging, and there is no single method recommended for combining the results of studies of a qualitative nature or of an observational quantitative design.

Meta-analysis

When reading systematic review papers in the past, you may have come across the phrase 'systematic review with meta-analysis' (for example, Jia et al., 2017; Lavelle et al., 2012). A meta-analysis is a statistical technique used to combine the quantitative data generated from RCTs. The result from a meta-analysis tells you what you might find if each individual study included in the review was merged with the others to create one large RCT.

All systematic reviews collating only RCT and quasi-experimental (or non-randomised controlled trial) data should consider undertaking a meta-analysis. There are numerous software packages available that can be used to perform meta-analysis and the most well known is RevMan (available for download from Cochrane). *The Cochrane Handbook for Systematic Reviews of Interventions* (Higgins and Green (eds) (2011)) also provides very detailed guidance on undertaking meta-analysis. It is important to note that due to differences in study methods and results, a feature frequently observed in public health research, it is not always possible or appropriate to follow this path.

If this approach is deemed to be inappropriate, narrative synthesis is recommended. Narrative synthesis involves presenting an overview of each study included in the review. This can contain more detail than the data extraction table can provide and includes the strengths and weaknesses of the study identified during critical appraisal.

Synthesising findings from observational studies

Some researchers have used meta-analysis methods to pool the findings of observational studies, but the general consensus is that this is poor practice (Greenland, 1994; Ioannidis et al., 2001). This is because observational studies do not randomise participants to different groups, resulting in possible differences between groups that are unknown to the original author or the reviewer, but that account for differences in the original study outcome. The results could, therefore, be due to these differences and not due to the variable of interest. These unknown differences are referred to as 'residual confounding' (see Chapter 1), and for this reason a narrative synthesis of the findings from observational studies is strongly recommended above meta-analysis.

Synthesising findings from qualitative studies

It is not possible to perform any form of statistical analysis on findings from qualitative studies. Combining evidence from qualitative studies is still in its relative infancy, and as yet there is no clear consensus recommending one specific approach. One approach to qualitative evidence synthesis that is gaining traction and support from public health researchers is meta-ethnography; this approach is discussed in more detail in Chapter 13.

Synthesising findings from mixed methods studies

Mixed methods systematic reviews are probably the most contentious form of review, in that there is debate surrounding the best approach for synthesising quantitative and qualitative data. There are three general frameworks put forward by Sandelowski et al. (2006) and presented in detail in The Joanna Briggs Institute *Reviewers' Manual* (2014).

One framework involves the completion of two evidence syntheses, conducted sequentially. This approach is unlikely to be utilised by someone new to evidence synthesis and for this reason it is not discussed further in this chapter. The other two frameworks are:

- *Segregated methodologies*: Quantitative and qualitative research evidence is identified and appraised separately, before being collated in a final mixed methods synthesis. Findings are categorised into 'agree' (quantitative and qualitative findings support each other), 'refute' (they contradict each other), or 'complement' (findings add to each other).
- *Integrated methodologies*: Both quantitative and qualitative data are synthesised together. This occurs either by converting quantitative data into themes, or converting qualitative data into a numerical format for statistical analysis.

Heterogeneity

Heterogeneity is a term that often unnerves people that are new to the concept of evidence synthesis. In lay language, heterogeneity simply means the degree to which studies included in a review are *different* to one another. Conversely, homogeneity is the degree to which studies included in a review are *similar* to each another. When conducting a review, it is the researcher's responsibility to consider whether the overall findings are valid or largely due to variation (heterogeneity) between included studies.

A useful tip for visualising the concept of heterogeneity is to think about fruit. This may sound surprising, but it does actually work! Apples and oranges are two variations of fruit. They differ in colour, texture, shape and taste, but they share the characteristic that they are both a fruit variety. It could be argued that apples and oranges are heterogeneous (because they differ in so many ways), but it could also be argued that they are homogenous (because ultimately, they are both fruits). When applying this concept to a systematic review, the researcher essentially needs to consider the ways in which studies are similar and ways in which they differ.

Purgato and Adams (2012) describe three types of heterogeneity that warrant consideration:

- *Clinical heterogeneity:* Differences in participants, interventions and outcomes studied.
- *Statistical heterogeneity*: Differences in the effects being studied.
- *Methodological heterogeneity*: Differences in study design and risk of bias.

Strengths and weaknesses of the systematic review

When interpreting the findings of a systematic review, it is always useful to ask yourself: Do you believe the findings? In order to answer this question, there is a need to consider how well the review and synthesis truly summarises the body of evidence reviewed. It might help to reflect upon the following:

- How thorough was the search strategy?

- What biases is the review at risk of (e.g. publication bias)?
- What could be done differently if the review were to be repeated in the future?

Strengths and weaknesses of the available evidence

In addition to considering the quality of the review itself, it is also important to reflect upon the strengths and weaknesses of the available evidence. This relates closely to the findings from the critical appraisal and data extraction tasks, in that it should provide an overview highlighting key strengths and weaknesses of the evidence assessed.

Generalisability of the findings of the review

The research question for each systematic review is often very specific to a group of people in a particular setting. Consideration of how the results may apply to different groups of people, in other settings and other circumstances is useful for exploring the generalisability of the review. For example, there may be reasons why the overall results of the review can only be applied to a specific group of people in a particular setting.

Implications of the review

Once all stages of the systematic review procedure are complete, it is useful to take the time to reflect upon the answer to the research question and to consider what the results mean for public health. This could include recommendations on what further research is required and how the findings can be used to influence and improve public health policy and practice.

A note on writing for publication

Developments in guidelines for standardised reporting of research studies have extended to systematic review. The Preferred Reporting Items for Systematic Reviews and Meta-Analyses (or PRISMA) is a checklist of items that should be followed in all systematic review (and meta-analyses) publications. A copy of the checklist is available to download from the Internet.

Conclusion

This chapter has explored the value and relevance of evidence synthesis for public health, with a specific focus on systematic reviews. The chapter includes critical reflection on systematic review methodology, and provides a step-by-step guide to undertaking a systematic review, from conception of the research question through to data synthesis processes and advice on writing up the results of a systematic review for publication.

Two alternative approaches to evidence synthesis, meta-ethnography and realist synthesis are explored in the next chapter.

Further reading

Higgins, J.P.T. and Green, S. (eds) (2011) *Cochrane Handbook for Systematic Reviews of Interventions Version 5.1.0* [updated March 2011]. Available from: http://handbook. cochrane.org.

Pope, C., Mays, N. and Popay, J. (2007) *Synthesizing Qualitative and Quantitative Health Research: A guide to methods.* Oxford: Oxford University Press.

The Joanna Briggs Institute (2014) *The Joanna Briggs Institute Reviewers' Manual 2014: Methodology for JBI Mixed Methods Systematic Review.* Adelaide, Australia.

13 EVIDENCE SYNTHESIS APPROACHES: META-ETHNOGRAPHY AND REALIST SYNTHESIS

━━━━━━━━ CHAPTER SUMMARY ━━━━━━━━

In this chapter we will introduce two less well-established approaches to public health evidence synthesis: **meta-ethnography** and **realist synthesis**. Meta-ethnography is an approach to **evidence synthesis** that involves the **synthesis of qualitative evidence**, while realist synthesis takes a theory-driven approach with the aim of developing **policy**. Through this chapter we will explore the principles and methods of both approaches and we will also consider how these alternative approaches to evidence synthesis can be used to address some of the criticisms associated with traditional systematic reviews (see Chapter 12).

Part 1: Meta-ethnography

Synthesising qualitative evidence – should we even attempt it?

An increased appreciation of the value and importance of qualitative research for enhancing public health knowledge has led to the development of various methods for synthesising qualitative evidence. For example, in Chapter 12 we briefly describe how traditional systematic review methods can be applied to undertake this task. However, as yet, there is no clear consensus in the literature recommending one specific approach. This is because there remains significant debate regarding appropriate terminology and methods that one might use for synthesising qualitative evidence. Furthermore, unlike quantitative research, qualitative studies are often small-scale, interested in theoretical development, and focused on single cases. Ultimately, as we have seen in Part II of this book, qualitative research is about providing analytical depth, not generalisability.

Given the differing epistemological foundations of qualitative compared with quantitative research and the variety of philosophical perspectives and methodological leanings within qualitative research (see Chapter 6), there is a fundamental question about whether it is even appropriate to attempt the task of qualitative evidence synthesis. Dixon-Woods et al. (2005) respond to this question in their review of methods for synthesising qualitative and quantitative methods, identifying a range of strengths associated with a variety of qualitative evidence synthesis methods:

- Can follow a systematic approach while preserving the properties of the original data.
- Can deal with diverse evidence types.
- Can be used for theory building.
- Can seek higher order theories.
- Can be explicitly orientated to testing of theory.

One approach to qualitative evidence synthesis that has received increased attention in recent years for its pragmatic methods is meta-ethnography (Noblit and Hare, 1988). It is this approach that is described and explored below.

Principles of meta-ethnography

Meta-ethnography has become more commonplace in recent years (Atkins et al., 2008), and it is the most widely cited approach for undertaking qualitative evidence synthesis (Campbell et al., 2011). Its predefined and structured methods are often said to resemble those used in quantitative systematic reviews, and, as such, the approach may be particularly appealing to those that are new to evidence synthesis or wanting to mimic the traditional systematic review approach. It also offers some reassurance to qualitative researchers who might be looking to follow a step-by-step process. Having said that, caution is advised when comparing the two approaches; quantitative reviews tend to focus on a specific problem to find a solution, whereas meta-ethnographic reviews seek to translate evidence from numerous qualitative studies to better understand a phenomenon or to identify gaps in the evidence base. Unlike traditional systematic reviews, which often attempt to quantify aspects of research according to statistical outcomes, meta-ethnography proposes a new approach in which meaning is preserved through the appreciation of original study data and the associated interpretations of these data.

Seven steps to undertaking a meta-ethnography

Noblit and Hare describe seven steps to undertaking a meta-ethnography, each of which is described in more detail below and in Table 13.1. The steps provide a useful framework for initiating a meta-ethnography and they have been praised for allowing researchers to collate qualitative evidence on a similar topic, to provide a new interpretation and summary of the evidence base, and to apply interpretations to improve existing policies and interventions or to generate new ones. However, it is important to recognise that since publication of the framework, some researchers have encountered difficulties in interpreting and applying the steps to qualitative research. This has resulted in some researchers utilising alternative approaches to reach the final step of evidence synthesis. In this chapter, we highlight a variety of methods used at each step of the process and we consider their strengths and weaknesses. In line with the overarching message of this textbook, we broadly advocate utilising the most pragmatic and practical methods to achieve research aims. You may wish to read two very helpful articles alongside this chapter. Atkins et al. (2008) and Britten et al. (2002) have both published worked examples in which they describe their experiences of applying meta-ethnography processes with regard to two health-related topics.

Table 13.1   Seven steps to meta-ethnography

Step	
1	**Getting started**
2	**Deciding what is relevant to the initial interest**
3	**Reading the studies**
4	**Determining how the studies are related**
5	**Translating the studies into one another**
6	**Synthesising translations**
7	**Expressing the synthesis**

Source: Noblit and Hare, 1988

Step One: Getting started

The importance of defining the scope of a review, regardless of methodological approach, cannot be underestimated. The careful and considered development of a research question is integral to good quality evidence synthesis. In Chapter 12 we describe the PICOS (Population, Intervention, Comparator, Outcome, Study design) framework, a well-used and useful strategy for formulating research questions. However, as meta-ethnography is concerned with qualitative and not quantitative evidence, it can be argued that the traditional PICOS framework has limited utility. As such, in recent years researchers have devised a variety of frameworks designed to aid the conceptualisation of qualitative research questions and many of these are available to view and download via the Internet. For example, there is the PICo framework (Population, phenomena of Interest, Context), which considers the population of interest, the phenomena (or issue) of interest, and the wider context within which the individual or group is located. There is also the SPIDER framework (Sample, Phenomenon of Interest, Design, Evaluation, Research type), which considers numerous aspects of research design and evaluation. An example, demonstrating the application of the PICo framework can be found in Box 13.1.

BOX 13.1   APPLICATION OF THE PICo FRAMEWORK

Research question: What are the experiences of community-based peer counsellors that promote exclusive breastfeeding (EBF) in sub-Saharan Africa?

- *Population:* Peer counsellors providing advice and support on exclusive breastfeeding
- *Phenomena of Interest:* Experience of providing advice and support on exclusive breast-feeding
- *Context:* Community-based interventions in sub-Saharan Africa

---

Step Two: Deciding what is relevant to the initial interest

The identification of strict eligibility criteria for meta-ethnography is contested, with some researchers advocating for traditional qualitative methods which may involve sampling to the point of data saturation (see Chapter 7) with researchers making their own judgements as to eligibility, while others suggest that a transparent and reproducible approach is important if the aim of the meta-ethnography is to be considered systematic. In light of limited guidance on how to establish saturation when undertaking an evidence review, we suggest that the breadth of the meta-ethnography is clearly defined in terms of eligibility criteria and search methods undertaken. If conducting a meta-ethnography for a student project, this is likely to be the most appropriate approach, as it will allow you to present clearly the boundaries of your work and demonstrate the comprehensive nature of the review you have undertaken. Having said that, a discussion of the merits of each of the different perspectives would be beneficial to demonstrate your critical understanding. At this point, it may be useful to refer back to Chapter 12, sections, *'Inclusion and exclusion criteria'* and *'Searching the literature'*, for guidance on how to search the electronic and grey literature.

As discussed in Chapter 12, traditional systematic reviews entail an explicit search for the 'best available' evidence related to a pre-defined topic. Studies that are of poor methodological quality are generally treated with caution, or excluded from the review altogether, due to their possible negative influence on the overall findings and conclusions of a systematic review. In the case of meta-ethnography, there remains debate about whether eligible qualitative studies *could* or *should* be assessed according to their quality.

Issues commonly observed in quantitative research, such as bias, are not always applicable to qualitative research and, as such, there is no consensus on which tools could and should be used to assess the quality of qualitative studies, if they are to be appraised at all. It is also important to acknowledge that reporting conventions for qualitative research may differ according to methodology. For example, ethnographic research is known for under-reporting methods in some journals. From our perspective, to generate trustworthy findings that are applicable and of value to public health policy and practice, an assessment of study quality is essential. Furthermore, if undertaking a meta-ethnography for a student project, evidence of skills in quality appraisal will showcase your critical analysis abilities.

In accordance with recommendations made in Chapter 12, the Critical Appraisal Skills Programme (CASP) tool, designed to assess the quality of qualitative studies, provides a good starting point. The CASP tool contains ten questions to determine qualitative study credibility and trustworthiness, and important features of qualitative research. Unlike traditional systematic reviews, where studies ranked poorly are removed from the final list of eligible studies, the removal of qualitative studies on poor quality reporting grounds from meta-ethnography is not advised. Researchers have suggested that the process of removing studies could be considered 'over-rigorous' and 'counterproductive' (Atkins et al., 2008: 5). Furthermore, the identification of, and reflection on, the findings from poor quality qualitative studies may still make an important contribution to the overall interpretation of findings reported.

Step Three: Reading the studies

Step Three is chiefly concerned with familiarising oneself with the eligible studies identified through your search of the literature. 'Familiarisation' in the case of meta-ethnography does not simply involve reading the studies, but also includes a consideration of original study aims and objectives, the study context, the quality of the research, and a reflection on the findings reported. At this stage we recommend utilising the data extraction process described in detail in Chapter 12: 'Data extraction'. Data extraction involves the recording of standardised information from each study included in a review. The process is objective and gives equal weighting to each study. As seen for traditional quantitative systematic reviews, the categories included on a data extraction form are likely to require tailoring from one review to the next. Guidance suggests that in the case of meta-ethnography, the data extraction form should include space for extracting information on metaphors, themes, interpretations, and concepts that emerged in the reporting of original studies. This may include extraction of specific verbatim quotations, although this may not always be possible if a large number of eligible studies has been identified. The broad purpose of this stage is to begin to determine how studies are (or are not) related to each other and to begin to contemplate how best to approach the synthesis of evidence.

Following the data extraction process, some advocates for meta-ethnography support the process of developing what are known as first-, second- and third-order constructs

(Schutz, 1971) to aid analysis of qualitative studies (see Table 13.2). However, other researchers have reported difficulties in applying these constructs effectively to their research. For example, in 2008 Atkins et al. published a paper reporting that first-order constructs were difficult to obtain as the full participant experience is rarely conveyed in a research article. It was also noted that the identification of second-order constructs was difficult to decipher as the findings reported in qualitative studies are often descriptive and do not offer much, if any, additional insight into the phenomena under investigation. Here, we recommend that the application of Schutz's constructs is taken on a case-by-case basis as the suitability of this method is likely to depend on the extent and quality of eligible evidence for each specific meta-ethnography.

Table 13.2 First-, second- and third-order constructs

Construct	Definition
First-order interpretation	Constructs that reflect participants' understandings, as reported in the included studies (usually found in the results section of an article).
Second-order interpretation	Interpretations of participants' understandings made by authors of these studies (and usually found in the discussion and conclusion section of an article).
Third-order interpretation	The synthesis of both first- and second-order constructs into a new model or theory about a phenomenon.

Source: Shutz, 1971, in Atkins et al., 2008

To illustrate how this might look in practice, let's return to the research question identified earlier in Box 13.1:

'What are the experiences of community-based peer counsellors that promote exclusive breast-feeding (EBF) in sub-Saharan Africa?'

Table 13.3 presents three hypothetical examples of synthesised first- and second-order constructs and shows how they could be used to generate a new theory about promoting exclusive breastfeeding in sub-Saharan Africa.

Step Four: Determining how the studies are related

Once all of the studies have been read and data extracted, it is helpful to map out all of the concepts and themes identified from each study onto one page. Visualising the concepts and themes in this way can aid identification and interpretation of new themes and ideas that may be relevant across studies, and it may highlight conflicting findings from

Table 13.3   First-, second- and third-order interpretations

First- and second-order interpretations	Third-order interpretations
Following training, EBF counsellors demonstrated: • improved knowledge of EBF, including benefits and risks • increased awareness of common EBF issues • ability to demonstrate EBF techniques.	Counsellors gained adequate knowledge and skills related to EBF.
Following training, EBF counsellors: • expressed satisfaction at knowledge gain • felt 'uplifted status' within the community • felt confidence in their abilities.	Counsellors were empowered by training and support.
EBF implementation affected by: • cultural and religious beliefs associated with EBF • fear of HIV diagnosis disclosure • fear of retribution in difficult social/political circumstances • access to women in isolated areas.	Counsellors are faced with a range of socio-environmental barriers and facilitators to successful intervention implementation.

study to study. If you have numerous eligible studies in your meta-ethnography then sometimes it can be hard to 'see the wood for the trees'; this mapping exercise can really help to drill down to identify the most important or relevant content within the studies included in your review.

Noblit and Hare (1988) describe three ways to approach this task:

- Reciprocal translation
- Line of argument
- Refutational translation

On first look, these typologies may sound rather intimidating, particularly if you are new to reviewing evidence. However, once explained in plain English, they are much easier to understand and apply in practice.

- *Reciprocal translation* is when a researcher identifies similar metaphors and concepts across studies. The findings from each individual study are understood in terms of how they relate to other studies eligible for inclusion.
- *Line of argument* is when a researcher takes all studies together to construct and interpret findings that go beyond the initial findings presented in each individual study. This typology

involves explicit identification of, and reflection on, the similarities and differences apparent across included studies.

- *Refutational translation* is when a researcher identifies concepts and themes across studies that directly refute or contradict each other. Notably, this typology is rarely used and published examples of how it has been applied in practice are rare.

Depending on the types of studies identified, it is possible to utilise more than one typology during analysis. Atkins et al. advise that researchers wishing to achieve a 'higher order interpretation' could develop a more in-depth theoretical understanding of a collection of studies if *reciprocal translation* is followed by *line of argument* analysis (Atkins et al., 2008: 7). For a real-world example we recommend Britten et al. (2002).

Step Five: Translating the studies into one another

Noblit and Hare's (1988) methods for translating studies into one another have been interpreted and applied in different ways by different researchers. In the original guidance, researchers are encouraged to compare the themes and metaphors (while also considering the study context) from study one to study two, and so on until all themes and metaphors are exhausted and a final translation emerges. In recent years, however, questions have arisen about how to actively apply this process in practice.

One article offers a pragmatic solution to undertaking study translation (Atkins et al., 2008). The three stages of study translation are described in brief below:

- Studies are initially arranged chronologically to encourage researchers to reflect upon changes over time in public health policy and practice and to consider how these changes may have influenced study findings.
- Next, themes and concepts from each study are examined, with the aim of merging and refining themes to reflect the broader body of evidence. To increase the credibility of findings, dual translation by two independent researchers is recommended. However, as highlighted in Chapter 12, independent assessment is not always possible, or appropriate for student projects. As such, we recommend single translation alongside explicit reporting of the approach taken, including consideration of the strengths and weaknesses of this approach.
- Finally, researchers are encouraged to reflect upon the socio-ecological context of each study and to consider how this might have influenced study findings. This is recognised as one of the more difficult tasks to complete as journal articles are traditionally constrained by a strict word limit, meaning that wider contextual details relating to a study are often missing. Available space is used instead to convey details on other features of the research that may be considered more important or relevant than context.

Step Six: Synthesising translations

It is widely acknowledged that the process of moving from translation to synthesis is not easy. In developing a synthesis of translations (this may also be referred to as *third-order interpretation* in the literature) lone researchers are encouraged to map themes derived from earlier analysis against any new interpretations that have emerged during the review process. Themes are merged to create final interpretations, which capture similarities and differences across studies while also preserving the original findings reported by authors.

Step Seven: Expressing the synthesis

The final stage of the meta-ethnography involves dissemination of the findings, considering the needs of the audience. Some researchers have suggested that it may be useful to generate a diagram of the findings. Providing a simplified visual representation of the findings may enhance their accessibility to a wider audience and highlight key messages for policy and practice. However, it is important to acknowledge that an over-simplification of findings may lose some of the contextual details surrounding the body of evidence, details that are considered integral to the credibility of qualitative research. As such, we recommend a joint approach that includes a summary diagram alongside a full and detailed description of the findings from the meta-ethnography. If conducting a meta-ethnography for a student project, a detailed description of the findings is essential.

A note on writing for publication

Reporting guidelines (eMERGe) designed to improve the reporting standards of meta-ethnographic reviews are available to download from the Internet (France et al., 2015). It is advisable to follow these guidelines if you intend to write up your findings for publication.

Part 2: Realist synthesis

The second part of this chapter is concerned with realist synthesis, a theory-driven and alternative approach to evidence synthesis. Realist synthesis attempts to better understand not only 'what works', something we might seek to examine through traditional systematic review methods, but to explore 'what works, for whom under what circumstances, how and why' (Pawson and Tilley, 2004). This relatively new approach to evidence synthesis is particularly appealing to public health professionals as it goes beyond traditional approaches and explicitly explores the contextual factors influencing how and why interventions are deemed to be effective, or not.

A critique of traditional systematic reviews

As explained in Chapter 12, systematic reviews are highly regarded in public health circles due to their collation of the best available evidence on a pre-defined topic. The evidence included in a good quality systematic review should be robust and have a low risk of bias, allowing researchers to draw clear conclusions from the data. Numerous examples of published systematic reviews from the literature have been used to make the case for the reallocation of funds, to identify gaps in the evidence base and, most importantly, to improve specific public health outcomes.

However, despite their benefits, the rigid and often uncompromising methods for conducting systematic reviews have been criticised for failing to recognise the complexity of interventions and their possible range of outcomes. Let's return to the example provided in Chapter 12: a systematic review examining the evidence for the effectiveness of insecticide-treated mosquito nets (ITNs) on reducing all-cause child mortality in sub-Saharan Africa. The findings of such a review may indicate a positive reduction in all-cause child mortality in sub-Saharan Africa as a result of the implementation of ITNs. This is good news! However, the findings are unlikely to tell us how ITNs work, in which specific contexts they are most effective, and how health-related outcomes may differ according to socio-economic groupings within sub-Saharan Africa. It is in response to these concerns that realist synthesis has emerged as an alternative approach to evidence synthesis.

Principles of realist synthesis

The term 'realist synthesis' first appeared in the published literature in 2002 (Pawson, 2002), and since then a number of key documents have been published (Pawson et al., 2004). The approach aims to generate evidence about interventions and their outcomes that goes further than evidence reported in systematic reviews. Simply put, realist synthesis methods can be used to begin to unpick how features of intervention design and implementation may influence a variety of intervention outcomes.

The purpose of realist synthesis is to articulate, test and refine 'programme theories' about how and why a programme (or intervention) works. Programme theories reflect the underlying assumptions about *how* an intervention is supposed to work *in a range of contexts* to lead to desired outcomes. Realist synthesis is, therefore, concerned with better understanding the relationship(s) between contexts, mechanisms and outcomes. The consideration of context and mechanism in realist synthesis is the key feature which sets it apart from traditional systematic reviews, where the outcome of interest is the main (and often only) focus of the review.

If you are just getting to grips with the concept of evidence synthesis, you may be pleased to learn that many of the essential steps followed when conducting a systematic review (as described in Chapter 12) are also involved when it comes to conducting a realist synthesis. Having said that, there are important philosophical and methodological distinctions between traditional systematic reviews and realist synthesis, and so it is important to ensure that you are familiar with each approach before pursuing your own synthesis.

Although realist synthesis as a method is newer and less well specified than the traditional systematic review there is an ever-increasing body of guidance on how to do them.

Key guidance documents include Pawson et al.'s (2004) *Realist Synthesis: An Introduction*, produced for the ESRC Research Methods programme, which gives a step-by-step guide to the stages of a realist synthesis. Wong et al. (2013) have published information on publication standards when conducting realist synthesis. Published examples of good quality realist syntheses of public health evidence include Kane et al. (2010), Wong et al. (2011) and Rycroft-Malone et al. (2012). It is worth looking at each of these documents alongside this chapter.

Important terminology

At first glance, the idea of undertaking a realist synthesis may seem rather daunting. Much of the terminology linked with the approach is likely to feel new and this is not something that instils confidence in one's abilities! However, as with most terminology, once it has been broken down and communicated in simpler language it is often easier to understand. Here, two central concepts of realist synthesis – 1) programme theories and 2) context, mechanisms and outcomes – are described.

Programme theories

From the realist perspective, programme theories are the ways in which intervention developers think an intervention is going to work to lead to desired outcomes. Programme theories are often unstated by researchers, and reflect underlying assumptions about how an intervention is supposed to work. When undertaking realist synthesis, the researcher seeks to identify a range of programme theories to understand how interventions work (or don't work) in a particular context and how this relates to intervention outcomes. Box 13.2 contains a simple example.

BOX 13.2 IDENTIFYING PROGRAMME THEORIES: AN EXAMPLE

Imagine you have been tasked with conducting a realist synthesis of a school-based peer-support intervention designed to reduce the incidence of sexually transmitted infections (STIs). What might you consider to be a programme theory or assumption about how this intervention works?

The influence of peers on young people's attitudes and behaviours is well researched in the literature. As such, you might theorise that a sexual health intervention developed and delivered through peers is going to work in a school setting because young people would rather listen and respond to their peers or 'people like me', than to other figures in their lives that they may not relate to in the same way, such as teachers or parents.

The example in Box 13.2 is just one programme theory (or assumption) about how the school-based peer-support intervention might work to reduce the incidence of STIs. When undertaking a full realist synthesis, you are encouraged to explore and identify as many programme theories as you can.

Context, mechanisms and outcomes (CMOs)

We have seen earlier on in this book that traditional systematic reviews are often concerned with identifying 'what works'. In other words, they may seek to clarify if a pre-specified intervention (e.g. a school-based peer-support intervention) has an impact on a pre-defined outcome (e.g. reducing STIs). Taking this example, you can probably see that it is useful to know if the school-based intervention is associated with a reduction in STIs as this would have important implications for future funding and improving public health outcomes. However, when approaching evaluations from a realist perspective, we would also want to know more about the setting within which an intervention is being implemented (context) and the features of the intervention that have influenced the outcomes (mechanisms). Taking this example, we might consider the existing sexual health provision in schools, if pupils have access to contraception, and if parents and teachers are jointly committed in their support for reducing STIs. These are all examples of intervention *context*. From a realist perspective, we would also want to know if sexual health knowledge, attitudes and behaviours have changed in response to the intervention. These are examples of intervention *mechanisms*. In realist synthesis, an appreciation of the context (C), mechanisms (M) and outcomes (O) of an intervention is essential if we are to better understand what works, for whom under what circumstances, how and why (Pawson and Tilley, 2004).

Six steps to undertaking a realist synthesis

Step One: Clarifying the scope of the review

Developing research questions and refining the purpose of the review

In Chapter 12 we explored how to develop a clear and coherent research question for undertaking a systematic review using the PICOs framework, and earlier in this chapter the PICo and SPIDER frameworks were introduced. Although for realist synthesis it is important to define the parameters of a review, the philosophical standpoint of the approach means that the process of identifying a research question is less well defined in the literature and can be more time consuming than other synthesis approaches. As we have seen, with realist synthesis it is not simply about examining whether an intervention works, it is also about considering the 'who', 'what', 'why', 'when' and 'how'.

Guidance recommends that a team of researchers and interested stakeholders develop the research questions. This is not always possible, but, as with other forms of evidence synthesis, it is important to discuss ideas with others to ensure that the scope of the proposed research is feasible to conduct in the time you have available. A pragmatic approach that stays true to the central principles of realist synthesis involves the development of a series of research questions that explicitly refer to programme theories, context and mechanisms. Let's take the above example that refers to a school-based peer-led intervention designed to reduce the incidence of STIs (Box 13.3).

BOX 13.3 DEVELOPING THE RESEARCH QUESTION FOR REALIST SYNTHESIS

Research question 1: What are the *programme theories* that best describe how school-based peer-led interventions might work to reduce the incidence of sexually transmitted infections (STIs)?

Research question 2: What are the most important *mechanisms* by which school-based peer-led interventions designed to reduce the incidence of STIs are thought to produce effective outcomes?

Research question 3: What *contextual* factors associated with school-based peer-led interventions designed to reduce the incidence of STIs augment or decrease the impact of these mechanisms?

The examples presented in Box 13.3 are less rigid than those we might see for a systematic review or meta-ethnography, but they do have clear boundaries, which help to ensure that focus is maintained as the research progresses.

Step Two: Articulating programme theories to be explored

The next step before conducting a full search of the evidence is to generate a list of key programme theories that might explain how and why an intervention works. This theory-driven process identifies the assumptions that underpin an intervention and involves the researcher drawing upon a range of sources, from published academic literature utilising a variety of study designs, to grey literature sources, to discussions with stakeholders or experts in the field. Some theories will be firmly rooted in the literature and based on robust data, while other assumptions may feel more anecdotal or based on your intuition. At this stage you should attempt to record all theories from all sources that are of interest. Ultimately, you will generate a long list of programme theories that may explain why an intervention is or is not successful. This initial list is unlikely to be exhaustive and will evolve as the review progresses.

Step Three: Searching for relevant evidence

When you have finished articulating programme theories to be explored, the next stage of the realist synthesis involves a comprehensive search of the literature. This stage of the realist synthesis is considered to be the 'official' search for evidence and will require detailed reporting in any write-up (see later in this chapter for guidance on reporting).

As we have seen previously, unlike traditional systematic reviews that involve a tightly constructed research question, realist syntheses tend to include a complex research question or many questions. This means that searching the literature to locate relevant and rigorous evidence requires extra thought. With realist synthesis a purposive approach, in which the researcher uses their judgement to search the evidence base, is advocated in the guidance. However, like meta-ethnography, there remains some debate about how wide to cast one's search net. Some suggest searching until a point of data saturation – a point when no new evidence adds to your understanding – while others suggest that a pragmatic reproducible search strategy is the best way forward. The approach you take will depend on the availability of literature related to your chosen topic area and your capacity to conduct a thorough search. With student projects, sometimes it is simply not possible to search until the point of data saturation, due to time and resource constraints. Either way, guidance encourages researchers to search in an iterative and interactive way, with frequent reference back to the research question(s) and initial programme theories to check that you remain on track.

The process of locating relevant and rigorous evidence via electronic databases and grey literature sources is the same as that used for systematic reviews and meta-ethnography. At this point, it may be useful to refer back to Chapter 12, sections *'Inclusion and exclusion criteria'* and *'Searching the literature'*, for advice on locating evidence, sifting and management of evidence.

Step Four: Assessing the quality of the evidence

As discussed earlier on in this book, the concept of 'quality' and how to assess it is widely contested. In systematic reviews, researchers are encouraged to think about quality in terms of freedom from bias or error (see Chapter 12). For meta-ethnography, quantitative concepts of bias and error do not apply, and so alternative quality assessment tools can be applied. With respect to realist synthesis, another approach to assessing the quality of the evidence base has emerged: the quality of evidence is considered according to *relevance* and *rigour* (Pawson, 2002: 22) (see Table 13.4).

Table 13.4 Relevance and rigour defined

Term	Definition
Relevance	Whether evidence can contribute to theory building and/or testing
Rigour	Whether the method used to generate that particular piece of data is credible and trustworthy

Guidance on assessing evidence according to relevance and rigour indicates that the process is far removed from completing a standard quality appraisal tool (e.g. CASP):

- A range of evidence utilising many study designs is likely to emerge through the realist synthesis process.
- It does not reduce the quality appraisal process to a series of 'yes/no' responses that may lose sight of the complexity of the original research question(s) under investigation.
- It accepts that the evidence base will have flaws but that the limitations will likely be overcome by information identified in other eligible documentation.

If undertaking realist synthesis for a research project, this would be the time to meet with your supervisor or project team to discuss your thoughts and approach to critical appraisal. If you are short of time and/or resources, you may lack confidence about how you have approached this task; this is where a supervisor or project team will be able to provide help and advice.

Step Five: Synthesising and interpreting the findings

Aspects of the data extraction process described in Chapter 12, section *'Data extraction'*, provide a useful starting point for understanding how to approach data synthesis. As a minimum, it is good practice to record the following details from each piece of evidence, where possible:

- Study details (author(s), year of publication, country of origin)
- Study methods (study design, number of participants, gender split, recruitment strategy, follow-up procedure(s))

Beyond this initial extraction, it is possible that bespoke forms will need to be developed depending on the range of evidence to be considered. Each researcher may approach this differently, but one approach could be to annotate and code each piece of evidence, highlighting sections or quotations that support or refute your initial programme theories and proposed context, mechanisms and outcomes (CMOs). Some researchers choose to do this by hand using lots of different colours to present their coding strategy while others prefer to use computer software packages such as NVivo to organise their thoughts (Blair, 2015). This is a matter of personal preference, and unfortunately none of these approaches is less time consuming than another.

At this stage you may find that potentially relevant documentation is cited in eligible documentation that you have not previously identified; this provides a good opportunity to widen your search and adhere to the iterative process supported when undertaking realist synthesis. As with systematic reviews and meta-ethnography, you will inevitably return to each document many times to clarify your understanding or to obtain additional information. Throughout this process, you must be sure to record your thinking. Your opinions, perceptions and possible changes over time in these are important and will help to generate a coherent synthesis. You will start to refine your programme theories as the data extraction process progresses, and it is likely that you will draw new assumptions from the data. Guidance indicates that findings can be used in a range of ways: 1) to explore programme theories, 2) to compare contested theories, 3) to consider programme theory in a range of settings, or 4) to examine expected intervention outcomes with actual outcomes.

Step Six: Drawing conclusions and making recommendations

A realist synthesis does not seek to provide a definitive explanation of the complexity of an intervention. Ultimately, realist synthesis begins with a list of programme theories and ends with a refined theory that aids understanding and explanation of 'what works, for whom under what circumstances, how and why' (Pawson and Tilley, 2004). When making recommendations to policy-makers, guidance on realist synthesis stresses the importance of highlighting contextual issues and how these may influence the outcomes of an intervention. At this point, we encourage looking back at Chapter 12, which provides guidance on content to include in the discussion section of your thesis, report or manuscript.

A note on writing for publication

Publication standards for realist synthesis (RAMESES) are freely available to download from the Internet (Wong et al., 2013). Following these guidelines is recommended if you intend to write up your work for publication.

Conclusion

This chapter has introduced two alternative and less well-established approaches to evidence synthesis; namely, meta-ethnography and realist synthesis. Meta-ethnography is explicitly focused on the synthesis of evidence from qualitative research, using predefined and structured methods, with the aim of translating evidence from qualitative studies to better understand a phenomenon or identify gaps in the evidence. Realist synthesis, on the other hand, aims to go beyond traditional approaches to evidence synthesis to explore the contextual factors that influence how and why interventions are deemed to be effective, or not. The principles and methods associated with these approaches have been critically explored in the context of public health, and advice and guidance has been given on their practical application.

Further reading

Atkins, S., Lewin, S., Smith, H., Engel, M., Fretheim, A. and Volmink, J. (2008) Conducting a meta-ethnography of qualitative literature: Lessons learnt. *BMC Medical Research Methodology*, 8: 21.

Britten, N., Campbell, R., Pope, C., Donovan, J., Morgan, M. and Pill, R. (2002) Using meta-ethnography to synthesise qualitative research: A worked example. *Journal of Health Services Research and Policy*, 7(4): 209–15.

Noblit, G.W. (1988) *Meta-ethnography: Synthesizing qualitative studies*. Newbury Park, CA: Sage.

Pawson, R. and Tilley, N. (2004) Realist Evaluation. Available from: www.community-matters.com.au/RE_chapter.pdf.

PART 4

APPLYING RESEARCH TO PUBLIC HEALTH PRACTICE

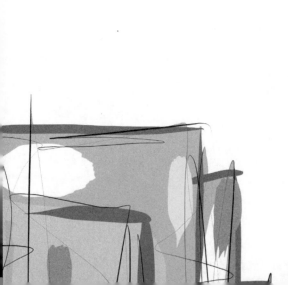

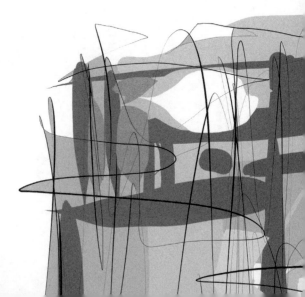

14 THE ETHICS OF PUBLIC HEALTH RESEARCH

════════════ CHAPTER SUMMARY ════════════

This chapter highlights how **ethical issues** are central to **public health research**. The core principles that underpin ethical research are explored, including some of the key challenges public health researchers encounter in seeking to tackle a **research problem**. Much-discussed, historical cases of global public health research are set in context, and the relationship between **medical ethics** and public health is explored.

Key ethical principles in research

The twentieth century saw the development of specific ethical principles, conventions and international declarations for scientific studies carried out with humans. Notably, this included the Nuremberg Code (1947) about the dangers and limits to human experimentation, the European Convention on Human Rights (1949), the Declaration of Helsinki (WMA 1964, revised 2013), the Belmont Report (1978) summarising core ethical principles, and the CIOMS International Ethical Guidelines for Biomedical Research Involving Human Subjects (2002). These have helped shape the ethical guidelines and codes of practice that are drawn up and developed today around research with human participants, particularly in the medical and health science fields.

BOX 14.1 RESEARCH GOVERNANCE/RESEARCH ETHICS?

Research governance refers to the broad range of regulations, principles and standards of good practice that ensure high-quality research. It is an umbrella term that relates to

(Continued)

(Continued)

matters of accountability, ownership and conduct of research. Attending to governance, therefore, means taking responsibility for the quality and impact of the research. Research activities involve varying degrees of 'risk' to any party involved or affected.

Research ethics are established principles governing the way all research is designed, managed and conducted. These include principles of dignity, rights, safety and wellbeing that must be considered, respected and actively managed. Research will normally be judged for its ethical quality in terms of whether it is justifiable, whether it is of adequate standard, whether it poses acceptable risks and how these are managed, whether it complies with statutory and regulatory protocols, whether data management and handling are compliant with national and international legislation, and whether the research is feasible.

Contemporary developments in research governance and ethics have arisen partly due to historical precedents, particularly the atrocities committed – in the name of research – by Nazi doctors during the Second World War, who were later tried for war crimes in the infamous Doctors' Trial known also as the 'medical case' (Annas and Grodin, 1992). Although the majority of this research was carried out by medical staff, the implications were seen more widely across the medical, health and social sciences. In the code of practice developed by the War Crimes Tribunal (*Nuremberg Code,* 1947) and further refined in the *Declaration of Helsinki* (WMA, 2013) a key set of principles were agreed upon, such as that no research should use human beings against their will, either by force/coercion or deception – research participation should be voluntary (Katz, 1992). Moreover, even if individuals provide informed consent, research should not expose them to undue risk of harm.

The ancient medical oath of *Hippocrates*, written in *c.*425 BC, stated that 'above all else [we should] seek to do no harm', and in the cases that led to the conventions described above, as well as many others that have been documented in the medical fields (Wooton, 2006), we can see that this approach was not taken. Today, research involving human participants in any research field is heavily regulated and governed by three core principles: *autonomy, beneficence* and *justice* (discussed later in the chapter).

Do no harm

Like medicine, public health takes as one of its central tenets that decisions should be evidence based. Just as a GP discussing treatment options with a patient should be using the best available evidence about likely outcomes to inform those discussions, we expect policy makers who decide how best to spend health and social care budgets to be using the best available evidence. This also applies to the wider determinants of health – housing, planning, transport, and environmental health. It is arguably of greater importance when discussing population rather than individual health, since it involves decisions about the expenditure of large amounts of public money. If these decisions are not evidence based then we can also argue that it is not ethical – we are not doing the best that we can for the population with the resources that we have. There is never going to be a bottomless pit of money for health and social care, and reductions in budgets simply mean we should be even more careful to make the best use possible of the resources that we do have.

We also expect a GP presenting us with treatment options to warn us about the possible side effects of any treatment, so that we can weigh that up in our decision-making about the best treatment for us as an individual. What is crucial here is the acknowledgment that interventions can have harmful effects. Policy-makers, too, should consider that their policies could have negative effects, some of them unforeseen. This is a very good reason for piloting any intervention programme before rolling it out on a wider scale. One of the problems with this, for public health, is that just as the benefits of interventions are often long term, so may the negative effects be, so it can be hard to pick them up in a pilot. A common side effect of public health interventions to be aware of is widening inequalities. This happens because of differential take-up of interventions – though they are often aimed at the least well-off, they may be taken up more readily by those that need the service least. An example of this would be initiatives such as *Sure Start* and *Book Start* in the UK.

BOX 14.2   DO PUBLIC HEALTH INTERVENTIONS WIDEN INEQUALITIES?

Sure Start, first implemented in 1999, provided early years support to young families through children's centres. Though initially targeted at the 20% poorest wards in England, it was hard to ensure that those who most needed support actually attended and benefited.

Book Start, founded in 1992, gives books to young children through health visitors and libraries. It is based on the premise that promoting reading from a young age will have important benefits in terms of development and future life chances. An evaluation has concluded that the intervention makes the most difference for those families that were not regularly reading with their child (Hines and Brooks, 2009: 24), but despite this it is most likely to have appealed to parents who already placed a high value on books.

Developing interventions that do not widen inequalities is a real challenge for public health.

Widening inequalities is one thing, but there are also interventions that do no good to any one, and actually do harm. We would not expect our GP to prescribe us a treatment if there was no evidence that it would improve our condition, and in fact there was evidence that it could do harm, but that can happen all too easily in policy making. A documentary broadcast in the USA in 1978, called 'Scared Straight', showed young delinquents brought face-to-face with convicted criminals, the idea being that this would encourage them to cease their anti-social behaviour. The idea was popular and led to a series of 'Scared Straight' interventions across the USA. Though early observational studies suggested positive effects, a meta-analysis of RCTs carried out in 2002 concluded that such programmes actively increased crime rates (Petrosino et al., 2002). Those who received the intervention were more likely to commit a crime than those who didn't.

In 2004, the Washington State Institute estimated that every dollar spent on these programmes incurred costs of $204 (Aos et al., 2004). Despite this, the programmes continued to be used. The systematic review was therefore updated in 2013 and showed similar results (Petrosino et al., 2013). The authors concluded that, 'programs such as "Scared Straight" increase delinquency relative to doing nothing at all to similar youths. Given these results, we cannot recommend this program as a crime prevention strategy. Agencies that permit such programs…must rigorously evaluate them, to ensure that they do not cause more harm than good to the very citizens they pledge to protect' (p.2).

This statement illustrates nicely the point made by Iain Chalmers, 'Because professionals sometimes do more harm than good when they intervene in the lives of other people, their policies and practices should be informed by rigorous, transparent, up-to-date evaluations' (Chalmers, 2003, p. 2).

Conflict of interest

There are other ways that professionals can do more harm than good, and often in partnership with industry and corporations that have a vested interest in limiting the impact of public health evidence in the areas of consumer behaviour, and in influencing policy making and implementation (Oreskes and Conway, 2010; White and Bero, 2010). Conflict of interest refers to the ways in which interests, particularly those around industry, interfere in the scientific objectivity, and values, of public health research. In the following we highlight high-profile examples (tobacco-control and soft drinks) of the corporate and industry influence on public health science, research and policy-making, but other industry sectors have been identified, such as chemicals, gambling, alcohol and pharmaceuticals (Babor and Robaina, 2013; Jernigan, 2011; Lexchin et al., 2003).

The tobacco industry

An important example where conflict of interest has been concealed, in an effort to manipulate the evidence base, is in the area of research relating to passive smoking (or second-hand smoke, SHS) and health. Although there has been a growing body of evidence since the 1970s that passive smoking is harmful to health, the literature on SHS reveals a particularly polarised debate. It has become clear following the release of internal tobacco industry documents (as a result of legal settlement in the USA) that the tobacco industry has fuelled controversy in this area by covertly sponsoring research aimed at undermining the links between SHS and ill-health (Drope and Chapman, 2001; Lee et al., 2004; Malone and Balbach, 2000). One example of tobacco industry activities is 'Project Whitecoat', in which the tobacco industry paid researchers, journal board members, and members of working groups to conduct and publish research showing no link between SHS and risk of disease, with the aim to maintain a debate on the issue and prevent smoke-free legislation (Dyer, 1998; Garne et al., 2005; McKee, 2000; Muggli et al., 2001; Ong and Glantz, 2000).

Researchers have assessed how the involvement of the tobacco industry has affected the evidence base relating to SHS and health. One study found that authors who were affiliated with the tobacco industry were more likely to publish reviews concluding that there was insufficient or no evidence linking SHS to ill-health: 94% of reviews by tobacco industry affiliated authors concluded that SHS was not harmful to health, compared with 13% of reviews by authors without tobacco industry affiliations (Barnes and Bero, 1998). Indeed, much of the criticism regarding the methodology of investigating associations between SHS and ill-health has come from industry-sponsored scientists, who claimed that a causal link is still unproven (Lee, 1994).

These examples underline the political nature of the evidence around the health effects of SHS, meaning caution must be exercised when assessing the evidence. Researchers should reveal any funding from the tobacco industry when submitting for peer-review publication, so that journals and reviewers can adequately assess any potential conflicts of interest.

The food and drink industry

There is emerging evidence that industry tactics comparable to those utilised by the tobacco industry (Glantz et al., 1998; Gruning et al., 2006) are also being used by the food and drink industry (Brownell and Warner, 2009; Stuckler and Nestle, 2012). In recent years, accusations have been levelled at the food and drink industry for funding and promoting research which suggests that the increasing global prevalence of overweight and obesity is a result of declining physical activity and not related to food and drink consumption (Barlow et al., 2018; O'Connor, 2015; Serôdio et al., 2018). A notable example comes from 2015, when the *New York Times* revealed that Coca-Cola invested $1.5 million in the creation of the Global Energy Balance Network (GEBN); a network promoting the message that there is no 'compelling evidence' for associations between sugar-sweetened drinks and obesity (O'Connor, 2015).

In 2018, further evidence suggesting a conflict of interest between Coca-Cola and researchers was published (Barlow et al., 2018; Serôdio et al., 2018). Findings from the review conducted by Serôdio and colleagues (2018) are presented in Box 14.3.

BOX 14.3 COCA-COLA AND CONFLICT OF INTEREST

Throughout 2015 and 2016 Coca-Cola, along with some of its subsidiaries and bottlers, released 'transparency lists'. These lists detailed the names of health professionals, scientific experts and research projects that have received sponsorship or financial support from Coca-Cola, or are associated with health and wellbeing partnerships supported by Coca-Cola (Coca-Cola Australia, 2016; Coca-Cola Deutschland, 2016; Coca-Cola España, 2016; Coca-Cola France, 2015; Coca-Cola Great Britain, 2016; Coca-Cola New Zealand, 2016).

In 2018, Serôdio and colleagues conducted a review of published articles, which cited funding from the Coca-Cola Company, and compared these data with the information reported in Coca-Cola's official transparency lists. Their aim was to establish the extent to which the transparency lists are comprehensive.

The review identified 389 articles authored by 907 authors. A comparison of these data with the transparency lists revealed that less than 5% of article authors (N=42) have been publically acknowledged by Coca-Cola. Secondly, findings revealed that many authors failed to report receipt of Coca-Cola funding. Finally, the review authors found that the majority of Coca-Cola's research support is focused on physical activity, with limited consideration of the role of diet in obesity (Serôdio et al., 2018).

Conducting ethical research

In the UK, public health research requires ethical approval from a recognised ethical committee before beginning the research. This would normally be sought by the principal investigator or lead researcher, either from a research ethics committee (REC) within a Higher Education Institution or attached to a statutory organisation such as the NHS or Ministry of Justice. The responsibility of an REC is to review proposed research that will involve either human participants or sensitive/secure secondary data to ensure it conforms to national and international ethical guidelines. Ethical review is legally mandatory in many countries, and host institutions therefore operate as legal guardians in this respect, essentially to protect human rights. The REC will thus determine whether a research project should proceed.

The ethical principles of autonomy, beneficence and justice underlie this process (see below), and researchers must therefore attend to these throughout their proposed research design. This means attending to issues of capability and competence, capacity to volunteer, potential coercion or deception, informed consent, providing full and comprehensible participant information, communicating potential or actual risks, harms or benefits, respecting confidentiality and privacy, assuring anonymity, being overt about tokens or payments, and ensuring transparency regarding conflicts of interest.

Public health research inevitably investigates sensitive issues affecting people in many different contexts and situations. There is therefore the likelihood of involving individuals or communities where there are significant, if not considerable, potential risks, which can arise from various forms of vulnerability. These might include limited ability to provide informed consent due to age or cognitive impairment; actual or perceived subordinate status within a social, institutional or organisational context; being in a dependent status (e.g. due to ill-health, disability or imprisonment); or having diminished or restricted access to resources or services (e.g. due to low income, lack of employment, low literacy, etc.). Such circumstances can mean that individuals or groups are more vulnerable to coercion or exploitation, especially where others are providing consent or access on their behalf. This means that consideration of how to access participants, to obtain informed consent, to recruit them into the research and to carry out data collection requires careful thought and planning. The notion of 'volunteering' must be carefully considered to ensure that participants are fully aware of what they are volunteering for and why. This can become problematic where a research project unavoidably involves people who have not volunteered or consented to be part of the study; for instance, in an ethnographic study where a situation is being observed in an ad hoc manner but not everyone who enters the 'field' has consented to be observed. Such situations therefore need to be thought through and addressed prior to the research commencing.

Attending to research ethics is an ongoing process, where researchers must continue to consider and apply principles of autonomy, beneficence and justice throughout research design. In other words, these principles apply whether at the recruitment stage, during data collection, in handling, analysing and interpreting data, and when exiting from the field. These principles govern our behaviour as researchers and therefore how we engage with participants and stakeholders at every stage of the process. Therefore, the consent form is not a mere tick box/through-the-gate exercise but should remain an operational document for the full course of the research and the standards that are signed up to should be readily adhered to.

BOX 14.4   WHAT IS INFORMED CONSENT?

- Research participants should be able to decide, free from coercion or undue influence and based on the information provided about the study, whether or not they would like to take part (this is enshrined in research ethics as a human right).
- Participants should be free to participate and, if needed, withdraw from research projects at any time without giving any reason. This may also include the decision to withdraw research data related to that participant that had already been collected.

(Continued)

(Continued)

- Research projects may have both foreseen and unforeseen risks and consequences (as well as benefits) for participants of which the researcher may be unaware and which the participants should be able to assess prior to taking part.
- Participants should have access to information about the project as a whole, including sources of help and support if they experience any ill effects connected to the study.

Public health methods and ethical conduct

One of the problems resulting from the dominance of the randomised drug trial in research ethics is that other standard methodologies do not fit the formulae and can then be dismissed too quickly as unethical. We suggest that a far more fruitful approach is to take seriously these methodologies and explore what ethical issues emerge in their use and discuss the best means to resolve them. For example, cluster randomised trials can be a useful way to assess such things as screening programmes or community interventions, such as attempts at mosquito vector control. Individual informed consent is not possible in at least some of these pieces of research. We suggest that this alone does not make them unethical. Similarly, cohort studies are an important method in public health, where a randomised trial might actually be considered unethical. Other research may focus on qualitative methods, such as questionnaires, focus groups or participant observation, or may involve reviewing and assessing policy changes for other reasons (e.g. a shortage of vaccine may result in changes to a vaccination schedule). It may be perfectly reasonable to conduct research to see if the reduced schedule is as effective as the established one.

Ethical conduct of public health RCTs

Randomised controlled trials (RCTs) raise several ethical issues. First, we should only carry out a trial if we genuinely don't know whether the new intervention leads to better outcomes than the standard treatment (known as 'equipoise'). Determining if this is the case is not straightforward, as different people will have different views (e.g. clinical experts, patient groups). Ideally, the best available evidence at any point in time should be summarised in a systematic review to reduce bias. If the review includes a meta-analysis with unequivocal results, then it is not ethical to do yet another trial. A classic example of this is a cumulative meta-analysis of RCTs of intravenous streptokinase in myocardial infarction patients. This retrospective analysis shows that as early as 1973 a meta-analysis could have demonstrated strong evidence ($p = 0.01$) of reduced mortality for those patients who received the intervention. As more trials were carried out, the strength of the evidence increased ($p = 0.001$ in 1977, $p = 0.0001$ in 1986), yet it was not until 1989 that the drug was licensed in the UK (Egger et al., 2001: 16). The trials carried out when there was already strong evidence of a benefit should not have been carried out – lives could have been saved if all patients received the intervention. If the review suggests that further research is needed (as is often the case), or if the existing evidence cannot be generalised to your population, then it is ethical to do another trial, but it is also important to learn lessons from any previous research about how best to conduct the trial.

A key element of an RCT is the choice of control group. This is usually 'standard treatment', and from an ethical point of view it is important that the control group do not get any less than 'standard treatment'. Consider a trial of a new smoking cessation intervention to be delivered to pregnant women by midwives. Given that midwives normally have conversations about smoking with women in their care, it would be unethical to ask them to refrain from discussing smoking cessation with women in the control group for the purposes of trialling the new intervention, as this would be a deviation from standard practice.

When planning a new trial, one of the problems faced by researchers is that RCTs are often seen by the public as being unethical, or akin to a postcode lottery. There are several ways that these ethical concerns can be addressed. Since many public health interventions are more easily delivered at the level of school, GP practice or ward for example, cluster randomisation can be used to alleviate the problems of perceived unfairness. A good example of this is a study to assess the effectiveness of an intervention to promote smoking cessation on hospital wards. Since it would be difficult from a practical point of view for healthcare professionals to offer differing levels of advice to patients in neighbouring beds on a ward, and it may cause questions about fairness from patients too, it is better to take a cluster randomisation approach, and to randomise wards within a hospital (Murray et al., 2013).

If resources are scarce, as is often the case, and the intervention cannot be delivered to everyone, then randomisation may actually be the fairest way of determining who gets the intervention, with the advantage that it allows assessment of the efficacy of the intervention compared with usual practice. An example of this is a study that offered places at a new, high-quality nursery to families living in a certain geographical area. There were not enough places for all eligible children, so allocation was randomised, and outcomes were compared for those families who were offered a place at the new nursery compared with the rest of the sample, who had to make their own childcare arrangements (Toroyan, 2003).

On the other hand, if resources allow, then an alternative strategy is to say that those who are randomised to the control group will be offered the intervention at the end of the trial, so that everyone is offered it eventually. Another way of ensuring that everyone gets the intervention at some point is to design a cross-over trial, in which case those who are randomised to the control group for the first phase of the study will switch to receive the intervention in the second phase of the trial (and vice versa). This is more appropriate for interventions that seek to alleviate symptoms than those that aim to cure a condition.

Similarly, they are more appropriate when the intervention does not have long-term effects, which would carry over from phase one into phase two.

As already discussed above, it is possible that an intervention we are testing because we hope it will be beneficial, might actually be harmful. RCTs should be managed according to a protocol, and this may include 'stopping rules'. These rules state in advance that at certain points in the trial (e.g. after half of the participants have been recruited), interim analyses will be run. If there is reliable evidence at this point that the intervention is doing more harm than good, then the trial will be stopped early to prevent more participants being harmed. A good example of this is a large multi-centre trial of corticosteroids as a treatment for head injury. Based on the first 10,000 patients, the interim analysis showed strong evidence that mortality was higher in those that received the intervention, so the trial was terminated early (CRASH Trial Collaborators, 2004). Other elements of the study protocol have a role in ensuring that the study is ethical. Sometimes, if there are multiple outcomes, there is a danger in the reporting of focusing on those that show most evidence of an improvement. Therefore, it is important that the primary and secondary outcomes are stated in the protocol, preferably published in advance.

Use of secondary data

Secondary data are widely used in public health research. If data already exist to answer a research question, then it is more ethical to use this data rather than collect new data, particularly when data collection places a burden on participants. Even if it does not involve participants (e.g. observation of mode of transport), it still requires resources, which could be better used. In the field of education, for example, schools collect vast amounts of data on the progress of individual children, and children themselves are subjected to an array of routine tests (such as standardised assessment tests, otherwise known as 'SATs'). To give children additional further tests for the purposes of research would be unethical unless it can be demonstrated that the existing secondary data is not sufficient to answer the research question.

While there are ethical considerations in sharing data, these can usually be addressed through Data Sharing Agreements, anonymisation of the data set to be shared, or even by the analysis being carried out at the institution where the data is held to avoid the data being transferred outside of that organisation. When accessing secondary data (for example, through the National Data Archive), the researcher is usually asked to abide by certain rules, such as acknowledging the contribution of the participants, informing the organisation which owns the data of any publications resulting from the data, storing the data securely and destroying it after a certain time period. It is also important to suppress small numbers (usually less than 5) in the reporting of routine data, to avoid individuals being identified. Advances in data linkage and pseudo-anonymisation mean that there is potential to combine data from a range of secondary sources (e.g. police data, education data, health data), creating comprehensive data sets that avoid instrusive and time-consuming data collection.

The final point is regarding the ethical use of secondary data for research, because the analysis must be congruent with the original purposes to which participants consented. If patients completed a survey and consented to their data being used for 'service improvement', then this might allow a range of analyses which conceivably contribute to service improvement, but if it was collected for a more specific purpose, or participants were assured that the data would not be shared beyond the organisation that collected it, this precludes reuse by other researchers.

Insufficiently powering studies

Many research studies are unethical because the design is not appropriate to answer the research question; ethical research is methodologically literate. In quantitative studies, often the problem is insufficient sample size. Even if a sample size calculation is performed, it may not take into account aspects of the design or analysis that increase the required sample size (such as a clustered design, or the number of covariates to be included in the analysis, or the intention to perform stratified analyses or test for interactions between variables). Another problem is that the required sample size may not be achieved due to problems with recruitment or attrition. If a study is not sufficiently powered (in other words, does not have a large enough sample to detect a difference or association if one exists) then it is not ethical, because it is using resources and subjecting participants to being in a study without having a reasonable chance of generating new knowledge.

This issue is not limited to RCTs, and applies equally to all the quantitative study designs (see Chapter 1). Over the years many under-powered studies have been conducted. To a certain extent, this problem can be overcome by carrying out a systematic review and meta-analysis which combines a number of under-powered studies, improving power and increasing precision of the estimates. However, it is worth bearing in mind that under-powered studies are more likely to produce negative results, and this may in turn lead to publication bias. In this case, small studies that do get published are biased in favour of the intervention, and this will affect any systematic review of these studies. So, a meta-analysis is not a panacea for under-powered studies.

Ethical challenges for qualitative studies

Autonomy

Autonomy in qualitative research is concerned with recognising and respecting people's capability and volition to become involved in research. It is about achieving genuine informed consent that is non-coercive and negotiated with trust. Qualitative research designs tend to be inductive and emergent, such that consent and informing or educating participants about the research can become an ongoing process as new angles are explored and opportunities arise. Consent is not a one-off procedure but is ongoing and may be renegotiated as the research proceeds. The research 'journey', whether at recruitment, sampling, data collection or data analysis stages, is a reflexive process whereby the researcher can have ongoing engagement with research participants or with others in the setting in evolving the methods and interpreting the emerging data. While research participants do not ordinarily have complete autonomy over research processes and outputs – except perhaps with participatory action research or where there is a strong PPI element – there is deliberate effort to represent participants' emic perspectives such that [1] research outputs are credible and dependable and [2] they are 'genuine' to participants and to the research context. This is a degree of autonomy that doesn't occur in quantitative research but that must be managed such that research processes and outputs are robust and the research has integrity.

Confidentiality and anonymity need careful management given that qualitative research tends to be highly specific and localised, and therefore individuals and settings can be identifiable if vigilance is not taken to anonymise them. This can be an issue within a research setting where, for instance, participants and non-participants know each other; an example might be in a prison where prisoners who volunteer as research participants are unable to conceal this. Similarly, in situations where status and identity demarcate individuals, this can have a bearing on an individual's willingness or reticence to participate in a research project if their anonymity cannot be assured. Privacy is an important dimension of confidentiality and can become compromised in situations where it is difficult not to be overheard or visible to others. Take again the example of a prisoner, who for security reasons must be interviewed in the presence of a prison officer. Furthermore, the interview setting could be an unnegotiated space where it is difficult to guarantee privacy. These are the kinds of scenarios that need careful planning and management.

Beneficence

A strong theme of qualitative research is to value the emic perspective of research participants and to seek to represent their subjective viewpoints. This is consistent with the principle of beneficence in endeavouring to support research participants, provide – to a degree – unconditional positive regard, and essentially to undertake the research for their benefit. Central to the ethos of qualitative research is building trusting relationship, with the intention of accessing participants' lived experiences or unique perspectives. The intimacy afforded through this process, however, brings a range of potential risks to both participants *and* researchers – vulnerability, emotional stress, disclosure, etc. – that need to be anticipated and managed. The potential harms of qualitative research tend to be emotional or psychological and therefore measures should be taken to provide support for potential occurrences, which may include having appropriate referral options and researcher debriefing. Indeed, in qualitative research, beneficence concerns participants *and* researchers given the investment in relationship building, reciprocity and the potential risks associated with intimacy.

A second aspect concerns the potential harms or benefits the research findings bring. This underlines the importance of ensuring the research process is robust, such that issues of trustworthiness (or validity and reliability) have been attended to throughout the research process. While findings should come as no surprise to participants, there is always the possibility that they could be controversial.

Justice

Another principle of qualitative relationship is equity – this means endeavouring to be fair when investigating the lives and experiences of others, in terms of managing the research relationship and interpreting the findings. Issues of bias and misrepresentation were discussed in Chapter 10, where techniques of rigour were described to build quality into the research design and process. Essentially, the qualitative researcher performs a facilitative role that is non-dominant and seeks to empower the research participant. In this sense, the researcher has an important duty of care in supporting participants and representing their perspectives with integrity.

Conclusion

This chapter has highlighted how ethical issues are central to robust public health research. There are core ethical principles that underpin public health research, as well as key challenges for researchers, particularly where researchers' interests intersect with professional, political or commercial partners.

Further reading

Oreskes, N. and Conway, E. (2010) *Merchants of Doubt. How a handful of scientists obscured the truth on issues from tobacco smoke to global warming*. London: Bloomsbury Press.
Serôdio, P.M., McKee, M. and Stuckler, D. (2018) Coca-Cola – a model of transparency in research partnerships? A network analysis of Coca-Cola's research funding. *Public Health Nutrition*, 21(9): 1594–607.

15 WRITING UP, DISSEMINATION AND PUBLICATION

===== CHAPTER SUMMARY =====

Postgraduate students often seek to **publish** and **disseminate** their work, whether this be the findings from a research study or maybe an assignment that has the potential to reach a wider audience. This chapter provides guidance and hopefully inspiration for students and novice researchers working in public health about the process of moving towards **publication**. The chapter will also address issues when **writing** up dissertations or doctoral theses. Students can often feel overawed by the task of getting their ideas and findings on paper – this chapter provides a series of tips for helping to overcome fears.

The writing process

Plan

Don't underestimate the importance of planning when undertaking a piece of writing. Planning is helpful in a number of ways, and there are different types of planning that serve different purposes. For example, a mind map can unlock ideas that might be covered in a piece of writing, and help you to identify links between different issues and a possible ordering of the key parts of your writing. From there, you may move to a more linear structure, identifying headings and sub-headings. If you are writing up your Masters dissertation, it's likely that the course leader will have provided you with a suggested chapter structure, possibly with approximate word counts for each section. This can be incredibly helpful in not only giving structure, but also breaking up the task of writing into manageable chunks. If a suggested structure is lacking, then one of the best things you can do is to seek out examples of other people's work. These days, selected good quality dissertations and most theses are hosted electronically on the university library, so it's very easy to see how other students have structured their work.

It's understandably off-putting to be faced with putting tens of thousands of words onto paper, so the more this can be broken down the better. It also helps to ensure that there is a proper balance across sections in terms of word count.

Once you have an idea of your structure, it's never too early to begin writing it. It may be that the structure will change, but there are ways to simplify the process of amending the structure of your written document. Probably the most common way if you write using Microsoft Word is to use its Styles feature. This enables you to create headings and varying levels of sub-headings, which you can then use as your structure for writing. Importantly, it allows you to move around the headings (and the text contained underneath it) simply by dragging from the Outline View window. This relatively simple way of organising your document before you put words to paper can be incredibly powerful in helping you to get the document written.

Write

You might think that planning and 'just write' might be a contradiction, but having an initial structure, whether this changes or not along the way, can free you to sit down and get those words onto the page. It is much easier to work with the words, once they are on a page, rather than merely locked in your head. Try not to worry too much about self-editing until you have got something down on paper. And then, it can be helpful to spend some time away from the words until you read them back. Giving yourself space for reflection can really help during the editing process. So, once you have your provisional structure, try to just sit down and free-type – bottom on chair, fingers on keyboard – and worry about editing later.

Another tip, which again goes hand in hand with structuring, is to write while you go along rather than leave all the writing until after the fieldwork (or deskwork, if conducting something such as a systematic review) has been completed. Writing as you go along has a number of benefits. First of all, it means that you are not left facing a blank screen and thousands of words after your fieldwork, which can help to avoid issues such as writers' block. Getting into a habit of writing as you go is also helpful in recording details, particularly relating to the research process, that you might forget if you leave the write up until later. Having that greater detail can make a real difference in the way you can reflect on your research in the document, and also demonstrate exactly what you did during your work in a level of detail that will do that work justice. One thing you can do is to maintain a reflective journal, which is where you can write down your thoughts and experiences during the research process. A practical tip is to carry the reflective journal with you, where possible, as ideas can emerge on a bus or train ride and it is useful to be able to write them down immediately. A lot of this material might never make it into your final document, but some of it will, and the rest will help you to clarify your thinking both during the research and when writing up.

Often, there is a formal structure that requires you to write material at early stages of your work. For example, MSc dissertations and doctoral research are often preceded by some form of protocol stage, usually followed by completion, submission and response to an ethics application (see Chapter 14 for more discussion on ethics). Both the protocol and ethics application stage entails outlining the aims and objectives of your research, background, methodology and methods (see Box 15.1 for example of content to include in a protocol). The material prepared for the protocol and ethics stages can then be used, or expanded on, in the final written document (see Box 15.2 for example dissertation structure). This is a really easy way of getting text into your document at an early stage and, if you have created a structure, it's simple to place the various pieces of text into the most appropriate place of your document.

BOX 15.1   SUGGESTED CONTENT TO INCLUDE IN A PROTOCOL

- A concise indicative title that describes succinctly the proposed study. The title should attempt to convey the essence of the research question or aim and the methodological approach.
- An introductory section that includes your aim(s), objectives, research question(s) and brief outline of the proposed research.
- A literature review, providing justification and rationale for the proposed study and the key contribution it will make. The literature review should develop the conceptual and theoretical framework, and identify gaps, challenges and questions raised by other research.
- The research design, with detailed explanation of and rationale for the methodology and methods. You must cite supporting methodology literature to explain and justify the methods; this means including conceptual and theoretical detail (i.e. definitions and explanations of methodology and methods) and practical details (in first person), explaining access, recruitment, sampling or case selection, data collection, data management and data analysis. You must also discuss verification techniques/reliability and validity. Each stage of the research design must be carefully described; for example, you must include proposed sample sizes (if appropriate), interviewing techniques, analysis approaches, etc. However, you do not need to develop fully piloted interview or questionnaire schedules, scales or instruments at this stage.
- Discuss any ethical or governance issues and procedures that will need to be addressed. What permissions/access will you need and how will you achieve these? What measures will you take in the research design to protect yourself and your participants from 'harm' or exploitation? How will you manage the data? You should consider issues of anonymity, confidentiality, privacy, respect, informed consent, safety, data protection and potential conflict/disclosure.
- A brief discussion of the proposed study's feasibility, providing a realistic timetable (e.g. a detailed Gantt Chart) and some discussion of the perceived strengths and limitations of the research.

BOX 15.2 SUGGESTED STRUCTURE OF PUBLIC HEALTH MASTERS DISSERTATION

- The declaration front sheet (available below).
- A title page.
- A contents page.
- An acknowledgements page.
- An abstract.
- A glossary of terms / abbreviations (if appropriate).
- An introduction.
- A review of the literature.
- The research design / methodology.
- The findings or results.
- A discussion chapter.
- Conclusion: This final section should summarise both the dissertation as a whole – reminding the reader of what you set out to achieve – and summarise and contextualise the findings. Here, you will present your key closing argument, revisiting the research question and objectives to consider to what extent they have been achieved. You should discuss how the strengths and weaknesses of the research process affected your outcomes.
- List of references.
- Appendices.

Deal with distractions

The ideal situation for writing is one that is free of distractions. You want to be able to focus on the task at hand, ideally getting into a 'flow-state', which is where the words come out onto the page easily and fast. The number one enemy here is distraction, and unfortunately there seem to be more distractions in life than ever – especially if you are working at a computer. So, turn off your email notifications and only check messages when your writing period is over. Work somewhere where you can't be disturbed, or ask people not to disturb you. This might be a room in your house, the university library, or your local library. Some people like to work in places such as cafes, and find background (or 'white') noise helpful in aiding concentration. Wherever you write, pick a place that works for you and make the most of your time there.

A good way to make the most of your time is to work in short, intense bursts, followed by a period of rest/relaxation. The Pomodoro Technique is a well-known method for facilitating more efficient writing, taking this approach (Cirillo, 2018). Twenty-five minute periods of writing, timed using a countdown timer, are separated by five-minute rest periods. This technique can help people to write faster in a more focussed way, free from distractions, knowing that following the relatively short period of time of activity, they can take a short break. You might find it helpful to arrange such sessions as part of a group, where you work in silence in the same room, and then come together to relax in between. The sense of community and peer support (and pressure!) can assist in giving people the added impetus to get their words down on paper. Such group sessions are increasingly prevalent in institutions – at our university a session called 'Shut Up and Write', open to staff and post-graduate students, takes just this approach.

However you choose to do it, try to write without fear of thinking 'is this good enough?'. Such thoughts may serve to block you from writing anything! Remember, once you have got your words down, you can work with them to improve your writing. But no one can work with a blank page.

Let me entertain you

You may not think that writing an academic publication, whether this be a dissertation, thesis, or journal paper, has anything in common with writing a novel. However, they have more in common than you might think. All these examples, to really be successful, should entertain the reader. Novels need a structure, just like academic works – a beginning, middle and end (generally speaking!). They should pique the reader's interest in some way, and make them want to keep reading – to keep turning those pages until the climax. A great novel is one where the reader can't put it down (or at least doesn't want to put it down), as the momentum of the story – the narrative drive – is almost irresistible. I'm not saying that your MSc dissertation, PhD thesis or journal paper needs to be as unputdownable as the latest bestselling thriller. It's unlikely you'll have a charismatic detective investigating the sinister circumstances of the body in the drawing room. But, you can still think about the opening of your work in a similar way. It needs to be intriguing, interesting and offer a reward for the reader. In crime fiction, the reward is often the uncovering of something that was hidden – the solving of a crime by unmasking a killer, finding a long-lost person, or making sense of mysterious happenings. In academia, the intrigue and interest can also come from offering a resolution to an unanswered question: your research question. Hopefully, the research question you set will be of interest to the reader, and your opening is to make the case for why it is of interest (the rationale), and, in effect, why the reader should bother to carry on reading. Obviously, in the case of a Masters dissertation or doctoral thesis, the examiner has a duty to carry on reading – it is their job! But in the case of a potential peer-reviewed publication, the readers of the journal, the peer reviewers, or before that the Editor, do not have any such responsibility. You need to think of how you can grab their attention and interest, and then set about taking them on the journey towards the climax of the work.

The most important thing is that the ending is satisfying. Have you ever been really engrossed in a novel, pulled in from page one by the intrigue, but then left feeling completely disappointed by the ending? Often this is because the intrigue set up at the beginning, the key question, hasn't (in the eyes of the readers at least, and they are the most important people!) been answered in a satisfying manner. It might be because there are loose ends that haven't been tied off, the ending feels rushed, or that the conclusion just doesn't feel right given what has come before. These factors can also affect how readers feel after experiencing your academic text.

To ensure that readers aren't left feeling that there has been unsatisfactory resolution to your work, you must first and foremost ensure that you have answered the overall research question that you set out at the start, along with any associated secondary questions. Make it very clear in your discussion chapter how you have answered these questions. If you have aims rather than research questions, you still need to revisit these and state how the aims have been met. This helps to ensure that the reader feels that the journey has reached its desired destination, with the required questions answered.

Pacing is very important in fiction, and ensuring that the novel has the right pace throughout the work can make a huge difference in the reader experience. It can be tempting to rush the end of a piece of academic work, either because the author is fed up with the work and desperate to get it finished, or because they are running out of steam or time, or possibly just out of the excitement at the thought of reaching the end of what has no doubt been a long and taxing process. The same is true in fiction writing. There are tricks to use that can help to avoid the ending to your work feeling rushed. One of the most effective ways is to not leave the two usual chapters that come at the end of a piece of academic work, the discussion and conclusions, until the end. It might seem the only logical option to work on your document in a linear fashion, but the truth is you can write in a non-linear way to some extent and build up your document. What can work very well is to complete your discussion and conclusions, before then finalising your introduction; but it's whatever works best for you, to ensure that the whole document has that consistent quality and feel to the reader.

Writing for publication

Why write for publication?

For many people, their academic writing will end at the point of submission. While for those undertaking a PhD it is expected that publications will arise, for those writing up an individual assignment or a dissertation as part of a course, there is no such assumption. Not everyone will want to write for publication, but it should certainly be considered and promoted for those who want to (or think they might want to). There are many benefits of writing up academic work for peer review publication. The first is the sense of achievement that you get from succeeding in having your work recognised in a journal. But just the process of doing so is beneficial itself, as it can really help to develop your writing skills – this is particularly useful if writing is part of your job, or a part of a job to which you aspire. Publishing your work can help it to reach a wider audience, contributing new knowledge, and maybe having an impact on policy, practice or research. It can also help to develop contacts and networks in the field, as people may contact you after reading your article (if you are the corresponding author it is usual that your email address will be included in the paper). This contact could lead to new partnerships, either for continued research or professional practice.

Achieving publication from your academic work can be hard work. It requires a certain level of commitment, as well as determination and persistence. The following sections provide advice for those aiming for publication, highlighting key issues to consider and suggesting techniques to help the process run as smoothly as possible.

When to write for publication

Deciding when to write for publication is a key decision if you are to maximise your chances of publishing your work. It depends on personal preference, and also on the nature of the work that you are wishing to write up for publication. For example, it would not be sensible to attempt to write up an assignment (as part of your Masters in Public Health, for example) for publication until this has been submitted and assessed by the teaching team. This way you can focus on the assignment task, which will likely require a slightly different focus than a published paper, and you will also receive helpful feedback from your lecturers that can be taken on board for writing up the assignment for publication. Unfortunately, this feedback may result in a realisation that the material may not be of sufficient quality for aiming for peer-reviewed publication. Or, alternatively, it might give you the confidence boost that will power you to your publication goals! Similarly, if you are intending to publish from your master's dissertation, it makes sense to wait until you receive your mark and feedback. Another advantage of waiting is that it will give you some time away from the work, both to reflect on what you did and found, and also just to give you a break from a piece of work that was likely quite intense and possibly draining. Having that bit of space to recuperate can then reinvigorate you for the task of converting your assignment or dissertation to a paper ready for submission to a journal.

The situation with a PhD is somewhat different. If you are undertaking doctoral studies, it is recommended that you do try and write up work for publication as you go. There are several reasons for this:

- First, if you succeed in publishing from your doctorate during the process, you can include those papers in your thesis. This is a form of validation of the quality and significance of your research, which should give you confidence going into the viva. It will also be looked upon favourably by your examiners.
- Second, undertaking a PhD is a long process, particularly if done on a part-time basis. You will find that if you leave all your publications until you have completed your doctoral studies, your early work may not feel as timely and relevant as it did three or four years ago. It's also

possible that if your topic is particularly high up the research and policy agenda, someone else might have published similar work in the meantime. Even if this isn't the case, revisiting work from several years ago will entail quite a bit of additional work, reviewing and updating references and generally refreshing your knowledge of the field. This may well be done anyway as part of your final preparations for your thesis submission, so it shouldn't be a reason on its own not to attempt to write up work from several years ago, but it is easier if done at the time.

- The final reason for trying to write up as you go along, is that if you save up possible papers until the end (and there may be several potential papers), you may find that this becomes too much of a task to complete or even contemplate. This could be a particular issue if you are starting a new job after the completion of your doctorate.

So, although it might feel tempting to wait until you know you have passed your viva, don't leave too many potential papers for this stage.

A final point, whether you are undertaking a Master's or a doctorate, is to discuss your plans to publish with your supervisor – they can help to advise on issues such as timing, framing of your potential paper, and potential journals to target (see next section).

Target the journal

One key piece of advice for those seeking to achieve publication is to identify a target journal for your piece of work. Deciding which journal to submit to can be based on several factors, and browsing a number of potential journals is highly recommended.

There are several reasons why it is a good idea to identify your target journal before you start writing. It can be a huge help when structuring your paper. Most journals provide guidelines to authors, including the maximum word length of different types of articles accepted by the journal (editorials, commentaries, research papers, etc.), suggested or required sub-headings, and sometimes topic areas that are of interest to the editors.

When preparing to write up a research paper, it is incredibly helpful to know beforehand the length that you will be aiming for. Maximum word counts can vary significantly between journals, and if you feel that your research requires more words to do it justice (for example, qualitative research can often need a longer article) then this can influence the journal that you target.

Similarly, the stated focus of a journal on their website might make you think again about whether it is a good place to target. Do look at the areas of interest, and whether the journal has published anything related to your research area. Don't be put off if you find that the journal has recently published research on the same, or similar, topic. It doesn't mean that they won't be interested in publishing more work in the area and, if anything, it is a positive finding as it shows that the journal is interested in the topic.

You will usually find that if you do submit your article and the topic of focus isn't considered within the remit of the journal, it will be returned to you speedily. Sometimes, a journal might recommend a sister journal that may be more appropriate. One option is to check with the journal before submission. Most journals provide contact details of the Editor(s) and it may be worth contacting them to check whether your research paper might be of interest. This is particularly the case if you are considering submitting an Editorial or other discursive piece, but could also be done for a prospective research paper. Editors might indicate whether an article's topic would fit within the area of interest of the journal, although it would be unusual for them to comment specifically about the chances of any article being accepted for publication, as that would depend on the feedback from peer reviewers. Another strategy is to research the interests of the Editor. Editors are usually fellow academics, so will have published papers, and the nature of their output might offer clues as to whether your paper might pique their interest. A final point to consider is to look at which journals are cited within your dissertation or thesis. This might reveal those journals that are more likely to be interested in your topic area.

Using guidelines to structure your paper

In recent years, a number of publication reporting guidelines have been developed to improve the quality and transparency of academic papers. Such guidelines ensure that authors report key information about their studies in a way that allows the reader:

- to understand what was done in the research
- to make informed judgements about whether the findings reported in the paper are fair and justified
- to replicate the research using the same practices or procedures that were utilised by the authors of the original research.

These guidelines can provide a very helpful template for those writing for academic publication, so it is well worth checking whether a set of guidelines exists for the type of study or paper that you are seeking to publish (e.g. randomised controlled trials, qualitative research, systematic reviews, etc). Copies of all recognised checklists are available to download from the Internet. One set of guidelines is the Preferred Reporting Items for Systematic Reviews and Meta-Analyses (PRISMA) (Liberati et al., 2009). The PRISMA checklist, at the time of writing, has 27 items that authors need to consider when writing up their paper, including how to present the methods and results. Other guidelines include the CONSORT Statement (for reporting randomised controlled trials) (Moher, 1998), STROBE (for reporting observational studies) (Vandenbroucke et al., 2007), and COREQ (for reporting qualitative research) (Tong et al., 2007). Table 15.1 presents publication reporting standards for a range of study types.

Journals increasingly require authors to follow the appropriate guidelines, so not only are these guidelines helpful for authors, but they are often necessary if publication is to be achieved in a journal of good standing.

Table 15.1 Publication reporting guidelines

Study type	Publication reporting guidelines	Reference
Randomised controlled trials	CONSORT Statement (Consolidated Standards of Reporting Trials)	Moher, D. (1998) CONSORT: an evolving tool to help improve the quality of reports of randomized controlled trials. Consolidated Standards of Reporting Trials. *JAMA, 279,* 1489–91.
Observational studies	STROBE (Strengthening the Reporting of Observational Studies in Epidemiology)	Vandenbroucke, J.P., von Elm, E., Altman, D.G., Gøtzsche, P.C., Mulrow, C.D., Pocock, S.J., Poole, C., Schlesselman, J.J. and Egger, M. (2007) STROBE Initiative. Strengthening the Reporting of Observational Studies in Epidemiology (STROBE): explanation and elaboration. *PLoS Med, 4* (10), e297.
Qualitative research	COREQ (Consolidated criteria for reporting qualitative research)	Tong, A., Sainsbury, P. and Craig, J. (2007) Consolidated criteria for reporting qualitative research (COREQ): a 32-item checklist for interviews and focus groups. *International Journal for Quality in Health Care, 19* (6), 349–57.
Systematic reviews and meta-analyses	PRISMA (Preferred Reporting Items for Systematic Reviews and Meta-Analyses)	Liberati, A., Altman, D., Tetzlaff, J., et al. (2009) The PRISMA statement for reporting systematic reviews and meta-analyses of studies that evaluate healthcare interventions: explanation and elaboration. *BMJ, 339.*
Meta-ethnography	eMERGe (Meta-ethnography Reporting Guidance)	France, E.F., Ring, N., Noyes, J., Maxwell, M., Jepson, R., Duncan, E., Turley, R., Jones, D. and Uny, I. (2015) Protocol-developing meta-ethnography reporting guidelines (eMERGe). *BMC Medical Research Methodology, 15,* 103.
Realist synthesis	RAMESES	Wong, G., Greenhalgh, T., Westhorp, G., Buckingham, J. and Pawson, R. (2013) RAMESES publication standards: realist syntheses. *BMC Medicine, 11,* 21.
Economic evaluation	CHEERS Statement (Consolidated Health Economic Evaluation Reporting Standards)	Husereau, D., Drummond, M., Petrou, S. et al. (2013) Consolidated Health Economic Evaluation Reporting Standards (CHEERS) statement. *BMJ, 346.*

Get and respond to peer feedback

Obtaining peer feedback can be very helpful in the publication process. If you are writing with others, then your co-authors will be an important source of this. You can seek feedback at all stages of the process, from conception of ideas, drafting of the paper, right through to final completion. If you are writing a paper based on your dissertation or doctoral research, then your co-authors will usually be supervisors, who will have the benefit of experience when it comes to writing for publication. They should, therefore, be able to offer you feedback from the right academic perspective. Do make use of your supervisors, and heed their comments. You may also seek feedback from friends and family, possibly fellow students on the course you are undertaking/have undertaken. This can also be helpful, particularly from the perspective of trying to ensure that your paper is written in plain English, free from jargon, and understandable to an educated reader but not necessarily a reader who knows a lot about your topic. Working with fellow students on papers can be a great way of providing peer support and motivation, and it can even be done in a group setting. Do be aware though not to fall into the trap of what has been termed the 'false feedback loop', where you seek feedback and make changes from those who are not necessarily the most appropriate people to critique your work. Close family members can definitely fall into this category; so although they can be helpful in providing lay feedback, do be cautious about using such people as your key respondents.

Believe in yourself and your work

One of the key issues that prevents students from attempting to publish their work is that they don't feel as though their work is good enough, or worthy enough, to be published in an academic journal. Even students who have achieved distinction level marks, based on impressive field-work and a well-written dissertation, can feel this way. It is of course understandable. To move from a position of consuming academic papers to producing them can be intimidating, and there is sometimes a misconception that such papers are solely the reserve of 'academics', who work in universities. The truth is that peer-reviewed journals will not discriminate against submissions that are led by postgraduate students or former students using work from their studies. Journals *will* be concerned about the quality of the research, the quality of the writing, and the added value of the work to existing literature/ evidence base. So, the issue to consider when thinking about whether to adapt your research into a peer-reviewed paper is whether academically it will appeal to journal editors and the wider readership. For a first opinion, ask your dissertation or PhD supervisor. It may well be that your research has a good chance of publication if it is framed in the right way – that is, you consider the best angle to present your research which both fills a gap in current knowledge around the subject, is of value to the subject area, and is interesting for the potential readers. Sometimes, your supervisor will suggest adapting the output for publication, in which case do take this as a big compliment and consider it seriously. There have been many instances where students have taken such a step and achieved publication in good quality journals – sometimes with accompanying press interest.

Be open to critique and comment

A slightly different, but connected issue is that there can be a fear of putting your work (and yourself) out there and being exposed to critique and comment. This includes feedback from reviewers at the review stage, and then responses from the wider readership and public once the paper is published. It's true that there will be an element of critique as part of the peer review process, but this should hopefully be constructive and help you to reach your goal of publication (see the next section on responding to reviewers). In terms of criticisms from the wider readership and public, this might occur if your publication relates to an issue where there is some controversy. If you are concerned about fielding emails from people about the publication, one solution would be to designate your supervisor or other co-author as the corresponding author. By doing this, their email address will be listed on the publication and they will become the first port of call for anyone seeking to make contact. Importantly, the corresponding author does not need to be the first author, so do not base authorship order on such concerns.

In these days of social media, there is an increased possibility that the findings from research studies are visible and discussed openly in public forums, such as Twitter. Again, this is more likely to be the case with more newsworthy, controversial topics, including those that catch the attention of traditional media outlets. If work is discussed publicly on social media platforms, do consider carefully whether and how to engage. A lot depends on the nature and tone of the communication, and person or organisation it is coming from. Engaging with people on social media can be very rewarding, but it can also be stressful. If you don't feel comfortable engaging in this way, then either let one of your co-authors reply or limit your engagement.

Respond to reviewers in the right way

As mentioned previously, subjecting your work to critique of peer reviewers can be a source of anxiety for those considering writing for publication. It's true that the peer review process can sometimes be a negative experience, if you are unlucky enough to be faced with an unreasonable reviewer. However, this would be a rare exception, as most of those who review articles on behalf of peer-reviewed journals do so in a fair-minded way. Remember that peer reviewers are not paid, and do reviewing on top of their day job, so their motivation should be largely altruistic. The whole concept of the peer review process is that it is peers who are reviewing the work of fellow peers, and the tone of feedback should be one of respect between colleagues. A good piece of peer-reviewed feedback will offer an opinion on the manuscript, backed up by evidence, with specific-enough comments and queries to enable the author to respond. It may be that the reviewers recommend that the article is not suitable for publication, which the editor then agrees with. In this situation, try not to feel too downhearted. If the critique has been provided in a constructive way, then you will be able to use the comments to improve your paper before submitting to another journal. And unless the paper was rejected purely on the basis of the topic not being suitable for the target journal (in which case it will often be rejected by the editor, without being sent out for peer review), then it is strongly advisable to take the reviewers' comments on board to strengthen the paper. It may be tempting to either send the paper straight back out for submission elsewhere, or maybe to give up on the paper, but making those changes could be the difference between achieving publication and not. A further word of warning – it is not unheard of for your paper to be allocated to the same reviewer, even if you submit to a different journal! And a reviewer receiving an unaltered paper that they have already reviewed and commented on for another journal, will not be pleased.

If you do receive comments from peer reviewers, and are invited to revise and resubmit your manuscript, what is the best approach? One key tip is to make things as easy as possible for the reviewers when they look at your resubmission, by responding to their comments in a point-by-point style (see Table 15.2 for example).

Table 15.2 Example: responses to reviewers

Reviewers' comments	Response from authors
Introduction needs more detail on the public health importance of green space, with more reference to the evidence base.	More detail has been added, including additional evidence detailing how access to green space can affect mental health and wellbeing and levels of physical activity (page 2).
Please can you give additional details on how the data collection tool was validated.	Additional detail has now been provided, explaining how the data collection tool was validated – including use of subject experts and the target population in the pre-testing and piloting stages (page 3).
There appears to be a typo in the third row, second column of Table 2. Should the figure read 3 rather than 30?	Thank you for spotting the typographical error in Table 2. This has now been corrected.
It would be helpful for you to structure your discussion using the suggested sub-headings for the journal (see author instructions on the journal's website).	We have now revised the discussion, following the recommended sub-heading structure for the journal.
We feel it would be helpful to include a clearer set of recommendations at the end of the discussion, particularly relating to planning policy in this area.	We have now included a number of recommendations, including relating to planning policy and increased provision of green space.

This can also make life easier for you, ensuring that you identify and respond to each comment. Structuring this in a table, with reviewers' comments in the left-hand column and your response in the right is a common way of achieving this. Do respond to all the comments, but that doesn't mean that you need to make all the changes that are suggested. Where changes can be made, and it makes sense to do so, then make changes. But where it is not possible, or where you feel that it doesn't make sense, then respond with a logical reason why the changes aren't being made. Most reviewers will accept that not all their suggestions might be possible to enact, but they will expect some form of response. Also, remember to share this task with your co-authors, who can advise on how best to respond to the reviewers.

Other means of dissemination

This chapter has focused on academic publication, but there are other ways of disseminating the findings and learning from your academic work. The most obvious way is to present your work at an academic conference, either via an oral presentation or a poster presentation. Some conferences also partner with a journal, meaning that your abstract will be included in a special edition of the partner journal, and therefore be referenced in electronic databases. When submitting for academic conferences, as with academic journals, it is vital to examine the event to determine whether your research might fit. Unlike academic journals, which are predominantly national or international in scope, conferences at regional or local levels might offer particular opportunities to present your findings if they are appropriate for that geographical area. Another possible area for dissemination is professional publications, such as newsletters for members of associations and accreditation bodies including those in public health. This can help your research to reach professionals and practitioners working in the field. And, finally, social media is now a great way to disseminate research findings, and connect with researchers, policy makers and practitioners in the field.

Conclusion

This chapter has provided guidance and, hopefully, inspiration for students and novice researchers working in public health about the process of moving towards publication. Although academic publication is sometimes thought of as restricted to those working in academia, it should be the aim of anyone who has conducted good quality research, at whatever academic level. The step from postgraduate research to publication can seem like a large leap, but with the right support and approach, it is certainly achievable. By following the advice given in this chapter, the perceived large leap can become a series of steps towards your goal.

Further reading

Liberati, A., Altman, D., Tetzlaff, J., et al. (2009) The PRISMA statement for reporting systematic reviews and meta-analyses of studies that evaluate healthcare interventions: explanation and elaboration. *BMJ*, 339.

Moher, D. (1998) CONSORT: An evolving tool to help improve the quality of reports of randomized controlled trials. Consolidated Standards of Reporting Trials. *JAMA, 279*: 1489–91.

Tong, A., Sainsbury, P. and Craig, J. (2007) Consolidated criteria for reporting qualitative research (COREQ): A 32-item checklist for interviews and focus groups. *International Journal for Quality in Health Care*, 19(6): 349–57.

REFERENCES

Abramson, J.H. and Abramson, Z.H. (1999) *Survey Methods in Community Medicine* (Fifth edition). Edinburgh: Churchill Livingstone.

Agarwal, B. (2010) Does women's proportional strength affect their participation? Governing local forests in South Asia. *World Development, 38*(1): 98–112.

Alreck, P.L. and Settle, R.B. (1995) *Survey Research Handbook* (Second edition). Illinois: Irwin.

Alvesson, M. and Sköldberg, K. (2009) *Reflexive Methodology* (Second edition). London: Sage.

Annas, G.J. and Grodin, M.A. (1992) 'Introduction', in G.J. Annas and M.A. Grodin (eds) *The Nazi Doctors and the Nuremberg Code: Human rights in human experimentation.* Oxford: Oxford University Press.

Aos, S., Lieb, R., Mayfield, J., Miller, M. and Pennucci, A. (2004) *Benefits and Costs of Prevention and Early Intervention Programs for Youth.* Olympia: Washington State Institute for Public Policy.

Aroni, R., Timewell, E., Alexander, L. and Minichiello, V. (1990) *In-depth Interviewing: Researching people.* Melbourne: Longman Cheshire.

Asad, T. (1973) *Anthropology and the colonial encounter.* London: Ithaca.

Atkins, S., Lewin, S., Smith, H., Engel, M., Fretheim, A. and Volmink, J. (2008) Conducting a meta-ethnography of qualitative literature: Lessons learnt. *BMC Medical Research Methodology, 8* (21).

Atkinson, P. (2017) *Thinking Ethnographically.* London: Sage.

Babor, T.F. and Robaina, K.(2013) Public health, academic medicine and the alcohol industry's corporate social responsibility activities. *American Journal of Public Health, 103* (2).

Banister, P. (2011) *Qualitative Methods in Psychology: A research guide* (Second edition). Maidenhead: McGraw-Hill/Open University Press.

Barbour, R. (2008) *Introducing Qualitative Research: A student guide to the craft of doing qualitative research.* London: Sage.

Barbour, R. (2013) *Introducing Qualitative Research: A student's guide* (Second edition). London: Sage.

Barbour, R.S. and Kitzinger, J. (eds) (1999) *Developing Focus Group Research: Politics, theory and practice.* London: Sage.

Barlow, P., Serôdio, P., Ruskin, G., McKee, M. and Stuckler, D. (2018) Science organisations and Coca-Cola's 'war' with the public health community: Insights from an internal industry document. *J Epidemiol Community Health, 72*: 761–3.

Barnes, D.E. and Bero, L.A. (1998) Why review articles on the health effects of passive smoking reach different conclusions. *Journal of the American Medical Association, 279*(19): 1566–70.

Barnett, E., Casper, M.L., Halverson, J.A., Elmes, G.A., Braham, V.E., Majeed, Z.A., Bloom, A.S. and Stanley, S. (2001) *Men and Heart Disease: An atlas of racial and ethnic disparities in mortality*. University of Michigan.

Beck, U. (1992) *Risk Society: Towards a new modernity*. London: Sage.

Bell, R. and Newby, H. (1977) *Doing Sociological Research*. London: Allen and Unwin.

Berlin, J.A. and Golub, R.M. (2014) Meta-analysis as evidence: Building a better pyramid. *JAMA, 312*: 603–5.

Bhopal, R. (2016) *Concepts of Epidemiology* (Third edition). Oxford: Oxford University Press.

Blair, E. (2015) A reflexive exploration of two qualitative data coding techniques. *Journal of Methods and Measurement in the Social Sciences, 6*(1): 14–29.

Bloom, H. (2007) *Mary Shelley's Frankenstein* (Updated edition). New York: Chelsea House.

Blumer, H. (1954) What is wrong with social theory? *American Sociological Review, 18*: 3–10.

BMJ (2018) *Editorial: Public Health at 170. 362.*

Boeke, A.J.P., Randwijck-Jacobze, M.E., de Lange-Klerk, E.M.S., Grol, S.M., Kramer, M.H.H. and van der Horst, H.E. (2010) Effectiveness of GPs in accident and emergency departments. *British Journal of General Practice, 60*(579): e378–e384.

Bonita, R., Beaglehole, R. and Tord, K. (2006) *Basic Epidemiology*. Geneva: World Health Organization.

Bornioli, A., Bray, I., Pilkington, P. and Bird, E. (2018) The effectiveness of a 20 mph speed limit intervention on vehicle speeds in Bristol, UK: A non-randomised stepped wedge design. *Journal of Transport and Health, 11*: 47–55.

Bowen, G.A. (2006) Grounded theory and sensitising concepts. *International Journal of Qualitative Methods, 5*(3).

Bowling, A. (2005a) 'Quantitative social science', in A. Bowling and S. Ebrahim (eds) *Handbook of Health Research Methods: Investigation, measurement and analysis*. Maidenhead: Open University Press.

Bowling, A. (2005b) Mode of questionnaire administration can have serious effects on data quality. *Journal of Public Health, 27*(3): 281–91.

Bowling, A. (2014) *Research Methods in Health: Investigating health and health services*. Fourth edition. Buckingham: Open University Press.

Bowling, A. and Ebrahim, S. (eds) (2005) *Handbook of Health Research Methods: Investigation, measurement and analysis*. Maidenhead: Open University Press.

Boynton, P.M. and Greenhalgh, T. (2004) Hands-on guide to questionnaire research: selecting, designing, and developing your questionnaire. *British Medical Journal, 29*(328): 1312–15.

Brannen, P. (1987) 'Working on Directors: some methodological issues.' in Moyser, G. and Wagstaffe, M. (eds) *Research Methods for Elite Studies*. London: Allen and Unwin.

Braun, V. and Clarke, V. (2006) Using thematic analysis in psychology. *Qualitative Research in Psychology, 3*(2): 77–101.

Bray, I., Kenny, G., Pontin, D., Williams, R. and Albarran, J. (2016) Family presence during resuscitation: Validation of the risk-benefit and self-confidence scales for student nurses. *Journal of Research in Nursing, 21*(4): 306–22.

Brewer, J.D. (2000) *Ethnography*. Buckingham: Open University Press.

Brion, M.J., Lawlor, D.A., Matijasevich, A., Horta, B., Anselmi, L., Araújo, C.L., Menezes, A.M., Victora, C.G. and Davey Smith, G. (2011) What are the causal effects of breastfeeding on IQ, obesity and blood pressure? Evidence from comparing high-income with middle-income cohorts. *Int J Epidemiol., 40*(3): 670–80.

Britten, N., Campbell, R., Pope, C., Donovan, J., Morgan, M. and Pill, R. (2002) Using meta-ethnography to synthesise qualitative research: A worked example. *Journal of Health Services Research & Policy, 7*(4): 209–15.

Brownell, K.D., and Warner, K.E. (2009) The perils of ignoring history: Big Tobacco played dirty and millions died. How similar is big food? *Milbank Q, 87*: 259–94.

Bryant, A. (2009) Grounded theory and pragmatism: the curious case of Anselm Strauss. *Forum: Qualitative Social Research, 10*(3), Art.2.

Bryman, A. (1988) *Quantity and Quality in Social Research*. London: Routledge.

Bryman, A. (2016) *Social Research Methods* (Fifth edition). Oxford: Oxford University Press.

Buchanan, D.R. (1992) An uneasy alliance: Combining qualitative and quantitative research methods. *Health Education Quarterly, Spring*: 117–35.

Bulmer, M. (1986) *The Chicago School of Sociology: Institutionalisation, diversity, and the rise of sociological research*. Chicago, IL: University of Chicago Press.

Burgess, R. G. (1984) 'Autobiographical accounts and research experience', in R.G. Burgess (ed.) *The Research Process in Educational Settings: Ten Case Studies*. Lewes: The Falmer Press, pp. 251–70.

Calvey, D. (2017) *Covert Research: The art, politics and ethics of undercover fieldwork*. London: Sage.

Campbell, R., Pound, P., Morgan, M., Daker-White, G., Britten, N., Pill, R., Yarley, L., Pope, C. and Donovan, J. (2011) *Evaluating meta-ethnography: Systematic analysis and synthesis of qualitative research*. NIHR Health Technology Assessment programme: Executive Summaries.

Caracelli, V. and Greene, J. (1993) Data analysis strategies for mixed-method evaluation designs. *Educ Eval Policy Anal, 15*: 195–207.

CASP (2018) Available from: https://casp-uk.net/ (accessed 7 December 2018).

Cassell, J. (1998) 'The relationship of observer to observed when studying up', in R.G. Burgess (ed.), *Studies in Qualitative Methodology*. London: JAI Press.

Chalmers, I. (2003) Trying to do more good than harm in policy and practice: The role of rigorous, transparent, up-to-date evaluations. *The Annals of the American Academy of Political and Social Science, 589*: 22–39.

Charmaz, K. (2003) Grounded theory: Objectivist and constructivist methods. In N. K. Denzin, & Y. S. Lincoln (eds), *Strategies for qualitative inquiry* (2nd ed.), pp. 249-291. Thousand Oaks, CA: Sage.

Charmaz, K. (2005) 'Grounded theory in the 21st century: Applications for advancing social justice studies', in N.K. Denzin and Y.S. Lincoln (eds), *The Sage Handbook of Qualitative Research* (Third edition). London: Sage, pp. 507–36.

Charmaz, K. (2014) *Constructivist Grounded Theory* (Second edition). London: Sage.

Ciliska, D., Thomas, H., and Buffet, C. (2012) *A Compendium of Critical Appraisal Tools for Public Health Practice* (Revised). (Available from: www.nccmt.ca/pubs/Compendium ToolENG.pdf).

Cirillo, F. (2018) *The Pomodoro Technique: The life-changing time-management system*. Virgin Digital.

Clifford, J. (1986) *Writing Culture*. Los Angeles, CA: University of California Press.

Closser, S., Rosenthal, A., Maes, K., Justice, J., Cox, K., Omidian, P.A., Mohammed, I.Z., Dukku, A.M., Koon, A.D. and Nyirazinyoye, L. (2016) The global context of vaccine refusal: Insights from a systematic comparative ethnography of the Global Polio Eradication Initiative. *Medical Anthropology Quarterly, 30*(3): 321–41.

Coca-Cola Australia (2016) List of health professionals and scientific experts. Available from: www.coca-colajourney.com.au/transparency/health-professionals-and-scientific-experts (accessed November 2018).

Coca-Cola Deutschland (2016) Partnerschaften mit Experten. Available from: www.coca-cola-deutschland.de/stories/partnerschaften-mit-experten (accessed November 2018).

Coca-Cola España (2016) Colaboraciones en salud, nutrición y actividad física y apoyo a través de becas a proyectos de investigación. Available from: www.cocacolaespana.es/prensa/coca-cola-anuncia-su-colaboracion-por-medio-de-becas-a-proyectos-de-investigacion-coca-cola (accessed November 2018).

Coca-Cola France (2015) Les experts avec lesquels nous avon travaillé. Available from: www.coca-cola-france.fr/Coca-Cola-et-la-science/les-principes-directeurs-de-notre-entreprise (accessed November 2018).

Coca-Cola Great Britain (2016) Our investments in wealth and wellbeing research and partnerships – Individuals. Available from: www.coca-cola.co.uk/blog/our-investments-in-health-and-wellbeing-research-and-partnerships (accessed November 2018).

Coca-Cola New Zealand (2016) List of health professionals and scientific experts. Available from: www.coca-colajourney.co.nz/transparency/health-professionals-and-scientific-experts (accessed November 2018).

Cohen, L., Manion, L. and Morrison, K. (2000) Research methods in education (5th ed.). London: Routledge/Falmer.

Collins, K.M.T., Onwuegbuzie, A.J. and Jiao, Q.G. (2007) A mixed methods investigation of mixed methods sampling designs in social and health science research. *Journal of Mixed Methods Research*, 1(3): 267–94.

Cotterill, P. (1992) Interviewing women: Issues of friendship, vulnerability, and power. *Women's Studies International Forum*, 15: 593–606.

Coyne, I.T. (1997) Sampling in qualitative research. Purposeful and theoretical sampling; merging or clear boundaries? *Journal of Advanced Nursing*, 26(3): 623–30.

CRASH Trial Collaborators (2004) Effect of intravenous corticosteroids on death within 14 days in 10 008 adults with clinically significant head injury (MRC CRASH trial): randomised placebo-controlled trial. *Lancet*, 364: 1321–8.

Creswell, J.W. (2005) *Educational Research: Planning, conducting, and evaluating quantitative and qualitative research* (Second edition). Upper Saddle River, NJ: Pearson Education.

Creswell, J.W. (2009) *Research Design: Qualitative, quantitative, and mixed methods approaches* (Third edition). London: Sage.

Creswell, J.W. (2013) *Qualitative Inquiry and Research Design: Choosing among five approaches* (Third edition). London: Sage.

Creswell, J.W. and Plano Clark, V.L. (2011) *Designing and Conducting Mixed Methods Research* (Second edition). London: Sage.

Creswell, J.W. and Plano Clark, V.L. (2018) *Designing and Conducting Mixed Methods Research* (Third edition). London: Sage.

Creswell, J.W. and Poth, C.N. (2018) *Qualitative Inquiry and Research Design: Choosing among five approaches* (Fourth edition). London: Sage.

Cunliffe, A.L. and Alcadipani, R. (2016) The politics of access in fieldwork: Immersion, backstage dramas, and deception. *Organizational Research Methods*, 19(4): 535–61.

Czaja, R. and Blair, J. (1996) *Designing Surveys: A guide to decisions and procedures*. London: Pine Forge Press.

Czarniawska, B. (2004) *Narratives in Social Science Research*. London: Sage.

da Costa, B.R. and Jüni, P. (2014) Systematic reviews and meta-analyses of randomized trials: Principles and pitfalls. *European Heart Journal*, 35(47): 3336–45.

Daivadanam, M., Wahlström, R., Sundari Ravindran, Thankappan, K.R. and Ramanathan, M. (2014) Conceptual model for dietary behaviour change at household level: A 'best fit' qualitative study using primary data. *BMC Public Health*, 14: 574.

Dawson, A. (2017) Driven to sanity: An ethnographic critique of the senses in automobilities. *The Australian Journal of Anthropology, 28*: 3–20.

Deegan, M.J. (2001) 'The Chicago School of Ethnography' in P. Atkinson, S. Delamont, A. Coffey, J. Lofland and L. Lofland (eds), *Handbook of Ethnography*. London: Sage.

Denzin, N. (2006) *Sociological Methods: A sourcebook* (Fifth edition). New Jersey: Aldine Transaction.

Denzin, N.K. and Lincoln, Y.S. (2013) *Strategies of Qualitative Inquiry* (Fourth edition). London: Sage.

Denzin, N.K. and Lincoln, Y.S. (2013) 'Introduction: The discipline and practice of qualitative research' in N.K. Denzin and Y.S. Lincoln (eds), *The Landscape of Qualitative Research* (Fourth edition). London: Sage.

Diamond, I. and Jefferies, J. (2009) *Beginning Statistics*. London: Sage.

Dickson-Swift, V., James, E.L. and Liamputtong, P. (2008) *Undertaking Sensitive Research in the Health and Social Sciences: Managing boundaries, emotions and risks*. Cambridge: Cambridge University Press.

Di Gregori, V., Franchino, G., Marcantoni, C., Simone, B. and Costantino, C. (2014) Logistic regression of attitudes and coverage for influenza vaccination among Italian Public Health medical residents. *Journal of Preventive Medicine and Hygiene, 55*(4): 152–7.

Dixon-Woods, M., Agarwal, S., Jones, D., Young, B. and Sutton, A. (2005) Synthesising qualitative and quantitative evidence: A review of possible methods. *Journal of Health Services Research & Policy, 10* (1): 45–53.

Donaldson, L.J. and Rutter, P.D. (2017) *Donaldson's Essential Public Health* (Fourth edition). Oxford: Radcliffe Publishing.

Douglas, J.D. (1976) *Investigative Social Research: Individual and team field research*. London: Sage.

Douglas, J.D. (1985) *Creative Interviewing*. London: Sage.

Dowdney, L., Woodward, L., Pickles, A. and Skuse, D. (1995) The Body Image Perception and Attitude Scale for children: Reliability in growth retarded and community comparison subjects. *International Journal of Methods in Psychiatric Research, 5*: 29–40.

Drope, J. and Chapman, S. (2001) Tobacco industry efforts at discrediting scientific knowledge of environmental tobacco smoke: A review of internal industry documents. *Journal of Epidemiology and Community Health, 55*: 588–94.

Dwan, K., Gamble, C., Williamson, P.R. and Kirkham, J.J. for the Reporting Bias Group (2013) Systematic Review of the Empirical Evidence of Study Publication Bias and Outcome Reporting Bias — An Updated Review. *PLoS One, 8*(7): e66844.

Dyer, C. (1998) Tobacco company set up network of sympathetic scientists. *British Medical Journal, 316*: 1553.

Edwards, P., Roberts, I., Clarke, M., DiGuiseppi, C., Pratap, S., Wentz, R. and Kwan, I. (2002) Increasing response rates to postal questionnaires: Systematic review. *British Medical Journal, 324*: 1183.

Effective Public Health Practice Project (1998a) Quality Assessment Tool For Quantitative Studies. Hamilton, ON: Effective Public Health Practice Project. Available from: https://merst.ca/wp-content/uploads/2018/02/quality-assessment-tool_2010.pdf.

Effective Public Health Practice Project (1998b) Dictionary for the Effective Public Health Practice Project: Quality Assessment Tool For Quantitative Studies. Available from: https://merst.ca/wp-content/uploads/2018/02/qualilty-assessment-dictionary_2017.pdf.

Egger, M., Davey Smith, G. and Altman, D. (eds) (2001) *Systematic Reviews in Health Care: Meta-analysis in Context*. London: BMJ Books.

Elliott, J. (2005) *Using Narrative in Social Research, Qualitative and Quantitative Approaches*. London: Sage.

Elmore, R. F. (1991) Comment on 'Towards rigor in reviews of multivocal literatures: Applying the exploratory case study method'. Review of Educational Research, *61*(3), 293–297.

ESRC (2018) ESRC Secondary Data Analysis Initiative. Available from: https://esrc.ukri.org/funding/funding-opportunities/secondary-data-analysis-initiative-sdai-open-call (accessed 7 December 2018).

Esser, M.B., Bao, J., Jernigan, D.H. and Hyder, A.A. (2016) Evaluation of the evidence base for the alcohol industry's actions to reduce drink driving globally. *Am. J. Public Health*, *106*: 707–1.

Evens, T.M.S. and Handelman, D. (eds) (2006) *The Manchester School*. New York: Berghahn.

Everitt, B.S. (2002) *The Cambridge Dictionary of Statistics*, 2nd Edition, CUP.

Fentiman, I.S., Wang, D.Y., Allen, D.S., De Stavola, B.L., Moore, J.W., Reed, M.J. and Fogelman, I. (1994) Bone density of normal women in relation to endogenous and exogenous oestrogens. *British Journal of Rheumatology*, *33*: 808–15.

Fielden, A., Sillence, E. and Little, L. (2011) Children's understandings of obesity, a thematic analysis. *International Journal of Qualitative Studies on Health and Well-Being*, *6*(3): 7170 –7183.

Fielding, N. (1993) 'Ethnography', in N. Gilbert (ed.), *Researching Social Life*. London: Sage.

Flick, U. (1998) *An introduction to qualitative research*. London: Sage.

Fontana, A. and Frey, J.H. (2005) 'The interview: From neutral stance to political involvement', in N.K. Denzin and Y.S. Lincoln (eds), *The Sage Handbook of Qualitative Research* (Third edition). London: Sage, pp. 695–727.

Foucault, M. and Gordon, C. (1980) *Power/knowledge: Selected interviews and other writings 1972–1977*. Hemel Hempstead: Harvester Wheatsheaf.

Fowler, F.J. (1993) *Survey Research Methods* (Second edition). London: Sage.

Fowler, F.J. (1995) *Improving Survey Questions: Design and evaluation*. London: Sage.

France, E.F., Ring, N., Noyes, J., Maxwell, M., Jepson, R., Duncan, E., Turley, R, Jones, D. and Uny, I. (2015) Protocol-developing meta-ethnography reporting guidelines (eMERGe). *BMC Medical Research Methodology*, *15*: 103.

Freire, P. (1970) *Pedagogy of the Oppressed*. New York: Continuum.

Gadamer, H.G. (1976) *Philosophical Hermeneutics*. Los Angeles, CA: University of California Press.

Gadamer, H.G (2006) *Truth and Method*, 2nd edition, translated by Joel Weinsheimer and Donald G. Marshall. New York: Continuum.

Gale, N.K., Heath, G., Cameron, E., Rashid, S. and Redwood, S. (2013) Using the framework method for the analysis of qualitative data in multi-disciplinary health research. *BMC Medical Research Methodology*, *13*: 117.

Galletta, A. (2013) *Mastering the Semi-structured Interview and Beyond: From research design to analysis and publication*. New York: New York University Press.

Gardner, M.J. and Altman, D.G. (1986) Confidence intervals rather than P values: Estimation rather than hypothesis testing. *Br Med J (Clin Res Ed)*, *292*(6522): 746–50.

Garne, D., Watson, M., Chapman, S. and Byrne, F. (2005) Environmental tobacco smoke research published in the journal Indoor and Built Environment and associations with the tobacco industry. *The Lancet*, *365*: 804–9.

Garner, P., Hopewell, S., Chandler, J., MacLehose, H., Akl, E.A., Beyene, J., Chang, S., Churchill, R., Dearness, K., Guyatt, G., Lefebrve, C., Liles, B., Marshall, R., Martinez Garcia, L., Mavergames, C., Nasser, M., Qaseem, A., Sampson, M., Soares-Weiser, K., Takwoingi, Y., Thabane, L., Trivella, M., Tugwell, P., Welsh, E., Wilson, E.D and

Schunemann, H.J. (2016) When and how to update systematic reviews: Consensus and checklist. *BMJ*, *354*: i3507.

GBD (2015) Mortality and Causes of Death Collaborators (2015) Global, regional, and national life expectancy, all-cause mortality and cause-specific mortality for 249 causes of death, 1980–2015: A systematic analysis for the Global Burden of Disease Study 2015. *The Lancet*, *388* (10053): 1459–544.

GBD (2015) GBD Diarrhoeal Diseases Collaborators (2017) Estimates of global, regional, and national morbidity, mortality, and aetiologies of diarrhoeal diseases: a systematic analysis for the Global Burden of Disease Study 2015. *The Lancet*, *17*(9): 909–48.

Geertz, C. (1973) *The Interpretation of Cultures: Selected Essays*. New York: Basic Books.

Giddens, A. (2009) *Sociology* (Sixth edition). Cambridge: Polity Press.

Gilbert, N. (2015) *Researching Social Life* (Fourth edition). London: Sage.

Glantz, S.A., Bero, L.A. and Slade, J. (1998) *The Cigarette Papers*. Berkeley and Los Angeles, CA: University of California Press.

Glaser, B.G. (1978) *Theoretical Sensitivity: Advances in the methodology of grounded theory*. Mill Valley, CA: Sociology Press.

Glaser, B.G. (1992) *Basics of Grounded Theory Analysis: Emergence vs. forcing*. Mill Valley, CA: Sociology Press.

Glaser, B.G. (1998) *Doing Grounded Theory: Issues and discussions*. Mill Valley, CA: Sociology Press.

Glaser, B. and Strauss, A.L. (1967) *The Discovery of Grounded Theory: Strategies for qualitative research*. London and New Brunswick: Aldine Transaction.

Global Burden of Disease Collaborative Network. Global Burden of Disease Study 2016 (GBD 2016) Results. Seattle, United States: Institute for Health Metrics and Evaluation (IHME), 2017. Available from: https://ourworldindata.org/grapher/mental-and-sub-stance-use-as-share-of-disease [Online Resource]. (accessed 24 April 2019).

Gluckman, M. (1964) *Closed Systems and Open Minds: The limits of naivety in social anthropology*. Chicago, IL: Aldine.

Goffman, E. (1956) *The Presentation of Self in Everyday Life*. New York: Doubleday Anchor Books.

Gordis, L. (2013) *Epidemiology*. Philadelphia: Saunders.

Gray, S., Pilkington, P., Pencheon, D. and Jewell, T. (2006) Public health in the UK: Success or failure? *Journal of the Royal Society of Medicine*, *99*(3): 107–11.

Greene, J. (2007) *Mixed methods into Social Inquiry*. San Francisco, CA: Jossey-Bass.

Greenfield, R., Busink, E., Wong, C.P., Riboli-Sasco, E., Greenfield, G., Majeed, A., Car, J. and Wark, P.A. (2016) Truck drivers' perceptions on wearable devices and health promotion: A qualitative study. *BMC Public Health*, *16*: 677.

Greenland, S. (1994) Invited commentary: A critical look at some popular meta-analytic methods. *Am J Epidemiol*, *140*: 290–6.

Gruning, T., Gilmore, A.B. and McKee, M. (2006) Tobacco industry influence on science and scientists in Germany. *Am J Public Health*, *96*: 20–32.

Guba, E.G. and Lincoln, Y.S. (2005) 'Paradigmatic controversies, contradictions, and emerging influences', in N.K Denzin and Y.S Lincoln (eds), *The Sage Handbook of Qualitative Research* (Third edition). London: Sage.

Guest, G. and Fleming, P. (2015) 'Mixed methods research', in G. Guest and E. Namey (eds), *Public Health Research Methods*. Thousand Oaks, CA: Sage, pp. 581–614.

Guyatt, G., Oxman, A.D., Akl, E.A., Kunz, R., Vist, G., Brozek, J., Norris, S., Falck-Ytter, Y., Glasziou, P., DeBeer, H., Jaeschke, R., Rind, D., Meerpohl, J., Dahm, P. and Schunemann,

H.J. (2011) GRADE guidelines: 1. Introduction-GRADE evidence profiles and summary of findings tables. *Journal of Clinical Epidemiology, 64*(4): 383–94.

Habermas, J. (1987) *Theory of Communicative Action*. Boston, MA: Beacon Press.

Hammersley, M. (1992) *What's Wrong with Ethnography?* London: Routledge.

Hammersley, M. and Atkinson, P. (2007) *Ethnography: Principles in practice*. London: Routledge.

Harding, S. (1991) *Whose Science? Whose Knowledge? Thinking from Women's Lives*. Milton Keynes: Open University Press.

Hardon, A., Hodgkin, C. and Fresle, D. (2004) *How to Investigate the Use of Medicines by Consumers*. World Health Organization and University of Amsterdam.

Hedges, B.M. (1979). Sampling minority populations. In *Social and Educational Research in Action* (Ed., M.J. Wilson) London: Longman, 245 – 261.

Hempel, S. (2018) *The Atlas of Disease: Epidemics, outbreaks and contagion in 50 maps*. London: White Lion Publishing.

Hennekens, C.H. and Buring, J.E. (1987) *Epidemiology in Medicine*. Boston: Little, Brown.

Hesse-Biber, S. (2010) *Mixed Methods Research: Merging theory with practice*. New York, NY: Guilford Press.

Higgins, J.P.T. and Green, S. (eds) (2011) *Cochrane Handbook for Systematic Reviews of Interventions Version 5.1.0* [updated March 2011]. Available from: http://handbook. cochrane.org.

Higgs, M. and Dulewicz, V. (2016) *Leading with Emotional Intelligence*. Basingstoke: Palgrave Macmillan.

Hill, A.B. (1965) The environment and disease: association or causation? *J. R. Soc. Med, 58*(5).

Hines, M. and Brooks, G. (2009). Bookstart National Impact Evaluation 2009. *Bookstart*. Available from: www.booktrust.org.uk/globalassets/resources/research/bookstart-national-impact-evaluation-2009.pdf

Holmes, S. (2013a) *Fresh Fruit, Broken Bodies: Indigenous Mexican farmworkers in the United States*. Berkeley, CA: University of California Press.

Holmes, S. (2013b) 'Is it worth risking your life?' Ethnography, risk and death on the U.S.-Mexico border. *Social Science and Medicine, 99*: 153–61.

Holstein, J. and Gubrium, J. (1995) *The Active Interview*. London: Sage.

Hseih, H-F. and Shannon, S.E. (2005) Three approaches to qualitative content analysis. *Qualitative Health Research, 15*(9): 1277–88.

Hulse, G.K., English, D.R., Milne, E., Holman, C.D. and Bower, C.I. (1997) Maternal cocaine use and low birth weight newborns: A meta-analysis. *Addiction, 92*(11): 1561–70.

Ioannidis, J.P.A., Haidich, A-B., Pappa, M., Pantazis, N., Kokori, S.I., Tektonidou, M.G., Contopoulos-Ioannidis, D.G. and Lau, J. (2001) Comparison of evidence of treatment effects in randomized and non-randomized studies. *JAMA, 286*: 821–30.

Jackson, A.Y. and Mazzei, L.A. (2012) *Thinking with Theory in Qualitative Research: Viewing data across multiple perspectives*. London: Routledge.

Jernigan, D.H. (2011) Global alcohol producers, science and policy: The case of the International Center for Alcohol Policies. *American Journal of Public Health, 102*(1). Available from: https://ajph.aphapublications.org/doi/pdf/10.2105/AJPH.2011.300269

Jia, Y., Li, F., Liu, Y.F., Zhao, J.P., Leng, M.M. and Chen, L. (2017) Depression and cancer risk: A systematic review and meta-analysis. *Public Health, 149*: 138–48.

Joanna Briggs Institute (2018) Critical Appraisal Tools. Available from: http://joannabriggs. org/research/critical-appraisal-tools.html (accessed 7 December 2018).

Jones, C.M., Taylor, G.O., Whittle, J.G., Evans, D. and Trotter, D.P. (1997) Water fluoridation, tooth decay in 5 year olds, and social deprivation measured by the Jarman score: Analysis of data from British dental surveys. *BMJ, 315*(7107): 514–17.

Kamberelis, G. and Dimitriadis, G. (2005) 'Focus Groups: Strategic articulations of peda-gogy, politics, and enquiry', in N.K. Denzin and Y.S. Lincoln (eds), *The Sage Handbook of Qualitative Research*. (Third edition). London: Sage, pp. 887–907.

Kane, S.S., Gerretsen, B., Scherpbier, R., Dal Poz, M. and Dieleman, M. (2010) A realist synthesis of randomised control trials involving use of community health workers for delivering child health interventions in low and middle income countries. *BMC Health Services Research, 10*: 286.

Katz, J. (1992) 'The Consent Principle of the Nuremberg Code: Its significance then and now', in G.J. Annas and M.A. Grodin (eds), *The Nazi Doctors and the Nuremberg Code: Human rights in human experimentation*. Oxford: Oxford University Press.

Kaur M. (2016) Application of mixed method approach in public health research. *Indian Journal of Community Medicine, 41*(2): 93–7.

Kirk, J. and Miller, M.L. (1986) 'Reliability and Validity in Qualitative Research.' *Qualitative Research Methods, Series 1. Sage University Paper*. London.

Kitta, A. and Goldberg, D.S. (2016) The significance of folklore for vaccine policy: Discarding the deficit model. *Critical Public Health, 27*(4): 506–14.

Koch, T. and Harrington, A. (1998) Reconceptualizing rigour: The case for reflexivity. *Journal of Advanced Nursing, 28*(4): 882–90.

Kozuki, N., Sonneveldt, E. and Walker, N. (2013) Residual confounding explains the asso-ciation between high parity and child mortality. *BMC Public Health, 13* (Suppl 3): S5.

Kuper, A. (1996) *Anthropology and Anthropologists: The Modern British School* (Third edition). London: Routledge.

Lancet (editorial) (2018) GBD 2017: A fragile world. *The Lancet, 392* (10159): 1683.

Last, J.M. (2001) *A Dictionary of Epidemiology*. Oxford: Oxford University Press.

Latour, B. (1988) *Science in Action: How to follow scientists and engineers through society*. Cambridge, MA: Harvard University Press.

Latour, B. and Woolgar, S. (1986) *Laboratory Life: The construction of scientific facts* (Second edition). Princeton, NJ: Princeton University Press.

Lavelle, H.V., Mackay, D.F. and Pell, J.P. (2012) Systematic review and meta-analysis of school-based intervention to reduce body mass index. *Journal of Public Health, 34*(3): 360–9.

Lee, P.N., (1994) *Environmental tobacco smoke, a commentary on some of the evidence provided by OSHA in support of their proposed rules*. Washington, DC: Occupational Safety and Health Administration

Lee, K., Gilmore, A.B. and Collin, J. (2004) Looking inside the tobacco industry: revealing insights from the Guildford Depository. *Addiction, 99*(4): 394–7.

Lexchin, J., Bero, L.A., Djulbegovic, B. and Clark, O. (2003) Pharmaceutical industry spon-sorship and research outcome and quality: systematic review. *BMJ, 326*: 1167.

Liberati, A., Altman, D., Tetzlaff, J., Murlow, C., Gotzche, P.C., Ioannidid, J.P.A., Clarke, M., Devereaux, P.J., Kleijnen, J. and Moher, D. (2009) The PRISMA statement for reporting systematic reviews and meta-analyses of studies that evaluate healthcare interventions: explanation and elaboration. *BMJ*, 339.

Lincoln, Y.S. and Guba, E.G. (1985) *Naturalistic Inquiry*. London: Sage.

Lincoln, Y.S. and Guba, E.G. (1989) Ethics: The failure of positivist science. *The Review of Higher Education, 12*(3): 221–40.

Lincoln, Y.S., Lynham, S.A. and Guba, E.G. (2013) 'Paradigmatic controversies, contradic-tions, and emerging confluences, revisited', in N.K. Denzin and Y.S. Lincoln (eds), *The Landscape of Qualitative Research*. London: Sage.

Lundh, A., Lexchin, J., Mintzes, B., Schroll, J.B. and Bero, L. (2017) Industry sponsorship and research outcome. *Cochrane Database Syst Rev., 2*:MR000033. doi: 10.1002/14651858. MR000033.pub3.

Lyons, L. and Chipperfield, J. (2000) (De)constructing the interview: a critique of the participatory model. *Resources for Feminist Research*, *28*(1/2): 33.

Lyons, R.A., Towner, N., Christie, D., Jones, S.J., Hayes, M., Kimberlee, R., Sarvotham, T., Macey, S., Brussoni, M., Sleney, J., Coupland, C. and Phillips, C. (2008) The advocacy in action study: a cluster randomized controlled trial to reduce pedestrian injuries in deprived communities. *Injury Prevention*, *14*(2).

Malin, B., Karp, D. and Scheuermann, R.H. (2010) Technical and policy approaches to balancing patient privacy and data sharing in clinical and translational research. *Journal of Investigative Medicine*, *58*: 11–18.

Malinowski, B. (1922) *Argonauts of the Western Pacific*. London: Routledge and Kegan Paul.

Malone, R.E. and Balbach, E.D. (2000) Tobacco industry documents: Treasure trove or quagmire? *Tobacco Control*, *9*: 334–8.

May, T. (1997) *Social Research: Issues, Methods and Process*. Milton Keynes: Open University Press.

Marshall, M.N. (1996) Sampling for qualitative research. *Family Practice*, *13*(6): 522–6.

Maxwell, J.A. (2013) *Qualitative Research Design: An interactive approach* (Third edition). London: Sage.

Mays, N. and Pope, C. (1995) Qualitative Research: Rigour and qualitative research. *BMJ*, *311*(6997): 109.

McCall, G. and Simmons, J. (1969) *Issues in Participant Observation*. New York: Addison-Wesley.

McCandless, D. (2012) *Information is Beautiful*. London: Harper Collins.

McClean, S. (2006) *Ethnography of Crystal and Spiritual Healing in Northern England: Marginal medicine; mainstream concerns*. Lewiston, NY: Edwin Mellen Press.

McKee, M. (2000) Smoke and mirrors: Clearing the air to expose the tactics of the tobacco industry. *European Journal of Public Health*, *10*: 161–3.

McLaughlin, J.C., Hamilton, K. and Kipping, R. (2017) Epidemiology of adult overweight recording and management by UK GPs: A systematic review. *British Journal of General Practice*, *67*(663): e676–e683.

McManus, S., Bebbington, P., Jenkins, R. and Brugha, T. (eds) (2016) *Mental Health and Wellbeing in England: Adult psychiatric morbidity survey 2014*. Leeds: NHS digital.

Menzel, J.E., Krawczyk, R. and Thompson, J.K. (2011) 'Attitudinal assessment of body image for adolescents and adults', in T.F. Cash and L. Smolak (eds), *Body image: A handbook of science, practice, and prevention*. New York, NY: Guilford Press, pp. 154–69.

Merriam, S.B. (2009) *Qualitative Research: A guide to design and implementation*. San Francisco, CA: John Wiley.

Mies, M. (1993) 'Towards a methodology for feminist research', in G. Bowles and R. Duelli-Klein (eds), *Theories of Women's Studies*. London: Routledge and Kegan Paul.

Miles, M.B. and Huberman, A.M. (1994) *Qualitative Data Analysis: An expanded sourcebook* (Second edition). London: Sage.

Moher, D. (1998). CONSORT: An evolving tool to help improve the quality of reports of randomized controlled trials. Consolidated Standards of Reporting Trials. *JAMA*, *279*: 1489–91.

Morse, J.M. (1998) 'Designing funded qualitative research', in N.K. Denzin and Y.S. Lincoln (eds), *Strategies of Qualitative Inquiry*. London: Sage.

Morse, J.M. (2015) Critical analysis of strategies for determining rigor in qualitative inquiry. *Qualitative Health Research*, *25*(9): 1212–22.

Morse, J.M. and Field, P. (1998) *Nursing research: the application of qualitative approaches*, 2nd edn, Stanley Thornes, Cheltenham.

Morse, J. and Niehaus, L. (2009) *Mixed Method Design: Principles and procedures*. Walnut Creek, CA: Left Coast Press.

Moses, J. and Knutsen, T.L. (2012) *Ways of Knowing: Competing methodologies in social and political research*. Second edition. Buckingham: Palgrave.

Muggli, M.E., Forster, J.L., Hurt, R.D. and Repace, J.L. (2001) The smoke you don't see: Uncovering tobacco industry scientific strategies aimed against environmental tobacco smoke policies. *American Journal of Public Health, 91*(9): 1419–23.

Murray, R.L., Leonardi-Bee, J., Marsh, J., Jayes, L., Li, J., Parrott, S. and Britton, J. (2013) Systematic identification and treatment of smokers by hospital based cessation practitioners in a secondary care setting: cluster randomised controlled trial. *BMJ, 347*: f4004.

NHS Digital (2018) *Prescribing*. Available from: https://digital.nhs.uk/data-and-information/areas-of-interest/prescribing (accessed 7 December 2018).

NIH *Study Quality Assessment Tools*. Available from: www.nhlbi.nih.gov/health-topics/study-quality-assessment-tools (accessed 7 December 2018).

Nielsen, J.M. (1990) *Feminist Research Methods: Exemplary readings in the social sciences*. Boulder, CO: Westview Press.

Noblit, G.W. and Dwight Hare, R. (1988) *Meta-ethnography: Synthesizing qualitative studies*. Newbury Park, CA: Sage.

Nunnaly, J. (1978) *Psychometric Theory*. New York: McGraw-Hill.

Nuremberg Code (1947) from Trials of War Criminals before the Nuremberg Military Tribunals under Control Council Law No. 10. Nuremberg, October 1946–April 1949. Washington, D.C.: U.S. G.P.O, 1949–1953.

Nzabonimpa, J.P. (2018) Quantitizing and qualitizing (im-)possibilities in mixed methods research. *Methodological Innovations*, 1–16.

Oakley, A. (1981) 'Interviewing women: A contradiction in terms', in H. Roberts (ed.) *Doing Feminist Research*. London: Routledge and Kegan Paul.

Okely, J. (2010) 'Fieldwork as free association and free passage', in M. Melhuus, J.P. Mitchell, and H. Wulff (eds) *Ethnographic Practice in the Present*. Oxford: Berghahn.

O'Connell Davidson, J. and Layder, D. (1994) *Methods, Sex and Madness*. London: Routledge.

O'Connor, A. (2015) Coca-Cola funds scientists who shift blame for obesity away from bad diets. *The New York Times, 9* August. Available from: well.blogs.nytimes.com/2015/08/09/coca-cola-funds-scientists-who-shift-blame-for-obesity-away-from-bad-diets/ (accessed November 2018).

O'Connor, A.M., Auvermann, B.W., Dzikamunhenga, R.S., Glanville, J.M., Higgins, J.P.T., Kirychuk, S.P., Sargeant, J.M., Totton, S.C., Wood, H. and Von Essen, S.G. (2017) Updated systematic review: Associations between proximity to animal feeding operations and health of individuals in nearby communities. *Systematic reviews, 6*: 86.

Office of the United Nations High Commissioner for Human Rights (2008) *The Right to Health. Fact Sheet No. 31*. Geneva: WHO.

Ong, E.K. and Glantz, S.A. (2000) Tobacco industry efforts subverting International Agency for Research on Cancer's second-hand smoke study. *Lancet, 355*: 1253–9.

ONS (2011) Census Data. Available from: www.ons.gov.uk/ons/guide-method/census/2011/census-data/2011-census-data-catalogue/census-data-quick-view/index.html

ONS (2015) Origin-destination Statistics on Migration for Local Authorities in the United Kingdom and on Workplace for Output Areas and Workplace Zones, England and Wales. Available from: https://webarchive.nationalarchives.gov.uk/20160106094447/http://www.ons.gov.uk/ons/rel/census/2011-census/origin-destination-statistics-on-migration-and-students-for-local-authorities-in-the-united-kingdom/index.html (accessed 7 December 2018).

Oppenheim, A.N. (2001) *Questionnaire Design, Interviewing and Attitude Measurement*. London: Continuum.

Oreskes, N. and Conway, E. (2010) *Merchants of Doubt. How a handful of scientists obscured the truth on issues from tobacco smoke to global warming*. London: Bloomsbury Press.

Orme, J., Powell, J., Taylor, P. and Grey, M. (2007) *Public Health for the 21st Century: New perspectives on policy and practice*. Buckingham: Open University Press.

Owen, R. (1982) Reader Bias. *JAMA*, 247(18): 2533–4.

Padgett, D.K. (2012) *Qualitative and Mixed Methods in Public Health*. Thousand Oaks, CA: Sage.

Painter, R.C., Roseboom, T.J. and Bleker, O.P. (2005) Prenatal exposure to the Dutch famine and disease in later life: An overview. *Reproductive Toxicology*, 20(3): 345-352.

Paley, J. (2017) *Phenomenology as Qualitative Research: A critical analysis of meaning attribution*. London: Routledge.

Pallant, J. (2016) *SPSS Survival Guide* (Sixth edition). Oxford: Oxford University Press.

Pardoe, I. (2012) *Applied Regression Modelling* (Second edition). Hoboken, NJ: Wiley.

Patton, M.Q. (1990) *Qualitative Evaluation and Research Methods*. London: Sage.

Patton, M.Q. (2002) *Qualitative Research and Evaluation Methods* (Third edition). London: Sage.

Patton, M.Q. (2015) *Qualitative Research and Evaluation Methods: Integrating Theory and Practice* (Fourth edition). London: Sage.

Pawson, R. (2002) Evidence-based policy: The promise of 'realist synthesis'. *Evaluation*, 8: 340–58.

Pawson, R. and Tilley, N. (2004) *Realist Evaluation*. Available from: www.community-matters.com.au/RE_chapter.pdf.

Pearce, M., Bray, I. and Horswell, M. (2017) Weight change in mid-childhood and its relationship with the fast food environment. *Journal of Public Health*, 40(2): 237–44.

Pels, P. and Salemink, O. (1999) *Colonial Subjects: Essays on the practical history of anthropology*. Ann Arbor, MI: University of Michigan Press.

Petrosino, A., Turpin-Petrosino, C. and Buehler, J. (2002) 'Scared Straight' and other juvenile awareness programs for preventing juvenile delinquency. *Cochrane Database Syst Rev*, (2): CD002796.

Petrosino, A., Turpin-Petrosino, C., Hollis-Peel, M.E. and Lavenberg, J.G. (2013) 'Scared Straight' and other juvenile awareness programs for preventing juvenile delinquency. *Cochrane Database Syst Rev*. Apr *30* (4): CD002796.

Petticrew, M. (2009) Systematic reviews in public health: Old chestnuts and new challenges. *Bull World Health Organ*, 87(3): 163.

Pilkington, P., Bird, E., Gray, S., Towner, E., Weld, S. and McKibben, M.A. (2014) Understanding the social context of fatal road traffic collisions among young people: A qualitative analysis of narrative text in coroners' records. *BMC Public Health*, 14(78): 1–8.

Plano Clark, V.L. and Badiee, M. (2010) 'Research questions in mixed methods research', in A. Tashakkori and C. Teddlie (eds), *SAGE Handbook of Mixed Methods in Social and Behavioural Research*. Thousand Oaks, CA: Sage, pp. 275–304.

Pope, C., Mays, N. and Popay, J. (2007) *Synthesizing Qualitative and Quantitative Health Research: A guide to methods*. Oxford: Oxford University Press.

Pope, C., Ziebland, S. and Mays, N. (2000) Qualitative research in health care: Analysing qualitative data. *BMJ*, 320.

Pope, D., Tisdall, R. and Middleton, J. (2015) Quality of and access to green space in relation to psychological distress: results from a population-based cross-sectional study as part of the EURO-URHIS 2 project. *European J Public Health*, 28(1): 35–8.

Public Health England (2010) Notifiable diseases and causative organisms: How to report. Available from: www.gov.uk/guidance/notifiable-diseases-and-causative-organisms-how-to-report (accessed 7 December 2018).

Public Health England (2018) Notifiable diseases: Weekly reports for 2018. Available from: www.gov.uk/government/publications/notifiable-diseases-weekly-reports-for-2018 (accessed 7 December 2018).

Public Health England (2018) *Statutory Notifications of Infectious Diseases*, Week 2018/12. Available from: www.gov.uk/government/uploads/system/uploads/attachment_data/file/694900/NOIDS-weekly-report-week12-2018.pdf (accessed 28 March 2018).

Purgato, M. and Adams, C.E. (2012) Heterogeneity: The issue of apples, oranges and fruit pie. *Epidemiol Psychtr Sci*, *21*(1): 27–9.

Reich, W. (2010) Three problems of intersubjectivity – And one solution. *Sociological Theory*, *28*(1): 40–63.

Reiners, G.M. (2012) Understanding the differences between Husserl's (descriptive) and Heidegger's (interpretive) phenomenological research. *Journal of Nursing and Care*, *1*(5): 1–3.

Resaland, G.K., Moe, V.F., Aadland, E., Steene-Johannessen, J., Glosvik, O., Anderson, J.R., Kvalheim, O.M., McKay, H.A. and Anderssen, S.A. (2015) Active Smarter Kids (ASK): Rationale and design of a cluster-randomised controlled trial investigating the effects of daily physical activity on children's academic performance and risk factors for non-communicable diseases. *BMC Public Health*, *15*: 709.

Riessman, C.K. (1993) *Narrative Analysis*. London: Sage.

Ritchie, J. and Lewis, J. (2003) *Qualitative Research Practice: A guide for social science students and researchers*. London: Sage.

Ritchie, J. and Spencer, L. (1994) 'Qualitative data analysis for applied policy research', in A. Bryman and R.G. Burgess (eds), *Analyzing Qualitative Data*. London: Routledge, pp. 173–94.

Rodeghier, M. (1996) *Surveys with confidence. A practical guide to survey research using SPSS*. SPSS Inc.

Rolfhamre, P., Grabowska, K., and Ekdahl, K. (2004) Implementing a public web based GIS service for feedback of surveillance data on communicable diseases in Sweden. *BMC Infectious Diseases*, *4*(17).

Rose, D. (2014) Patient and public involvement in health research: Ethical imperative and/or radical challenge? *Journal of Health Psychology*, *19*(1): 149–58.

Rothman, K.J. (2012) *Epidemiology; An introduction* (Second edition). Oxford: Oxford University Press.

Rudge, J. and Gilchrist, R. (2005) Excess winter morbidity among older people at risk of cold homes: A population-based study in a London borough. *Journal of Public Health*, *27*(4): 353–8.

Ryan, G. W. and Bernard, H. R. (2000) 'Data management and analysis methods', in N.K. Denzin and Y.S. Lincoln (eds), *Handbook of Qualitative Research* (Second edition). Thousand Oaks, CA: Sage, pp. 769–802.

Rycroft-Malone, J., McCormack, B., Hutchinson, A.M., DeCorby, K., Bucknall, T.K., Kent, B., Schultz, A., Snelgrove-Clarke, E., Stetler, C.B., Titler, M., Wallin, L. and Wilson, V. (2012) Realist synthesis: Illustrating the method for implementation research. *Implementation Science*, *7*: 33.

Saldana, J. (2016) *The Coding Manual for Qualitative Researchers*. London: Sage.

Sandelowski, M. (1995) Sample size in qualitative research. *Research in Nursing & Health*, *18*(2): 179-183.

Sandelowski, M. (1997) 'To be of use': Enhancing the utility of qualitative research. *Nursing Outlook*, *45*: 125–32.

Sandelowsi, M. (2000) Combining qualitative and quantitative sampling, data collection, and analysis techniques in mixed methods studies. *Research in Nursing & Health*, *23*(3): 246–55.

Sandelowski, M., Voils, C.I. and Barroso, J. (2006) Defining and designing mixed research synthesis studies. *Res Sch, 13*(1): 29.

Schuman, H. and Presser, S. (1996) *Questions and Answers in Attitude Surveys: Experiments on question form, wording and content.* London: Sage.

Sebrié, E., Sandoya, E., Hyland, A., Bianco, E., Glantz, S.A. and Cummings, K.M. (2012) Hospital admissions for acute myocardial infarction before and after implementation of a comprehensive smoke-free policy in Uruguay. *Tobacco Control, 22*(e1): e16–20.

Serôdio, P.M., McKee, M. and Stuckler, D. (2018) Coca-Cola – a model of transparency in research partnerships? A network analysis of Coca-Cola's research funding. *Public Health Nutrition, 21*(9): 1594–607.

SIGN (2018) Critical appraisal notes and checklists. Available from: www.sign.ac.uk/checklists-and-notes.html (accessed 7 December 2018).

Silverman, D. (2015) *Interpreting Qualitative Data* (Fifth edition). London: Sage.

Silverman, R.M. and Patterson, K.L. (2015) *Qualitative Research Methods for Community Development.* London: Routledge.

Smith, J.A. and Osborn, M. (2007) 'Interpretative phenomenological analysis', in J.A Smith (ed.) *Qualitative Psychology: A Practical Guide to Research Methods.* London: Sage, pp. 53–80.

Smith, J.A., Flowers, P. and Larkin, M. (2009) *Interpretive Phenomenological Analysis.* London: Sage

Spradley, J.P. (1979) *The Ethnographic Interview.* London: Routledge.

St. Pierre, E.A. and Jackson, A.Y. (2014) Qualitative data analysis after coding. *Qualitative Inquiry, 20*(6): 715–19.

Stefan, C., Bray, F., Ferlay, J., Liu, B. and Maxwell Parkin, D. (2017) Cancer of childhood in sub-Saharan Africa. *Ecancermedicalscience, 11*: 755.

Stott, H., Cramp, M., McClean, S. and Turton, A. (2018) Exploring altered body perception and comfort after stroke: An interpretive phenomenological analysis. *Clinical Rehabilitation, 32*(10): 1406–17.

Strauss, A. and Corbin, J. (1998) *Basics of Qualitative Research Techniques and Procedures for Developing Grounded Theory* (Second edition). London: Sage Publications.

Stuckler, D. and Nestle, M. (2012) Big food, food systems, and global health. *PLoS Med, 9*, e1001242.

Suri, H. (2011) Purposeful sampling in qualitative research synthesis. *Qualitative Research Journal, 11*(2): 63–75.

Tashikkori, A. and Creswell, J.W. (2007) Editorial: Exploring the nature of research questions in mixed methods research. *Journal of Mixed Methods Research, 1*(3): 207–11.

Tashakkori, A. and Teddlie, C. (eds) (2010) *Handbook of Mixed Methods in Social and Behavioural Research.* Thousand Oaks, CA: Sage.

Thapa, S., Hannes, K., Buve, A., Bhattarai, S. and Mathei, C. (2018) Theorizing the complexity of HIV disclosure in vulnerable populations: A grounded theory study. *BMC Public Health, 18*: 162.

The Coca-Cola Company (2015a) List of Health Professionals and Scientific Experts. Available from: www.coca-colacompany.com/transparency/list-of-health-professionals-and-scientific-experts (accessed November 2018).

The Joanna Briggs Institute (2014) *The Joanna Briggs Institute Reviewers' Manual 2014: Methodology for JBI Mixed Methods Systematic Review.* Adelaide, Australia.

Thomas W.I. and Znaniecki, F. (1918) *The Polish Peasant in Europe and America: Monograph of an immigrant group.* Vol. *1.* Boston, MA: The Gorham Press.

Thornberg, R. (2012) Informed grounded theory. *Scandinavian Journal of Educational Research, 56*(3): 243–59.

Thornton, A. and Lee, P. (2000) Publication bias in meta-analysis: Its causes and consequences. *Journal of Clinical Epidemiology, 53*: 207–16.

Tilford, S., Green, J. and Tones, K. (2003) *Values, Health Promotion and Public Health*. Report commissioned by the Health Development Agency, Leeds Metropolitan University.

Tong, A., Sainsbury, P. and Craig, J. (2007) Consolidated criteria for reporting qualitative research (COREQ): A 32-item checklist for interviews and focus groups. *International Journal for Quality in Health Care, 19*(6): 349–57.

Toyoran, T., Roberts, I., Oakley, A., Laing, G., Mugford, M. and Frost, C. (2003) Effectiveness of out-of-home day care for disadvantaged families: Randomised controlled trial. *BMJ, 327*: 906.

Tripepi, G., Jager, K.J., Dekker, F.W., Wanner, C. and Zoccali, C. (2007) Measures of effect: Relative risks, odds ratios, risk difference, and 'number needed to treat'. *Kidney International, 72*, 789–91.

Tufte, E.R. (1983) *The Visual Display of Quantitative Information*. Cheshire, CT: Graphics Press.

Tuhiwai Smith, L. (1999). *Decolonizing methodologies*. London: Zed Books Ltd.

Twibell, R.S., Siela, D., Riwitis, C., Wheatley, J., Riegle, T., Bousman, D., Cable, S., Caudill, P., Harrigan, S., Hollars, R., Johnson, D. and Neal, A. (2008) Nurses' perceptions of their self-confidence and the risks and benefits of family presence during resuscitation. *American Journal of Critical Care, 17*(2): 101–11.

Tyndall, J. (2010) AACODS Checklist. Flinders University. Available from: http://dspace.flinders.edu.au/dspace/ (accessed 7 December 2018).

Vandenbroucke, J.P., von Elm, E., Altman, D.G., Gøtzsche, P.C., Mulrow, C.D., Pocock, S.J., Poole, C., Schlesselman, J.J. and Egger, M. (2007) STROBE Initiative. Strengthening the Reporting of Observational Studies in Epidemiology (STROBE): Explanation and elaboration. *PLoS Med, 4*(10): e297.

Wager, E. and Wiffen, P.J. (2011) Ethical issues in preparing and publishing systematic review. *Journal of Evidence-Based Medicine, 4*(2): 130-4.

Van Ewijk, R. (2011). Long-term health effects on the next generation of Ramadan fasting during pregnancy. *Journal of Health Economics, 30*(6), 1246-1260.

de Vaus, A.D. (2002) *Surveys in Social Research* (Fifth edition). London: UCL Press.

de Viggiani, N., Daykin, N., Moriarty, Y. and Pilkington, P. (2013) *Musical Pathways: An exploratory study of young people in the criminal justice system engaged with a creative music programme*. Bristol: University of the West of England.

Weisberg, H.J., Krosnick, J.A. and Bowen, B.D. (eds) (1996) *An Introduction to Survey Research, Polling, and Data Analysis* (Third edition). London: Sage.

Wherton, J., Sugarhood, P., Proctor, R., Hinder, S. and Greenhalgh, T. (2015) Co-production in practice: How people with assisted living needs can help design and evolve technologies and services. *Implementation Science, 10*: 75.

White, J. and Bero, L.A. (2010) Corporate manipulation of research: Strategies are similar across five industries. *Stanford Law and Policy Review, 21*: 105–34.

Willig, C. and Stainton Rogers, W. (2012) *The SAGE Handbook of Qualitative Research in Psychology*. London: Sage.

WMA (World Medical Association) (1964[2013]) *Declaration of Helsinki – Ethical Principles for medical research involving human subjects*. Available at www.wma.net/policies-post/wma-declaration-of-helsinki-ethical-principles-for-medical-research-involving-human-subjects

Wong, G., Greenhalgh, T., Westhorp, G., Buckingham, J. and Pawson, R. (2013) RAMESES publication standards: Realist syntheses. *BMC Medicine*, *11*: 21.

Wong, G., Pawson, R. and Owen, L. (2011) Policy guidance on threats to legislative interventions in public health: A realist synthesis. *BMC Public Health*, *11*: 222.

Wooton, D. (2006) *Bad Medicine: Doctors doing harm since Hippocrates*. Oxford: Oxford University Press.

Wright, J., Sim, F. and Ferguson, K. (2014) *Multidisciplinary Public Health: Understanding the development of the modern workforce*. Bristol: Policy Press.

WHO (1978) *The Alma-Ata Declaration on Primary health care*. Geneva: WHO.

WHO (1981) *Global strategy for Health for All by the Year 2000. 16th plenary session of the World Health Assembly, 1981*. Geneva: WHO.

WHO Europe (1986) The Ottawa Charter for Health Promotion. First International Conference on Health Promotion, Ottawa, Canada. Geneva: WHO Europe. Available from: www.euro.who.int/__data/assets/pdf_file/0004/129532/Ottawa_Charter.pdf?ua=1 (accessed 1 February 2019).

WHO (1991) Sundsvall Statement on Supportive Environments for Health. Third International Conference on Health Promotion, Sundsvall, Sweden. Geneva: WHO. Available from: www.who.int/healthpromotion/milestones_ch3_20090916_en.pdf (accessed 1 February 2019)

World Health Organization & World Trade Organization (2002) World Trade Agreements and Public Health. WTO & WHO. Available from: www.who.int/media/homepage/en/who_wto_e.pdf (accessed 1 February 2019).

World Health Organization (2018) WHO methods and data sources for country-level causes of death 2000–2016. Global Health Estimates Technical Paper WHO/HIS/IER/GHE/2018.3, Geneva: WHO.

WHO & WHO Commission on Social Determinants of Health (2008) Closing the gap in a generation: Health equity through action on the social determinants of health: Commission on Social Determinants of Health final report. Geneva: World Health Organization.

WHO International (2018) Global Health Observatory data. Available from: www.int/gho/mortality_burden_disease/causes_death/en (accessed 27 November 2018).

Whyte, W.F. (1943) *Street Corner Society*. Chicaho, IL: University of Chicago Press.

Additional resources

a) Systematic reviews

Bambra, C. (2011) Real world reviews: A beginner's guide to undertaking systematic reviews of public health policy interventions. *Journal of Epidemiology and Community Health*, *65*; 14e 19.

Boland, A. (2014) *Doing a Systematic Review: A student's guide*. London: Sage.

Carande-Kulis, V.G., et al. (2000) Methods for systematic reviews of economic evaluations for the guide to community preventive services. *Am J Prev Med*, *18*(1S): 75–91.

Deville, W.L., Buntinx, F., Bouter, L.M., Montori, V.M., de Vet, H.C.W., van der Windt, D.A.W.M. and Bezemer, P.D. (2002) Conducting systematic reviews of diagnostic tests: Didactic guidelines. *BMC Medical Research Methodology*, *2*: 9.

Gough, D., Oliver, S. and Thomas, J. (2012) *An Introduction to Systematic Reviews*. London: Sage.

Gough, D., Thomas, J. and Oliver, S. (2012) Clarifying differences between review designs and methods. *Systematic Reviews, 1*: 28.

Harden, A. (2010) *Mixed-methods systematic reviews: Integrating quantitative and qualitative research.* Focus: A Publication of the National Center for the Dissemination of Disability Research (NCDDR). Technical Brief No. 25.

Harden, A. and Thomas, J. (2007) Methodological issues in combining diverse study types in systematic reviews. *International Journal of Social Research Methodology, 8*(3): 257–71.

Joanna Briggs Institute (2014) *Joanna Briggs Institute Reviewers' Manual 2014: The Systematic Review of Prevalence and Incidence Data.* Adelaide, Australia: The Joanna Briggs Institute.

Khan, K.S., Kunz, R., Kleijnen, J. and Antes, G. (2003) Five steps to conducting a systematic review. *J R Soc Med, 96*: 118–21.

Khan, K., Kunz, R., Kleijnen, J. and Antes, G. (2011) *Systematic Reviews to Support Evidence-based Medicine* (Second edition). London: Royal Society of Medicine.

Moher, D., Liberati, A., Tetzlaff, J. and Altman, D.G. (2009) The PRISMA Group. Preferred Reporting Items for Systematic Review and Meta-Analyses: The PRISMA Statement. *PLoS Med, 6*(6): e1000097.

Stroup, D., Berlin, J.A., Morton, S.C., Olkin, I., Williamson, G.D. Rennie, D., Moher, D., Becker, B.J., Sipe, T.A., and Thacker, S.B. (2000) Meta-analysis of observational studies in epidemiology. *JAMA, 283*(15): 2008–12.

Wager, E. and Wiffen, P.J. (2011) Ethical issues in preparing and publishing systematic reviews. *Journal of Evidence-Based Medicine, 4*(2): 130–4.

Wong, G., Greenhalgh, T., Westhorp, G., Buckingham, J. and Pawson, R. (2013) RAMESES publication standards: Meta-narrative reviews. *BMC Medicine, 11*: 20.

b) Meta-ethnography and realist synthesis

Booth, A. (2001) *Cochrane or cock-eyed? How should we conduct systematic reviews of qualitative research?* Paper presented at the Qualitative Evidence-based Practice Conference, Taking a Critical Stance. Coventry University, 14–16 May 2001.

France, E.F., Ring, N., Thomas, R., Noyes, J., Maxwell, M. and Jepson, R. (2014) A methodological systematic review of what's wrong with meta-ethnography reporting. *BMC Medical Research Methodology, 14*: 119.

France, E.F., Wells, M., Lang, H. and Williams, B. (2016) Why, when and how to update a meta-ethnography qualitative synthesis. *Syst Rev, 5*: 44.

Hannes, K. and Lockwood, L. (2011) *Synthesizing Qualitative Research: Choosing the right approach.* Oxford: Wiley Blackwell.

Jamal, F., Fletcher, A., Harden, A., Wells, A., Thomas, J. and Bonell, C. (2013) The school environment and student health: A systematic review and meta-ethnography of qualitative research. *BMC Public Health, 13*: 798.

Jones, M.L. (2004) Application of systematic review methods to qualitative research: Practical issues. *Journal of Advanced Nursing, 48*(3): 271–8.

Kane, S., Gerretsen, B., Scherpbier, R., Dal Poz, M. and Dieleman, M. (2010) A realist synthesis of randomised control trials involving use of community health workers for delivering child health interventions in low and middle income countries. *BMC Health Services Research, 10*: 286.

Major, C. Howell and Savin-Baden, M. (2012) *Introduction to Qualitative Research Synthesis.* Abingdon: Taylor and Francis.

Malpass, A., Shaw, A., Sharp, D. et al. (2009) 'Medication career' or 'Moral career'. The two sides of managing antidepressants: A meta-ethnography of patients' experiences of antidepressants. *Social Science and Medicine, 68*: 154–68.

Pawson, R. (2006) *Evidence Based Policy, A Realist Perspective*. London: Sage.

Pawson, R., Greenhalgh, T., Harvey, G. and Walshe, K. (2004) *Realist Synthesis: An introduction*. ESRC Research Methods Programme, University of Manchester RMP Methods Paper 2/2004.

Pope, N., Mays, C. and Popay, J. (2007) *Synthesizing Qualitative and Quantitative Health Research*. Maidenhead and New York: Open University Press.

Toye, F., Seers, K., Allcock, N., Briggs, M., Carr, E. and Barker, K. (2015) Meta-ethnography 25 years on: Challenges and insights for synthesising a large number of qualitative studies. *BMC Medical Research Methodology, 14*: 80.

INDEX

Page numbers in *italics* refer to Figures and page numbers in **bold** refer to Tables and Boxes.